T0311782

Dressings for Advanced Wound Care

Textile Institute Professional Publications
Series Editor: Helen D. Rowe for the Textile Institute

Care and Maintenance of Textile Products Including Apparel and Protective Clothing
Rajkishore Nayak and Saminathan Ratnapandian

Radio Frequency Identification (RFID) Technology and Application in Fashion and Textile Supply Chain
Rajkishore Nayak

The Grammar of Pattern
Michael Hann

Standard Methods for Thermal Comfort Assessment of Clothing
Ivana Špelić, Alka Mihelić Bogdanić and Anica Hursa Sajatovic

Fibres to Smart Textiles: Advances in Manufacturing, Technologies and Applications
Asis Patnaik and Sweta Patnaik

Flame Retardants for Textile Materials
Asim Kumar Roy Choudhury

Textile Design: Products and Processes
Michael Hann

Science in Design: Solidifying Design with Science and Technology
Tarun Grover and Mugdha Thareja

Textiles and Their Use in Microbial Protection: Focus on COVID-19 and Other Viruses
Jiri Militky, Aravin Prince Periyasamy and Mohanapriya Venkataraman

Dressings for Advanced Wound Care
Sharon Lam Po Tang

For more information about this series, please visit: www.crcpress.com/ Textile-Institute-Professional-Publications/book-series/TIPP

Textile Institute Professional Publications

The aim of the *Textile Institute Professional Publications* is to provide support to textile professionals in their work and to help emerging professionals, such as final year or Master's students, by providing the information needed to gain a sound understanding of key and emerging topics relating to textile, clothing and footwear technology, textile chemistry, materials science and engineering. The books are written by experienced authors with expertise in the topic and all texts are independently reviewed by textile professionals or textile academics.

The textile industry has a history of being both an innovator and an early adopter of a wide variety of technologies. There are textile businesses of some kind operating in all counties across the world. At any one time, there is an enormous breadth of sophistication in how such companies might function. In some places where the industry serves only its own local market, design, development and production may continue to be based on traditional techniques, but companies that aspire to operate globally find themselves in an intensely competitive environment, some driven by the need to appeal to followers of fast-moving fashion, others by demands for high performance and unprecedented levels of reliability. Textile professionals working within such organisations are subjected to a continued pressing need to introduce new materials and technologies, not only to improve production efficiency and reduce costs, but also to enhance the attractiveness and performance of their existing products and to bring new products into being. As a consequence, textile academics and professionals find themselves having to continuously improve their understanding of a wide range of new materials and emerging technologies to keep pace with competitors.

The Textile Institute was formed in 1910 to provide professional support to textile practitioners and academics undertaking research and teaching in the field of textiles. The Institute quickly established itself as the professional body for textiles worldwide and now has individual and corporate members in over 80 countries. The Institute works to provide sources of reliable and up-to-date information to support textile professionals through its research journals, the *Journal of the Textile Institute*[1] and *Textile Progress*,[2] definitive descriptions of textiles and their components through its online publication *Textile Terms and Definitions*,[3] and contextual treatments of important topics within the field of textiles in the form of self-contained books such as the *Textile Institute Professional Publications.*

References

1 http://www.tandfonline.com/action/journalInformation?show=aimsScope&journalCode=tjti20
2 http://www.tandfonline.com/action/journalInformation?show=aimsScope&journalCode=ttpr20
3 http://www.ttandd.org

Dressings for Advanced Wound Care

Sharon Lam Po Tang

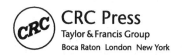

CRC Press
Taylor & Francis Group
Boca Raton London New York

CRC Press is an imprint of the
Taylor & Francis Group, an **informa** business

First edition published [2021]
by CRC Press
6000 Broken Sound Parkway NW, Suite 300, Boca Raton, FL 33487-2742

and by CRC Press
2 Park Square, Milton Park, Abingdon, Oxon, OX14 4RN

Library of Congress Cataloging-in-Publication Data
Names: Tang, Sharon Lam Po, author.
Title: Dressings for advanced wound care / authored by Sharon Lam Po Tang.
Description: First edition. | Boca Raton, FL : Taylor and Francis, 2021. |
Series: Textile professional institute publications | Includes
bibliographical references and index. | Summary: "The book starts by
helping the reader understand what advanced wound care is and the market
size. It then explains how different types of wounds may require
different environments to heal and how dressings can help in creating
the right environment. It gives an overview of the various dressing
technologies that are available to help manage wounds that are difficult
to heal. It provides recent clinical evidence that support how well (or
not) the technologies work, and also discusses on how such technologies
are launched in the market. Finally, the book will highlight the current
trends that may be directing the future of the advanced wound dressing
sector"-- Provided by publisher.
Identifiers: LCCN 2021004563 (print) | LCCN 2021004564 (ebook) | ISBN
9780367204402 (paperback) | ISBN 9780367204433 (hardback) | ISBN
9780429261497 (ebook)
Subjects: LCSH: Disposable medical supplies industry. | Bandages and
bandaging--Technological innovations. | Wounds and injuries--Economic
aspects.
Classification: LCC HD9995.D562 T36 2021 (print) | LCC HD9995.D562
(ebook) | DDC 338.4/76778--dc23
LC record available at https://lccn.loc.gov/2021004563
LC ebook record available at https://lccn.loc.gov/2021004564

ISBN: 978-0-367-20443-3 (hbk)
ISBN: 978-0-367-20440-2 (pbk)
ISBN: 978-0-429-26149-7 (ebk)

Typeset in Palatino
by SPi Global, India

To my husband, Duncan, and my father, Gary

In remembrance of Dennis Keith Gilding

Contents

Author Biography

Sharon Lam Po Tang has a BA(Hons) in Textile Design and an M.Sc. in Textiles from the University of Leeds, UK. Her Ph.D. in technical textiles, also from the University of Leeds, was on the topic of melt-blown cellulosic nonwovens, developed with potential uses in filtration and medical devices. She has worked in academia as a research fellow at the School of Textiles and Design of Heriot-Watt University, before joining the industry with Convatec, exploring a range of textiles and related technologies and working on the development of new wound dressings. Following Convatec, Sharon joined the Durex innovation team at SSL International before transitioning to Reckitt-Benckiser's footcare innovation team. She is currently self-employed and is still based in the UK.

Preface

Advanced wound care is a very complex field, and covers a wide range of products, equipment, therapies and techniques. This book looks at a specific section of this industry (the wound dressing side), and provides more depth and clarity on the numerous options available and their suitability for different care requirements. As a young professional in the industry, I remember being marked by the discrepancy between academic teaching, academic research and industry realities in this field. This book aims at bridging some of these gaps, linking where possible commercial examples and clinical evidence with the three core elements of wound dressing design: the base materials, the form these materials are made into and active ingredients that are subsequently added. A basic introduction to wounds and their requirements also helps to provide more relevance to materials and technologies discussed.

For those entering the wound care industry, or interested to do so, whether from the healthcare side, or the product development side, this book is intended to provide a good foundation of the dressing aspect of wound management. It can act as a reference point to understand the various solutions available on the market or under development, explaining the range of materials and technologies being used. For those concerned mostly with the development aspects of novel wound dressings, in addition to being a source of reference for different materials and technologies, the book also provides key elements to consider for launching a new product. Many of these elements are underestimated without the hindsight of experience, or are evolving as business models around the world are changing. This includes for example the regulatory aspects, the innovation process and the need to incorporate patient and carer needs in the design of the product.

My hope in writing this book is that it can be a useful tool, particularly for our new innovators of the future, to navigate the diverse field of advanced wound care and to provide food for thought on the development of new solutions for wound care.

1

Introducing Advanced Wound Care

1.1 Wound Care Today

Like all living species, humans have always been subjected to wounds of all types and severities, whether by accident, by disease, by consequence and even caused on purpose. From a young age, we are accustomed to seeing or getting minor wounds, and either leaving them to heal by themselves or administering basic medical care at home. A layman, having likely experienced multiple minor wounds himself in his lifetime, could perhaps describe a wound as being an injury, a tear, cut, or break in the skin surface. This could be with or without further damage to the underlying tissues and bones.

For a broader definition of a wound, it could be described as *any form of damage or break in the continuity of a living tissue.* The damage may be caused by physical/mechanical aggression, chemical aggression, or by radiation or thermal aggression. It may result in the wound being 'open' (with the skin being cut, torn, or broken), or 'closed' (where the injury occurs without an apparent break in the skin). It also includes wounds that are purposefully created under controlled conditions, such as during surgery. Thus, wounds come in all shapes and forms, from the minor cuts, bruises, grazes and burns, to complex 'dirty' wounds where tissue has been randomly torn or damaged and exposed to an unfavourable environment.

Under normal, healthy and clean conditions, most minor wounds should heal by themselves, and need little attention. The body naturally engages into various stages of wound healing as soon as it becomes aware of an injury: (1) haemostasis, (2) inflammation, (3) proliferation and (4) remodelling/maturation. When there is any breach in tissue continuity, blood vessels and capillaries, haemostasis starts via several mechanisms which lead to the coagulation of blood, and fibrin and clot formation at the site of injury. Inflammation, which starts in parallel and continues for longer, is noticeable by swelling, redness and pain. It is caused by blood vessels releasing fluids, which among other things contain neutrophils and macrophages, to help get rid of damaged cells, debris and pathogens. The inflammation phase reduces when new and living cells begin to accumulate at the site. The third stage, proliferation then occurs, with the formation of new granulation tissue from the base of the wound to replace the original clot. This granulation tissue eventually completely covers the wound area with its mix of connective tissues made of collagen, extracellular matrix and microscopic blood vessels. Towards the end of the proliferation phase, re-epithelialisation occurs to resurface the wound site and restore the skin's barrier function. Finally, the last stage of remodelling or maturation starts when the previously formed granulation tissue, and the newly formed micro blood vessels are gradually degraded when no longer needed. The collagen is remodelled from the immature Type III to the mature Type I and is reorganised and crosslinked in a more orderly way and eventually the wound is fully closed.

While the above stages have been simplified for a basic understanding, the details and the multiple mechanisms within each stage are complex and may occur simultaneously. The process is also made more complicated when additional factors come into play, such as the age, nutritional status, or behaviour of the injured person, the size, depth and severity of the wound, the environmental conditions, the position of the wound, the medications being used, the presence of systemic diseases, etc. Naturally, the more complex the situation is, the more care is required to keep the wound protected and help it heal.

The primary objective of basic wound care is to get the wound to progress through the above normal stages and eventually safely close or heal. To help this process, it is now well understood that wound beds need to be kept moist (not wet), as this is a better environment for the multitude of activities that need to take place in the wound healing stages. Today, wound care (particularly where more complex cases are concerned) has expanded to be more holistic, not simply concentrating on the injury site only. It is commonly accepted that healing may be compromised with nutritional deficits and is influenced by lifestyle choices such as eating, exercising, smoking and drinking habits. The whole picture needs to be looked at before prescribing the best course of treatment.

With regard to *advanced wound care*, it can be viewed as care that enables *faster healing* or healing with *other better outcomes* than what can be achieved with standard wound care. Some of the outcome measures that may be considered when discussing advanced wound care are given in Table 1.1. By way of examples, rather than simply concentrating on getting a wound to close, advanced wound care may consider products and procedures that will also minimise pain and odour during the treatment period, efficiently manage exudate and/or result in less scarring in the future. Some consider advanced wound care to be the interventions that they turn to when standard wound care has failed, for example in the case of the management of chronic or non-healing wounds (Greer et al. 2012). In these cases, the advanced interventions may sometimes be significantly more complex in

TABLE 1.1

Examples of outcome measures for advanced wound care

Outcome	Advanced wound care objectives
Time to healing	Faster healing or healing of chronic wounds
Scar formation	Reduced or no scarring
Pain	Reduced or no pain
Infection	Prevention and management of infection
Odour	Odour minimisation or control
Exudate management	Moist wound healing, no maceration, no pooling of excess fluid
Lifestyle	Enables as lifestyle as close to normal as possible (mobility, independence, dignity)

administering, more costly, less frequently used, more experimental or a combination thereof.

Advanced wound care is intrinsically linked with advances in technology, but not all new technologies would automatically lead to faster healing or other better healing and wellbeing outcomes. Although the theoretical principles may apply in the early stages of development and trials, clinical evidence remains the main determinant of whether any of the outcomes in Table 1.1, or indeed other positive clinical outcomes not mentioned here, are achieved.

1.2 The Current Global Advanced Wound Care Market

The size of the advanced wound care market varies to some extent depending on the precise definition of the terms and the inclusion criteria by the researching body. Overall, in the later years of the 2010s, the global size of the market was about USD 8–9 billion, and by the mid-2020s, this was expected to be around USD 13–14 billion before the COVID-19 global pandemic hit. Specifically, Fortune Business Insights (2019) estimated the global market size to be about USD 9.3 billion in 2017, predicted to grow by a CAGR of 4.8% to USD 13.5 billion by 2025. Allied Market Research (2019) estimated the size to be USD 8.5 billion in 2018, predicted to grow at a more optimistic CAGR of 6.5% to USD 13.9 billion in 2026. BIS Research (2019) valued the market size at USD 8.9 billion in 2018, growing to USD 11.1 billion by 2024 at a CAGR of 3.6%. These figures were generated prior to the general economic downturn caused by the 2020 pandemic, and are therefore now not likely to be achieved within the timescale predicted. In particular, it can be expected that North America and Europe will exhibit more conservative growth in the short term, if any, and the high increases expected in the mid-2020s in some emerging markets such as Brazil will be considerably cut down due to the economic downturn. With the focus of healthcare providers on dealing with COVID-19 patients, one of the most impacted sectors has been surgical wound care, due to many elective surgeries having been postponed or cancelled in 2020 and beyond. However, given the nature of the industry, it can be anticipated that there will be eventual recovery and growth in the future.

There is an agreement that North America takes the lead in the market share, at about 40%, with a revenue of USD 3.9 billion in 2017 (Fortune Business Insights, 2019). This is thought to be because of the favourable health care insurance system, higher income and large presence of businesses developing advanced wound care products in the country. Other demographic and health drivers outlined in Section 1.3 also contribute to this large market share. Europe is the second market share leader, but the Asia-Pacific region is expected to see the highest growth in the future, due to a combination of population surge, increasing disposable income and healthcare spending budget, prevalence of some chronic diseases and a growing ageing population. The economic buoyancy of China and India despite the pandemic also reinforces this potential growth.

In terms of sub-sectors within the advanced wound care market, chronic wounds, advanced dressings, surgical wound care, active wound care products (which includes skin substitutes and growth factors) and therapy devices (such as negative pressure wound therapy (NPTW)) have the biggest shares or predicted growth in the next few years (Data Bridge Market Research, 2019; Allied Market Research, 2019).

1.3 Growth Drivers and Enablers for the Industry

Growth in the advanced wound care sector is driven largely by demographic and health factors and partly by socio-economic trends. The last few decades have exhibited certain global trends which shape the wound care sector, the directions of growth and the likely future developments (Figure 1.1).

1.3.1 The Ageing Population

One single major player in the wound care market is the global ageing population (Table 1.2). There are two main elements that contribute to the increase in the proportion of the geriatric population: (a) we live longer due to advances in healthcare and better lifestyle management and (b) the fertility rates are dropping, and have been particularly low in developed, high-income countries.

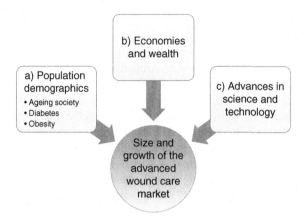

FIGURE 1.1
Growth drivers for the advanced wound care market

TABLE 1.2

The global ageing population in numbers

	2019	Predicted 2050
No. of persons aged 65 and over globally	703 million	1.5 billion
Eastern and South-Eastern Asia	261 million	573 million
Europe and Northern America	200 million	296 million
% of the global population aged 65 and over	9%	16%
No. of persons aged 80 or over globally	143 million	426 million
Ratio of persons aged 65 and over to those between 20 and 64 (working age) – globally	12:100	17:100
Europe and North America	30:100	49:100
Australia and New Zealand	27:100	42:100

Source: United Nations (2020).

The geriatric population faces some wound care challenges. As we get older, our skin and its ability to heal are gradually compromised both by intrinsic ageing factors and exposure to the external environment, particularly UV light. As summed up by Gosain and DiPietro (2004), a number of changes occur in the skin with age, including a reduction of protein and collagen content, of elasticity, cutaneous blood flow, lymphatic drainage and even a diminished perception of pain and pressure. From a wound care perspective, some of the physiological activities during the various stages of wound healing are reduced or slowed down with age, for example, decreased capillary permeability at injury site, declined macrophage function, reduced proliferative response and re-epithelialisation, and also lower tensile strength at incision wounds (Gosain & DiPietro, 2004). The older person's skin is therefore inherently more fragile and more prone to wounds, but also needs more care to heal – even without the presence of comorbidities and lifestyle risk factors such as smoking, obesity or nutritional deficiencies.

In addition to the challenges of older skin, there are a number of health and fitness changes associated with age which indirectly affect the wound care requirements. Among them, those of most relevance to the wound care market are changes in the immune system, which weaken the body's capacity to fight infection, cardiovascular diseases, which can inhibit blood, oxygen and nutrition at the wound site, and diabetes, which has many complications in itself (Jaul & Barron, 2017). Physically, the loss of muscle and bone strength, frailty and reduction in mobility can lead to greater risks of falls. These can all contribute to a greater risk of wounds, deterioration of wounds, slowing down of the body's natural healing process, or stalling it altogether. Diminished mobility leads to the additional challenge of not being able to properly self-care, not only to prevent injury, but also after an injury has occurred.

Other cognitive and psychological issues such as natural cognitive ageing and dementia can further aggravate the situation. Some older patients may struggle to protect themselves from injury, or maintain a healthy level of nutrition and appropriate physical activity to sustain their strength, or even understand the medical requirements if they are injured. Some may find it difficult to follow instructions regarding their health and wounds if they are at home, especially if they live on their own. As a result, with the ageing population, both the incidence of wounds can increase and the wound care duration and requirements can increase, due to the healing of the wound being compromised intrinsically or extrinsically.

1.3.2 Diabetes

In the previous section, diabetes was mentioned as a possible risk factor for the ageing population. According to the International Diabetes Federation (IDF, 2019), one in five adults over the age of 65 has diabetes. It is not however exclusively an older person ailment, and the IDF highlights that about 1.1 million under 20 years olds live with the disease and this number is on the increase. Diabetes, which is linked to the rise in obesity and overweightness in the population has been on a steady increase in the last few decades, and because of this, has sadly become an important growth driver for the wound care market. The prevalence of diabetes in adults worldwide nearly doubled between 1980 and 2014 to about 422 million, and is expected to rise to 642 million by 2040 (World Health Organization, 2016; Diabetes.co.uk, 2019). The increases are seen to be faster in low and middle-income countries

TABLE 1.3

Effects of diabetes

Physiological variables	Effects
Elevated blood sugar	Stiffening of arteries, narrowing of blood vessels
	Decreasing function of red blood cells to carry nutrients to affected tissues
	Lower efficiency of white blood cells to fight infections
	Immune cells become less effective and increase risk of infection and slow wound healing
Narrowing of blood vessels	Poor circulation leading to decreased blood flow and oxygen to a wound
	Nerves in the body become affected
Affected nerves	Diabetic neuropathy, loss of sensation, leading to patients not feeling when there is a minor injury or infection, which can then lead to deteriorate

Source: Wound Care Centers (2014).

than in higher income countries, with the largest numbers being in China, India, USA, Brazil and the Russian Federation (Diabetes.co.uk, 2019).

Diabetes is a chronic disease where the body does not produce enough of the hormone that regulates blood sugar (insulin), or does not effectively use it. The healthcare burden for the disease globally is high, standing at an estimated USD 760 billion (International Diabetes Federation, 2019) – of which a small proportion is linked to the advanced wound care sector. One of the several risks or complications of diabetics is to develop a foot ulcer, and it is estimated that 15–20% of diabetics may develop one during their lifetime (Chun et al., 2019). As well as the ulceration risks, the disease can lead to a number of other complications (Table 1.3), which slow down wound healing if an ulcer is formed or after surgery and affect the duration and cost of the appropriate care. For ulcers that deteriorate and cannot be healed, the unfortunate consequence is amputation. Globally, the size of the market for the treatment of diabetic foot ulcers (DFU) was valued at USD 3.6 billion in 2017, with North America and Europe taking the largest shares (Grand View Research, 2019). The CAGR is anticipated to be about 8.2%, with the Asia Pacific markets expected to have the highest growth rate.

1.3.3 Excessive Weight and Obesity

According to the World Health Organization (2020), since 1975, the number of overweight or obese people has nearly tripled. Carrying a bit of excess weight might once have been considered a sign of higher income, but today, this problem permeates across income levels, applies across the world, and

TABLE 1.4

WHO statistics on obesity and overweight population

	Total	%
Overweight and obese adults (2016 data)	1.9 billion	39%
Americas		63%
Europe		59%
Eastern Mediterranean		49%
Obese adults (2016 data)	650 million	13%
Overweight and obese under 5 years old children (2018 data)	40 million	
Overweight and obese 5–19 years olds (2016 data)	340 million	15%

Source: World Health Organization (2017, 2020).

is seen rising in low- and middle-income countries. An interesting observation is that obesity is correlated with income but this correlation differs in the overall country income level (Ameye & Swinnen, 2019). It tends to increase with income in poor countries, but in the richer countries, the poor are the most obese.

The two main causes of excess weight are an increase in availability and consumption of high calorific content food (partly also helped by a reduction in the price of such foods), and an increasingly sedentary lifestyle, particularly in towns and cities. As the requirements of jobs change in the world, a higher level of desk-based or even home-based work has been observed, which naturally limits the physical activity levels. This is seen to happen progressively as a nation moves from low-income, manual manufacturing labour to high-income service-led. As seen in Table 1.4, a sizeable proportion of adults and children are overweight or obese, which puts them at risk of developing weight-associated illnesses such as cardiovascular disease, diabetes, certain cancers and musculoskeletal disorders. In turn, these diseases can lead to higher risk of incurring wounds and having wound healing difficulties.

Obesity itself has been shown to impair wound healing and is linked to an increase in the risk of infection, pressure and venous ulcers, and wound care complications, including at surgical sites (Guo & DiPietro, 2010; Pence & Woods, 2014). It is thought that deviations in the inflammatory stage are the main underlying cause of delayed wound healing. In the case of surgical wounds, factors such as specific features of the fatty tissues, vascular insufficiencies, changes in the cells, oxidative stress, alterations in immune mediators and nutritional deficiencies have been highlighted (Pierpont et al., 2014). A higher rate of infection has been noticed in obese patients, and wound dehiscence can occur due to the increased tension on the wound edges (Guo & DiPietro, 2010). A summary of potential problems caused by overweightness and obesity is given in Table 1.5.

TABLE 1.5

Obesity and the wound risks associated with

Obesity factors	Wound risk
Poor and inadequate blood supply to subcutaneous fatty tissue	- Wound healing complications - Increased risk of pressure ulcers or pressure-related injuries
Increased wound tension after surgery	- Increased wound tissue pressure - Reduced micro-perfusion - Reduced availability of oxygen to the wound
Reduced mobility	- Increased risk of pressure-related injuries
Skin folds	- Provide an environment of growth for micro-organisms - Can contribute to infections - Skin to skin friction can cause ulceration
Stress, anxiety, depression	- Can weaken the immune response

Source: Guo and DiPietro (2010).

1.3.4 Economies and Wealth

Advanced wound care is currently a sector that is mostly concentrated in the higher-income countries, predominantly North America as was highlighted in Section 1.2. As income and wealth eventually start to grow again in this zone after the 2020 COVID-19 global pandemic recovery, it is expected to continue to be an influential driver of the demand for advanced wound care in the future. Likewise, despite the expected temporary decrease in wealth in Europe, particularly the UK, caused by the pandemic (Credit Suisse Research Institute, 2020), it is believed that this area too will continue to play an important part in the demand for advanced wound care now and in the future. Eventually, as the world all over recovers, gets wealthier and has easier access to medical advances, pockets of demand will spread out more, particularly towards emerging markets. Prior to the 2020 pandemic, global wealth was predicted to rise by 27% over the period 2019–2024, with the low- and middle-income countries responsible for 38% of the growth (Lluberas & Shorrocks, 2019). As seen in Table 1.6, annual growth was expected to be significantly higher in low-income countries. These higher growth areas are key target markets for advanced medical manufacturers, as they are opportunities for business growth from new markets. Notably, emerging markets such as China, Russia, India, Mexico, Saudi Arabia and Brazil, as they transition away from their low-income economies, generally aspire to higher standards of living, including higher standards of medical care. While previous economic reports estimated the growth of emerging markets to be bigger in the next few years, the negative impact of COVID-19, particularly in South America may be felt for longer before emerging markets are able to grow to the levels predicted. China and India appeared to have managed to be

TABLE 1.6

Pre-2020 estimated annual wealth growth to 2024

Region	Annual growth
World	4.9%
Low-income countries	7.4%
Middle-income countries	5.9%
High-income countries	4.4%

Source: Lluberas and Shorrocks (2019).

less economically affected (Credit Suisse Research Institute, 2020), and therefore will likely drive the growth for advanced wound care in the emerging markets.

Wealth generation influences the healthcare industry on two levels. Nationwide, the country starts to invest more in healthcare for the general population. On the individual level, the wealthy start to expect more out of their private medical care. The total purchasing power of the individually wealthy may be quite influential in shaping the advanced wound care sector: the number of millionaires is expected to grow by 34% globally between 2019 and 2024: by 55% in China, 56% in India, 47% in Asia-Pacific, 37% in Africa, 35% in Europe, 27% in Latin America and 24% in North America (Lluberas & Shorrocks, 2019).

With the impact of the 2020 pandemic, global wealth is unlikely to each the figures estimated, and growth – if any – will be sluggish for the first few years, taking example from the 2008 financial crisis. Economists worldwide predict a major recession in the wake of the pandemic (Surico & Galeotti, 2020). Geographical Europe is likely to be quite hardly hit, with an already sluggish growth predicted, topped with the enormous impact of the pandemic, and with the consequences of Brexit disruptions. However, healthcare in these old-world economies tends to be a social and economic priority closely linked to their lifestyle and standards of living. These markets are likely to continue to be significant, despite perhaps reducing investment levels in this area. China is expected to recover fairly quickly from the pandemic and is more likely to be the main key growth driver. It will still remain a major new market in volume and in value for many advanced wound care sub-sectors.

1.3.5 Other Growth Drivers

Several other growth drivers are worth mentioning in the global advanced wound care equation. On the healthcare aspect, medical advances occur rapidly and continuously provide more opportunities to save lives, whether by pharmaceutical treatment, by surgery or other means. By prolonging life, the inevitable result is the rise in the geriatric population, which leads to its own issues as discussed above. Although statistics on the growth rate of surgical operations being conducted globally are not clear, some reports refer to the surgical wound care segment expanding, due to increasing number of surgical procedures globally (Data Bridge Market Research, 2019; Fortune Business Insights, 2019). Certainly, there is consensus that there are large numbers of people in low-income countries who are unable to access surgical treatment. There are global efforts to address this imbalance, which will eventually and gradually increase the number of surgical operations across the world (German Global Surgery Association and Program in Global Surgery and Social Change at Harvard Medical School, 2018). Putting aside the number of procedures, surgery can also lead to more wound complications with the prevalence of diabetes, obesity, and of course with older patients. Delayed healing or infections are well-known risks, and as such, they increase the need for advanced wound care products.

From an innovation perspective, the development of new technologies for wound care is generally also very dynamic, boosted by national and international collaborations, interdisciplinary research, clinical evidence and funding. Despite the large market size, public funding on wound care specifically does not tend to be very big. However, there are pockets of small funding available from organisations and businesses, from various angles, e.g., the materials, technology, or clinical aspects. Internally, medical devices businesses have appeared to invest more on research and development than their counterparts in other industries (Stirling & Shehata, 2016). This is because for many of them, innovation and new product development is high on their agenda for business growth (Table 1.7).

One of the main outcome measures for innovation is the number of new products launched. However, the number of patents granted is also an indication of the activity levels in an area and highlights the dynamism and potential future growth in the sector. In a review of patents on wound

TABLE 1.7

2015 survey on R&D and innovation in medical devices companies

	Percentage
The business strategic focus:	
Engineering/innovation led	55%
Sales led	29%
Top 3 strategic priorities in the next 1–2 years:	
Sales growth	53%
Development of new products	49%
Reducing cost structure	35%

Source: Stirling and Shehata (2016).

healing submitted to the US, Europe and China patent offices, Gwak and Sohn (2017) show that the number of patents on the subject matter has continuously increased from the late 1980s. The review shows that one of the most popular topics in wound healing was 'films for dressing', followed by growth factors, antibacterial materials and NPWT. Unsurprisingly, the key medical devices companies hold the lion share of the patents applied and granted, particularly in the films and NPWT topics.

Finally, the degree of penetration of new technologies, or technologies that are no longer proprietary will also contribute to the size of the advanced wound care market. For example, it was mentioned above that 'growth factors' was an area of high activity in the patent world. This type of advanced technology (along with other biologics for example), has a higher degree of penetration in the US at the moment. Gradually, it may capture more of the market size in the rest of the world, particularly Europe in the first instance (Paquette & Stadler, 2019). Another example is successful technologies that have run out of their patent protection: generic versions will be made at a lower price point, which pushes for more innovation to compete, and also expands the reach of the generics to countries that previously would not have been able to afford them.

References

Allied Market Research. (2019). *Advanced Wound Care Market by Product (Infection Management, Exudate Management, Active Wound Care and Therapy Devices), Application (Chronic Wounds and Acute Wounds) and End User (Hospitals and Community Health Service Centers): Global Opportunity Analys.* Pune: Allied Market Research.

Ameye, H., & Swinnen, J. (2019). "Obesity, Income and Gender: The Changing Global Relationship." *Global Food Security* 23: 267.

BIS Research. (2019). *Global Advanced Wound Care Market.* Fremont: BIS Research Inc.

Chun, D.-I., Kim, S., Kim, J., Yang, H.-J., Kim, J. H., Cho, J.-H., Yi, Y., Kim, W. J., & Won, S. H. (2019). "Epidemiology and Burden of Diabetic Foot Ulcer and Peripheral Arterial Disease in Korea." *Journal of Clinical Medicine* 8 (5): 748.

Credit Suisse Research Institute. (2020). *Global Wealth Report 2020.* Credit Suisse.

Data Bridge Market Research. (2019). *Advanced Wound Care Market – Trends and Forecast to 2027.* Pune: Data Bridge Market Research.

Diabetes.co.uk. (2019). *Diabetes Prevalence.* 15 January. Accessed March 23, 2020. https://www.diabetes.co.uk/diabetes-prevalence.html

Fortune Business Insights. (2019). *Advanced Wound Care Market Size, Share and Industry Analysis, by Product (Advanced Wound Dressings, Wound Care Devices & Active Wound Care), by Indication (Diabetic Foot Ulcers, Pressure Ulcers, Surgical Wounds, Others), by End User, and Regional Forecast.* Pune: Fortune Business Insights.

German Global Surgery Association and Program in Global Surgery and Social Change at Harvard Medical School. (2018). *Global Surgery & Anaesthesia Statistics: The Importance of Data Collection*. New York: The G4 Alliance.

Gosain, A., & DiPietro, L. A. (2004). "Aging and Wound Healing." *World Journal of Surgery* 28: 321.

Grand View Research. (2019). *Diabetic Foot Ulcer (DFU) Treatment Market Analysis Report by Treatment (Biologics, Wound Care Dressings, Therapy Devices), by Ulcer Type (Ischemic, Neuro-Ischemic, Neuropathic), and Segment Forecasts 2019–2025*. San Francisco: Grand View Research.

Greer, N., Foman, N., Wilt, T., Dorrian, J., Fitzgerald, P., MacDonald, R., & Rutks, I. (2012). *Advanced Wound Care Therapies for Non-Healing Diabetic, Venous and Arterial Ulcers: A Systematic Review*. Washington, DC: Department of Veterans Affairs, Health Services Research & Development Service.

Guo, S., & DiPietro, L. A. (2010). "Factors Affecting Wound Healing." *Journal of Dental Research* 89 (3): 219.

Gwak, J. H., & Sohn, S. Y. (2017). "Identifying the Trends in Wound-Healing Patents for Successful Investment Strategies." *PLoS One* 12 (3): 1–19.

International Diabetes Federation. (2019). *IDF Diabetes Atlas* (9th ed.). Brussels: International Diabetes Federation.

Jaul, E., & Barron, J. (2017). "Age-Related Diseases and Clinical and Public Health Implications for the 85 Years Old and Over Population." *Front Public Health* 5: 335.

Lluberas, R., & Shorrocks, A. (2019). "Wealth Outlook." In *Global Wealth 2019*, by Credit Suisse Research Institute, 37. Credit Suisse.

Paquette, S., & Stadler, L. (2019). *EWMA 2019: Insights and Innovation in Advanced Wound Care*. 30 July. Accessed March 28, 2020. https://blog.smarttrak.com/ ewma-2019-insights-and-innovation

Pence, B. D., & Woods, J. A. (2014). "Exercise, Obesity and Cutaneous." *Advanced Wound Care (New Rochelle)* 3 (1): 71.

Pierpont, Y. N., Dinh, T. P., Salas, R. E., Johnson, E. L., Wright, T. G., Robson, M. C., & Payne, W. G. (2014). "Obesity and Surgical Wound Healing: A Current Review." *ISRN Obesity*: 638936.

Stirling, C., & Shehata, A. (2016). *Collaboration – The Future of Innovation for the Medical Device Industry*. 133166-G. KPMG International Cooperative.

Surico, P., & Galeotti, A. (2020). *The Economics of a Pandemic: The Case of COVID-19*. London Business School. Accessed March 28, 2020. https://sites.google.com/ site/paolosurico/covid-19

United Nations. (2020). *World Population Ageing 2019*. New York: United Nations.

World Health Organization. (2016). *Global Report on Diabetes*. Geneva: World Health Organization.

World Health Organization. (2017). *Global Health Observatory Data Repository*. 27 September. Accessed March 25, 2020. https://apps.who.int/gho/data/view. main.GLOBAL2461A?lang=en

World Health Organization. (2020). *Obesity and Overweight Key Facts*. 3 March. Accessed March 25, 2020. https://www.who.int/news-room/fact-sheets/ detail/obesity-and-overweight

Wound Care Centers. (2014). *How Diabetes Affects Wound Healing*. 24 March. Accessed March 24, 2020. https://www.woundcarecenters.org/article/living-with-wounds/how-diabetes-affects-wound-healing

2

Understanding Wounds and Their Requirements

2.1 The Variability of Wounds

In Chapter 1, the process of wound healing was summarised into the four stages of haemostasis, inflammation, proliferation and remodelling/maturation. As a natural process, a degree of variation can be expected within these stages, and some overlap is also likely to occur. Wounds, as are patients, are all individually shaped and formed, and as such no two wounds are going to be identical, nor behave in the exact same way.

The depth of a wound through the skin also affects how easy it is to heal. The skin is made of three main layers – the outermost epidermis, the middle dermis and the hypodermis, which contacts the underlying connective tissues. The epidermis provides the main barrier function, and a breach in this layer means that bacteria and other environmental contaminants can easily penetrate the body. The dermis contributes to restoring the epidermis and is another protective layer, which also provides sensation and thermoregulation and contains sweat glands, and in some areas, hair. The hypodermis, underneath the dermis, mainly contains adipose tissue and sweat glands and is responsible for the production of vitamin D and triglycerides. The type and severity of damage to the three layers or to the underlying tissue affect the outcomes of the wound.

Despite the innumerable variations wounds may present themselves in, for the benefit of wound care guiding principles, they can still be broadly categorised into different groups. The two main ones are acute and chronic wounds, each with their own sub-categories. Wound care can be facilitated for each sub-category, with the right choice of dressing and other treatments.

2.2 Acute Wounds

An acute wound is one that occurs suddenly or reasonably rapidly. It can be caused by mechanical, irradiation, electrical, thermal and chemical damage. The wound can in some cases be closed, i.e., showing no break in the outer layers of the skin, for example, bruises caused by sudden compression such as a fall or a bump into a hard surface. By contrast, an open wound is one where there is a breach in the skin, sometimes accompanied by bleeding.

It is expected that acute wounds, unless complications (such as infections) occur, will progress through the stages of wound healing in a predictable time frame. The first three stages normally take from a few days (in the case of minor superficial epidermal wounds) to several weeks, after which the wound's edges, if any, are closed and the tissue has more or less regenerated. The remodelling or maturation phase, during which the skin regains its strength, can last for months, or even up to two years (Richardson, 2004).

2.2.1 Wounds Caused by Traumatic Mechanical Damage

Traumatic wounds caused by mechanical damage present themselves in many different ways, which are summed up in Table 2.1. The complexity of the wound damage is affected by a combination of various factors including the forces involved at impact/contact, the depth of the injury through the skin, whether underlying tissue has been affected, the position of the wound, the age of the patient and whether or not contaminants are involved.

In terms of care, the main objective of treating an acute traumatic wound is to ensure it stops bleeding, that it is not infected, to clean it where necessary and for as long as necessary, to repair the damage to the tissue, closing the

TABLE 2.1

Types of open acute wounds caused by mechanical damage

Type	Description
Abrasion	Rubbing off of the superficial layers of the skin against a rough or abrasive surface such as the road. If superficial, bleeding is minimal but the wound may be wet due to the inflammatory stage.
Laceration	An irregular, jagged cut or tear of the skin, caused by a sharp object such as tool, knife or machinery. For deep lacerations, bleeding can be very profuse.
Incision	A straight edge cut caused by a sharp blade such as a knife cut.
Puncture	Caused by a long and pointy object such as a nail, bullet, spear. If deep, they can go through the skin and muscle tissues and reach other internal organs.
Avulsion	Partial or complete tearing away of parts of the skin and its surrounding tissues. These normally occur during violent accidents or blows and also lead to profuse bleeding.

gap between the edges if required and finally to dress the wound to protect it against contaminants. For minor open wounds, this is generally done at home, but for severe or deep wounds going through all three layers of the skin, professional help is required. The outcomes of the wound (e.g., how fast it heals, if there are any scarring and if there is any limitation to movement or function after healing), may depend very much on the speed and quality of treatment.

Acute traumatic wounds are at greater risk of infection if there are foreign bodies in the wound, if they are deep and difficult to clean, if they were caused by human or animal bites and/or if patients do not get the wound treated quickly (Richardson, 2004). Where the wound is contaminated with debris or dead tissue, a surgical debridement may need to be conducted by a professional, and a layer of topical antibiotic can be applied as a precautionary measure. In some cases, oral antibiotics or antitetanus therapy may be prescribed prophylactically too, and normally, the wound will not be closed (if needed) until resistance to infection is established. Infections are one of the possible complications of most wounds, and even where all the necessary steps have been taken to clean the wound after injury, subsequent contamination when the patient is recovering can also lead to infections.

For small lacerations, abrasions or even small punctures, the wound's edges may be brought together and held with just a dressing. If the wound is deeper, the edges may require some support such as sutures, staples, adhesive tape or glue to close or reduce the gap and facilitate healing, allowing for any drainage if necessary. A dressing is generally applied on top to protect the wound from contamination and act as a physical barrier while the skin's integrity is broken. The role of the dressing in acute wounds is mostly protective, assuming that the wound will naturally heal.

In some instances, where there is significant tissue loss, it may not be possible to bring together the edges without creating further damage. In these cases, the wound bed is cleaned, covered with a dressing and if healing occurs naturally, granulation tissue will grow from the bed up and close the wound gradually. Wound healing via this route, also called secondary intention, is slower and is likely to result in a broader scar. Dressings in such cases play an additional role to that of a surface barrier; they need to provide or create the right environment to enable the wound to close.

2.2.2 Surgical Wounds

Surgical wounds are incisions through the whole skin depth and underlying tissues that are created by a highly trained professional for the purpose of conducting a planned clinical procedure on the body. They are normally conducted under sterile and controlled environment and are precise cuts with clean edges. As such, they are normally considered acute wounds, with a predictable healing timeframe. Nevertheless, depending on the position of

TABLE 2.2

Classification of surgical wounds according to the Centers for Disease Control and Prevention (CDC)

Class	Description
Class I	**Clean:** an uninfected operative wound, primarily closed (if necessary, with closed drainage). Does not enter the respiratory, alimentary, genital or uninfected urinary tracts. Shows no inflammation. Surgical wounds that follow a non-penetrative trauma should be included in this category if they meet the criteria.
Class II	**Clean-contaminated:** Operative wounds under controlled conditions and without unusual contaminations in the respiratory, alimentary, genital and urinary tracts. Operations that involve the biliary tract, appendix, vagina and oropharynx are also in this category if there is no evidence of infection or major break in technique.
Class III	**Contaminated:** Open, fresh, accidental wounds with contact with non-sterile material, or surgical procedures with major breaks in sterile techniques (for example open cardiac massage), or gross spillage from the gastrointestinal tract. Also includes incisions where dry necrotic tissue occurs.
Class IV	**Dirty/infected:** Surgical wounds with devitalised tissue, or an existing clinical infection, or perforated viscera.

Source: World Health Organization (2018a).

the incision and what the wound is going to be in contact with, some surgical wounds can be contaminated or dirty, and can have unexpected healing rates.

The classifications in Table 2.2 were developed in order to help understand and mitigate the risks of surgical site infections after an operation. Infections are the most likely cause of a non-healing surgical wound and the main concern that drives post-operative and wound care. The probability of incurring one depends on the surgical wound class (the higher the class in Table 2.2, the higher the risk), the patient's health and also on the environmental and geographical conditions in which the patient is treated. Perhaps not surprisingly, higher income countries tend to fare better in keeping surgical site infections at bay compared to low and middle income developing countries (Collaborative GS, 2017; Sawyer & Evans, 2018). Despite this, surgical site infections are in the topmost frequent types of hospital acquired infections in Europe and the US (World Health Organization, 2018a, 2018b). The tell-tale signs are inflammation of the area (the wound looking red, feeling hot and being swollen), pain, fever and/or draining fluids that are not clear or have a smell.

In high-income countries, care for surgical wounds tends to follow planned protocols to minimise complications. A surgery is normally conducted under strict environmental controls, where the operation room and its equipment and tools have been properly sterilised or decontaminated. Surgical and nursing staff are fully trained and equipped with the right tools, protective equipment and materials. All necessary precautions prior to the operation and after the operations are taken in order to keep any open wound as clean as possible. This includes completing pre-operative preparations for the patient (cleaning, removal of hair, nutrition, etc.) and having post-operative procedures in place such as extra oxygenation, physiological and blood sugar monitoring and control, proper hydration, adequate nutrition and so on. The WHO's guidelines provide detailed information on steps towards reducing surgical site infections (World Health Organization, 2018a).

With all the controls in place, the treatment for surgical wounds is to either close the incision with staple, sutures or adhesives, or to leave it unclosed to heal depending on the surgery. Dressings for surgical wounds are critical to prevent or manage infection. It is essential that they perform their barrier function. For wounds that are not closed, as well as protecting against infection, dressings need to provide an adequate environment to enable the body to heal itself, or to enhance the healing process. For instance, the dressing should not be desiccating, which would hamper the re-epithelialisation process, neither should it allow the wound to macerate if there is a lot of drainage. In recent years, dressings have played an important role in the prevention of surgical site infections. The use of negative pressure wound therapy prophylactically (pNPWT) has even been recommended in the WHO guidelines, as a way to prevent surgical site infections on primarily closed high-risk wounds, taking resources into consideration. More on NPWT is discussed in Chapter 5.

2.2.3 Burns

Burns are wounds to the skin caused primarily by excessive heat, but also by radiation, radioactivity, electricity, friction and chemicals. The most common types of burns are heat- and radiation-related damage, for example, sunburn, hot liquid burns (scalds), hot contact burns and flame burns. One particular aspect of burns, unlike previous acute wounds, is that the damage can continue even after the source has been taken away. Heat and chemicals can continue to travel across the skin layers for some time and cause further damage, if the appropriate measures are not taken. Another aspect to consider is that some of the sources of damage can easily lead to large areas of injury, for example, radiation, hot liquids, flames and chemicals. The severity of the burn and its treatment are affected by the source of the damage, the depth to which the skin and underlying tissues have been compromised (Table 2.3), the age of the patient, and the location of the injury and the size of the burn. Burn size is defined as a percentage of the total body surface area (TBSA) and burn patients are diagnosed as having a minor, moderate or major injury based on the % TBSA (Table 2.4). Age is a significant factor in determining risk, as the skin of younger and older people tends to be thinner and weaker, making it more easily damaged across the layers.

One of the main first aid steps is to immediately cool or irrigate the wound with copious amounts of water, in the case of thermal and chemical burns.

TABLE 2.3

Categorisation of burn wounds

Burn type	Description
Superficial	First-degree burn: Limited to the superficial layers of the skin's epidermis; the total barrier function of the skin may not be compromised fully, but the wound is tender, painful, red and hot.
Superficial partial thickness	Superficial second-degree burn: involves the upper layer of the dermis (papillary dermis). Presents with pain, redness that blanches when pressure is applied and clear blistering, moist skin and has a high risk of infection. May heal on its own.
Deep partial thickness	Deep second-degree burn: affects the lower layer of the dermis (reticular dermis), and can quickly evolve into a third-degree or full-thickness burn. Presents with pain, red and white skin that does not blanch readily, bloody blisters and moist skin.
Full thickness	Third-degree burn: Involves all the epidermis, the dermis and the hypodermis. Presents as whitish or charred black, and is painless.
Fourth degree	Subdermal burn: destruction of all the layers of the epidermis, dermis, hypodermis, and subcutaneous tissues, reaching out to muscles, fat, tendons and bones.

TABLE 2.4

Burn injury severity

Severity	Description	Care setting
Minor burn injury	Partial-thickness burns*: • Children and older persons: <10% TBSA • Adults: <15% TBSA Full-thickness burns*: <2%	Outpatient
Moderate burn injury	Partial-thickness burns: • Children and older persons: 10–20% TBSA • Adults: 15–25% TBSA Full-thickness burns: 2–10% TBSA	In-patient during initial care
Major burn injury	Partial-thickness burns: • Children and older persons: >20% TBSA • Adults: >25% TBSA Full-thickness burns: >10% TBSA Burns involving the face, eyes, ears, hands, feet or perineum that may result in impairment; burns caused by caustic chemical agents, high voltage electricity, complicated by inhalation injury or trauma, or sustained by high-risk patients.	Specialised burns unit

Source: Vorstenbosch and Buchel (2019).
* Where the burn is not a risk to the eyes, ears face, hands or perineum.

Skin with superficial burns such as sunburns tends to heal itself spontaneously in less than a week and no specific treatment is required, although a moisturiser or soothing lotion can help. For superficial partial-thickness burns, where the epidermis is damaged, large amounts of fluids are released in blisters due to the damage in the microvessels, but as the blood flow is adequate and the risk of infection is low, healing is also generally spontaneous (DeSanti, 2005). To help, the wound needs to be cleaned and debris removed; a dressing that can cope with the fluids while not sticking to the wound bed can be used, with or without a soothing or antibacterial ointment.

In deep partial-thickness burns, dead tissue cells adhere to the viable tissue and blood flow is compromised, making the risks of infection and conversion to a third-degree burn higher. If there are some viable epithelial appendages, healing may occur naturally albeit at a slower rate than with superficial wounds. The removal of any dead tissue (debridement) to clean the wound is necessary and should be conducted by a professional under sterile environment. To minimise the risk of infection, the use of an antimicrobial ointment or cream such as silver sulfadiazine, or the application of an antimicrobial dressing are common. When dressings are used, they have to be changed in order to manage the fluids and prevent infection. This may be a painful experience for partial-thickness burns as the nerve endings are exposed and may still be sensitive. Another point to note for deep partial-thickness burns is that the risks of negative outcomes such as scarring and skin contraction are higher compared to superficial wounds. Where the burn is over a joint, contraction of the skin can subsequently limit the patient's range of motion. These need to be taken into consideration in selecting the appropriate treatment and follow-up. A variety of burn-specific wound dressings have been developed over the years, addressing the various concerns of partial-thickness burn care: pain management, exudate management, minimisation of scarring and prevention of infections. Most advanced wound dressings for burns provide a moist wound environment to promote healing and minimise pain upon removal.

For third-degree or full-thickness burns, as all the layers of the skin are destroyed and no epidermal cells are present to regenerate, debridement and skin grafting are normally necessary unless the burn is very small (<1 cm). This approach is also recommended on partial-thickness burns to minimise scarring if the severity of the wound or the patient's condition suggests that the wound will take longer than 21 days to heal spontaneously (Vorstenbosch & Buchel, 2019). For burns of less than 30% TBSA, the wound is excised and can be closed using split-thickness skin grafts from unburnt areas on the patient (an autograft). The donor site area is then cared for using a suitable dressing to cover, protect and promote healing. For burns over 40% TBSA, as there is insufficient healthy skin to cover the burn area without compromising the overall body status, it is common to use allografts,[1] xenografts[2] or artificial skin substitute or templates such as Integra™. The skin replacement material is critical to reduce pain (particularly in partial-thickness burnt areas), prevent evaporative heat and moisture loss and protect against contaminants and bacteria (Chiu & Burd, 2005; Vorstenbosch & Buchel, 2019).

In patients with over 30% TBSA partial-thickness or full-thickness burns, significant complications occur in parallel, which necessitates treatment at a specialist burns unit. A systemic rather than local inflammation response occurs at this level. Excessive fluids are lost through vascular permeability. Perfusion and oxygen delivery to the body are consequently impaired. Other risks increase, e.g., hypothermia due to increased evaporative water loss, lower pulmonary function, excessive blood loss and hypovolemic shock (Vorstenbosch & Buchel, 2019). Shock is also possible for fourth-degree burns because of the large inflammatory response, which may even affect the major organs. Normally, fourth-degree burns require extensive debridement and complex reconstruction of specialised tissues, often resulting in some form of subsequent disability if not amputation.

2.2.4 Specific Challenges for Acute Wounds

The three main types of acute wounds described above have each some specific needs (Table 2.5), other than the common point of rapid healing. Speed is essential as the longer the skin is compromised, the longer the chance of exposure to bacteria and contaminants. In addition, the faster a patient can return to a kind of normality in their life, the better it is from a mental health perspective. The common challenge for all three types of wounds, and the one that is most likely to result in delayed healing, is infection. For traumatic wounds, infection can occur because the wound has not been properly cleaned, for surgical wounds because they are contaminated by body fluids or skin bacteria, and for burns, because large areas of the skin, which act as a bacterial barrier, are affected. Ways of preventing and managing infections have been highlighted for each wound type and in Chapter 6, antimicrobial additives that are used in flexible materials for infection management are discussed.

TABLE 2.5

Key challenges for acute wounds

Trauma wounds	Surgical wounds	Burns
Excessive bleeding	Surgical site infection	Fluid and heat loss
Contamination from debris		Exudate management
Infection		Infection
		Scarring
		Contraction of skin, leading to reduced movement

2.3 Chronic Wounds

In contrast with acute wounds, chronic wounds are those that do not appear to move predictably or in a timely manner through the stages of the healing process. Typically, it is thought that chronic wounds stall in the inflammatory or proliferative phases. The reasons commonly evoked are insufficient oxygen or nutrients to the wound, or the presence of an infection, or an imbalance in the wound bed environment, generally characterised by too much elastase and matrix metalloproteinases (MMPs) and too little growth factors. With this protease imbalance, the degradation of proteins on the wound bed is in excess and cells are unable to proliferate as required. With an infection, the wound stays in the inflammatory stage as it tries to fight the infection. With a lack of sufficient oxygen, the cellular functions and other activities required to progress the wound slow down. The outcome of all of the above is that the wound can become stuck and does not progress through the healing cycle.

Chronic wounds are mostly, but not exclusively, seen in the older population. This is because the rate of healing of wounds is significantly impacted by existing comorbidities, which are more probable with age. The most common types of chronic wounds are often situated in the lower limb area, or in areas where there are pressures onto the skin, such as the back of the body when a person is bed-ridden or wheel-chair bound.

2.3.1 Common Types of Chronic Wounds

Venous leg ulcers are one of the most common types of chronic wounds and could account for between 75 and 80% of all lower-extremities chronic wounds (Berenguer Pérez et al., 2019). Venous disease, which is characterised by the valves of veins not working correctly, leads to backflow in blood vessels. If not properly managed, this results in pooling, swelling, inflammation, damage to blood vessels walls and breakdown in the skin. In parallel, the swelling prevents the damaged tissue from being properly irrigated with oxygen, nutrients and growth factors. Ischemia (a restriction of blood supply to a tissue resulting in lack of oxygen to the tissue) followed by reperfusion (when flow is restored) causes reperfusion injury and its associated inflammatory response, which could then lead to tissue damage and ultimately an ulcer. Generally, this presents itself as an irregular, large but shallow wound in the gaiter area of the leg, which can be accompanied by pain and oedema and a large amount of exudate. The wound needs an appropriate dressing to manage the fluids, alongside compression therapy to manage the venous insufficiency. It is thought that for the majority of patients with venous leg ulcers, the application of high compression bandaging, with simple dressings, is enough to stimulate the body to get rid of unwanted debris, manage the moisture and kick-start the healing process (Moffatt et al., 2004). The compression therapy part of the treatment returns blood flow to a manageable level and this may be sufficient for the wound to progress naturally. While most uncomplicated venous ulcers do not have much necrotic tissues, some of the complex ones could contain devitalised tissues and/or a fibrinous base, which need to be debrided. This is done either using instruments or enzymatic or larval preparations, before following up with a suitable dressing and graduated compression therapy.

Significantly less frequently seen than venous leg ulcers, arterial ulcers are caused by arterial insufficiency, where the lower extremities suffer from poor perfusion. Tissues on bony prominent areas such as the toes, or outer ankle gradually become oxygen-deprived and if damaged, breakdown into painful full-thickness ulcers that have a punched-out appearance with smooth edges. Restoration of proper blood circulation through a surgical procedure, and management of the wound with the correct dressing type are essential treatment procedures.

Diabetic foot ulcers are quite common, as pointed out in Chapter 1. They tend to happen on the plantar aspect of the foot and can form by a combination of factors, including repetitive irritation or rubbing, damage caused by foot deformities, repetitive injury, and dry calloused skin. When combined with poor circulation and neuropathy – a common condition which develops with diabetes – these irritations can lead to extended and repetitive micro-damage to the skin. Eventually, the damage turns into an ulcer. Despite being partial or full-thickness, because of the patient's neuropathy, the wound is often painless, which can make it remain undetected for too long. Poor perfusion and a susceptibility to infection complicate the healing process further. As with venous leg ulcers, regular debridement of any hard skin, devitalised tissues and bacteria, and a suitable dressing are all necessary, along with proper foot care and reduction of pressure on the affected area. Managing the wound exudate levels and preventing infection for those at higher risk are essential too, as are moving and repositioning the patient, to prevent the formation of pressure sores if the patient is bed-ridden or otherwise immobilised.

The fourth type of chronic wounds, pressure ulcers or bedsores, occurs because of extended periods of pressure, shear or friction on the skin, generally due to a lack of sufficient movement. This can happen for example when a patient is on bed rest, or in a wheelchair and is not moved frequently enough. They often appear where there is a bony prominence such as the ankles, heels, coccyx, sacrum, shoulder blades, back of the head, spine, etc. The body's weight, via the bones, leads to gradual damage to the skin and tissue, primarily because of compromised blood flow to the area. As with other chronic ulcers, reperfusion injury also occurs and damages the tissues. At Stage 1 of a pressure ulcer, the skin feels different to surrounding tissue, possibly more tender. The damage at this point is only superficial, affecting only the epidermis. At Stage 2, blisters can occur, and a shallow, painful ulcer is formed with a reddish base. Stage 3 sees further progress into a full-thickness wound, often with bad odour and signs of infection, and finally at Stage 4, underlying tissues are affected and the skin may look black, with signs of infection, such as odour, exudate and heat. Depending on the stage of the pressure ulcer, the wound may have to be cleaned and debrided (surgery may even be needed in the case of some Stage 4 ulcers), and dressed with a suitable dressing. Regular moving and repositioning of the patient is essential during the treatment, and also as an ongoing preventative routine.

Of note, are non-healing surgical wounds, which are not normally considered chronic wounds per se. Most acute wounds heal within a few weeks. A small percentage of surgical wounds fail to heal in their predicable and timely manner, and may appear to be stalled in one of the stages of wound healing. This is often linked to surgical site infections, damage to the blood supply to the surgery area, or the presence of other comorbidities such as diabetes, which delay the wound healing process.

2.3.2 Wound Healing Delay Factors

The examples of chronic wounds given above indicate that for many of such wounds, a pre-existing illness or condition (physical or mental) is a high-risk factor. The reasons for wounds to stall and not progress however extend beyond this. Some are patient-related, others are wound-related, environment-related or care-related, or a mixture of all, as illustrated in Figure 2.1.

2.3.2.1 Patient-Related Factors

From a patient's perspective, age, weight, nutrition, lifestyle choices, mobility and mental status can have an impact on whether a wound is likely to heal in a predictable manner or not. The skin of older patients is more fragile and may take longer to heal and repair. Even though ageing does not reduce the quality of healing, it has been associated with an altered inflammatory response which leads to delayed healing (Guo & DiPietro, 2010). Overweight and obese patients are faced with extra risks of infection due to bacteria lodging in between skin folds, the complications of excessive fatty tissues, which are not properly vascularised, and in some cases, the challenges of poor mobility creating more pressure and repetitive damage on existing wounds. It is important to note that even overweight and obese patients may suffer from nutritional deficiencies alongside any other health conditions they might have. While for the underweight patient, the body does not receive enough nutrients to be able to properly heal a wound, for the overweight or obese one, the body may be getting too much of the wrong type of food and not enough of the right nutrients necessary for the healthy physiological processes, again leading to poor healing quality and speed.

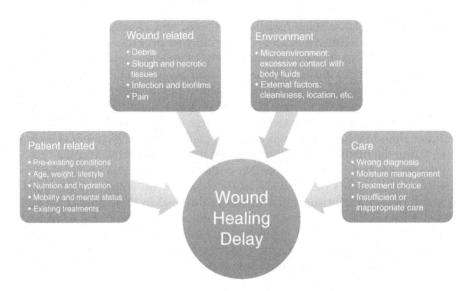

FIGURE 2.1
Wound healing delay factors

The detailed nutritional requirements for a patient are as complex as the wound healing process is itself. Deficiencies have systemic effects such as affecting the immune system and the susceptibility to infection, or localised effects such as slowing down collagen synthesis or fibroblast proliferation at the wound. One study by Heyman et al. (2008) showed that there was an improvement in the overall healing of pressure ulcers when patients took a high-energy, protein-enriched supplement with arginine, vitamins C and E, and zinc. Guo and DiPietro (2010) summarise that although the detailed nutritional requirements of a wound are not fully understood, deficiencies in proteins, carbohydrates, arginine, glutamine, polyunsaturated fatty acids, vitamins A, C and E, magnesium, copper, zinc and iron can contribute to a delay in wound healing. It is worth also noting that nutrition should also cover the right level of hydration for the body to function properly. Nutritional and hydration deficiencies can occur because of poverty, a lack of education on the subject matter, a lack of motivation, inadequate care, or simply because of the patient's lifestyle choices. Indeed, how people choose to live their life in other aspects, such as alcohol consumption, use of recreational drugs or smoking are also factors that can influence the body's ability to deal with wounds appropriately.

One of the most frequent existing illness that becomes a significant risk factor is diabetes, which has already received several mentions in this book previously. How this disease can lead to delayed wound healing is linked to several effects it could have on the body. The Wound

TABLE 2.6

How diabetes affects wound healing

Effect of diabetes	Effect on wound healing
Elevated blood sugar level	Stiffens arteries and narrows blood vessels: reduces blood flow and oxygen to wounds (may also be a cause of wound formation). Decreases function of red blood cells that carry nutrients to tissue; lowers white blood cells efficiency to fight infection.
Affected nerves and neuropathy	Patients cannot feel minor injuries such as a developing blister, infection or surgical wound problem, and the wound can deteriorate before it is noticed. They are also more at risk of causing repetitive trauma to the same injury site due to not having the pain warning.
Lowered efficiency of immune system	Increased risk of infection; if left untreated (for example combined with neuropathy above), can lead to gangrene, sepsis or bone infection.

Source: Wound Care Center (2014).

Care Center (2014) explains it up nicely in layman's terms, which is now summed up in Table 2.6.

Other diseases or conditions that affect the blood circulation and can cause ischemia are also risk factors for delayed wound healing. With decreased blood flow, oxygen, nutrition and immune cells delivery to the wound site is decreased, leading to a slower rate of healing. Wounds normally start off being deprived of adequate oxygen levels due to vascular disruption and high consumption of oxygen by the cells at the site of injury. This short-term status stimulates wound healing to kick-start and does not pose a major problem in many wounds. However, sustained hypoxia is detrimental to the healing process as oxygen is needed for all the activities to carry on. Insufficient oxygen levels also increase the risk for infection, as it has been linked to reduced levels of reactive oxygen species (ROS), an important bacteria-fighting element on the wound bed.

Examples of conditions that can exhibit ischemia include hypotension, vascular impairment, oedema, anaemia, hypoxia, peripheral vascular disease, coronary artery disease, cardiopulmonary and oxygen transport disorders (Wound Source, 2019). The presence of malignant cells, as in the case of cancers, can also affect the body's ability to deal with a wound. In addition to this, cancer treatments and chemotherapeutic drugs themselves are known to impede cell growth and can therefore negatively impact wound healing too. The same applies for a number of other treatments or medications – some have side effects that affect the integrity of the skin; others such as anti-inflammatory medication, can interfere with the inflammatory phase of healing.

Patients who are unable to move properly or regularly may be unable to care for the wound as it should. This could be as simple as not being able to keep the wound clean themselves, or to prevent it from being under pressure for prolonged periods. Physical disability, mental disability and illness can all lead to the same mobility issues, and in some cases also with compliance issues, an unwillingness or inability to follow the basic required routine of care.

2.3.2.2 Wound-Related Factors

From a wound perspective, factors that can lead to a delay include the presence of debris and necrotic tissue, infection and pain. Slough, eschar, dead tissue, biofilms and even dressing residues can hamper the wound healing process as the body still wants to keep the wound in the inflammation stage to get rid of the unwanted material. As a result, it does not progress significantly onto the next stage and new granulation tissue cannot be formed. Likewise, for infections, when the body is aware of the excessive presence of microorganisms, it concentrates efforts on trying to get rid of them, and as a result, the wound remains in the inflammation stage. A prolonged inflammation has a number of consequences that complicate the wound healing process and render it difficult to progress. Levels of MMPs, which degrade the extracellular matrix, increase; protease inhibitors decrease; growth factors degrade rapidly; and the proliferation phase cannot be engaged successfully (Guo & DiPietro, 2010).

Pain at the wound site, or elsewhere, or during dressing changes can have a debilitating psychological effect by affecting the quality of life, and may end up affecting oxygenation and susceptibility to infection (Wound Source, 2019). Pain, which is a combination of physical sensations, psychological processes and socio-cultural beliefs, often induces stress and anxiety, both of which can in turn interfere with the efficiency of the immune system and the wound healing process itself. Woo (2012) summed up several studies linking wound healing and pain or stress levels, indicating that pain, stress and distress were negatively correlated to the rates of various processes during wound healing.

2.3.2.3 Environmental and Care-Related Factors

Finally, the environment and care that the patient is able to receive can help a wound to heal properly, or hinder it from doing so too. An environment that is unclean may lead to infections that delay healing. If the patient is not cleaned and cared for properly – for example, if the wound is allowed prolonged contact with bodily fluids such as perspiration, urine, exudate or even saliva, the skin around the wound can become inflamed, leading to further delays. Patients who are not mobile need to be regularly moved and turned, otherwise excessive pressures on existing wounds, or on surrounding areas will worsen their condition.

If the wound is managed with the wrong treatment, its healing time will certainly be affected. Misdiagnosis of the aetiology of the wound, particularly for the more rarely seen ones, can lead to the wrong treatment and medication approach, which can hinder rather than encourage the healing process. From a wound surface perspective, it is widely accepted now that moist wound healing is the golden standard in treatment of any wound. The aim is to prevent desiccation of the wound bed and maintain an optimum environment for the numerous activities happening in the wound healing process. Mismanagement of the moisture levels can have detrimental effects. If the wound is allowed to get too dry, cell division and migration may slow down. If the wound has an excessive amount of exudate, which is not contained properly, the fluids can lead to 'maceration' causing more damage to the wound bed. If fluid is not contained onto the wound bed area, and is allowed to spread sideways, it can impact on the peri-wound area (i.e., the healthy skin surrounding the wound) and cause the wound to increase in size.

2.3.3 Key Challenges for Chronic Wounds

Caring for a chronic wound commonly involves a routine of debridement or cleaning of the wound, followed by applying a dressing and changing it when necessary. This process is repeated again and again, but does not necessarily get the wound to progress from its stalled position. The symptoms are simply being managed. For the wound to heal, one of the biggest challenges is to understand the root cause of the chronicity, and determine a way to eliminate this cause if possible. If a treatment plan includes strategies to deal with the root cause, e.g., with surgery, lifestyle changes, systemic medication, etc., then the chances of success in healing the wound are improved and the chances of future recurrence could be reduced.

There are difficulties that are associated with the fact that chronic wounds are long-term events, that they occur mostly in elderly patients and often have to be managed in the community. While there are disparities in the length of time chronic wounds take to heal, it has been reported that 50% take more than a year, 20% take over two years, and 10% never heal (Berenguer Pérez et al., 2019). As the patient experiences the wound and changes within the wound over a long period of time, breaks in the continuity of care can occur. This can complicate matters, making it difficult for a proper holistic and historical understanding of the wound. When managed in the community, chronic wounds also have the challenge of needing a degree of compliance from the patient, and an adequate level of care from both the professional and non-professional care providers. Assuming that the root cause of the delay is understood correctly, in some cases unfortunately, it is not possible to completely eliminate the cause. The objective may still be to heal the wound, but the risk of recurrence could remain high in those cases, and preventative measures must be part of the daily routine. Sometimes, the strategy would then turn into how best to manage the wound itself, the patient and the care to give the patient as good a quality of life as possible.

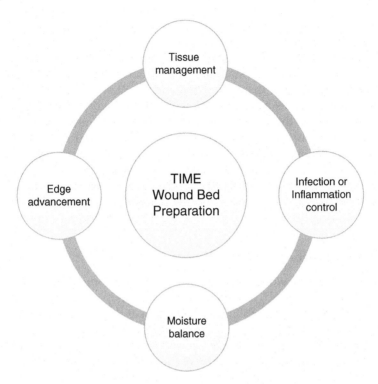

FIGURE 2.2
TIME model for wound bed preparation

The wound bed preparation model, with the four elements of TIME can be a comprehensive tool for caring for chronic wounds, particularly for the difficult cases (EWMA, 2004). The four aspects of the model to consider are (a) Tissue management, (b) Infection or inflammation control, (c) Moisture balance and (d) Epithelial (edge) advancement (Figure 2.2). They each address the different issues that can cause wounds to remain chronic and altogether, but not necessarily in a linear fashion, the four elements aim to optimise the wound bed by reducing inflammation, infection, excess exudate, and correcting the abnormalities that are causing the wound to stall.

In tissue management, the first element of the TIME model, the objective is to assess for non-viable or deficient tissue, and remove any necrotic, non-vascularised debris, to encourage the build-up of healthy tissue. This debridement procedure may be required repeatedly to maintain a positive environment for the cell growth. The right level of debridement is critical. Done too much, the wound can experience more damage leading to further delays. The opposite does not have sufficient effect on the wound, leaving it in the same stalled state.

Debridement is also a step to physically remove any bacteria and biofilms present, giving a start in addressing any long-standing infection and inflammation issues, the second aspect of the TIME model. A number of additional infection and inflammation control measures are available to support this aspect of the model, both from a systemic or localised approach. Some are discussed in Section 2.4.1, and other strategies involving additives in the dressings are discussed in Chapter 6.

Moisture balance, the third aspect, is about the need to maintain a moist wound healing environment, while managing excess exudate. In particularly with chronic wounds, exudate can contain excessive amounts of proteinases (e.g., MMPs), which can impair the proliferation stage. It has also been reported that even when proteinases are in balance, excessive plasma fluids can lead to trapping of macromolecules and growth factors in the tissues, leading to delays in healing (EWMA, 2004).

The last aspect of the TIME model is to consider what could help in the epithelial or edge advancement, i.e., the restoration of the skin function and closing of the wound. This process of cell generation and growth may be affected by various factors, including the supply of oxygen, mismanagement of exudate, lack of cell responses to growth factors, and so on. It is important to consider as well the health of the peri-wound skin. While it may be reasonably healthy and well perfused, this area may still be quite sensitive and any breakdown in the tissue can deteriorate the wound by enlarging the affected area. Excessive contact of exudate or other body fluids onto the surrounding skin can cause damage, as can the use of the wrong type of product, e.g., an adhesive that is too harsh for the skin.

While the TIME model gives a pathway to follow in assessing and addressing the underlying causes of chronicity in wounds, the big challenge after preparing the wound bed to optimise healing, is finding the right treatment that will trigger the wound to get back on track and continue to progress through the wound healing process. As wounds and patients are all unique, a holistic approach may have to be taken, looking at all aspects of health and wound care altogether. Advanced wound care is now such a vast area of expertise that it can be difficult to navigate to find the appropriate treatment without too much trial and error. The most recent developments on the market involve not only dressing the wound, but proactively stimulating it, whether biologically (e.g., with enzymes or growth factors), chemically (e.g., with anti-infectives or oxygen), physically (e.g., with negative pressure therapy), or even using irradiation as with light therapy or electrically, as with bioelectric dressings. Many clinicians advocate decisions based on clinical evidence. However, as wounds can respond differently to the same treatment, the outcome can still be different to those observed in prior clinical data and another treatment route may need to be investigated.

2.4 Infected Wounds

Bacteria and other microorganisms are present all around us and on our skin, which when intact, acts as a protective barrier. It is quite common for a range of bacteria to be active on a wound site (contamination), without the wound being infected. Wounds can test positive for bacterial cultures without as such exhibiting any classic signs of infection. Likewise, in some patients, the clinical signs of infections may be absent or reduced in intensity, despite the clear presence of infection, e.g., in the case of some diabetic patients who have poor supply to the feet or severe neuropathy. A clinical and holistic diagnosis is therefore important to support evidence from any surface cultures and vice versa.

Infection presents itself with symptoms such as bad odour, ongoing inflammation (redness, pain, swelling, hotness, fever), presence of debris and pus or cloudy exudate or increased amounts of exudate. Further symptoms also include the presence of an abscess, unanticipated delayed healing, friable and bleeding granulation tissue, and wound breakdown (Collier, 2004). At this stage when infection sets in, the body's immune system is already overwhelmed by the number or type of pathogens present, and cannot cope anymore (Figure 2.3). It is worth pointing out that in the stage before infection sets in, when a wound is critically colonised, the wound healing process can start to be affected.

The outcome of critical colonisation or an infection in the wound is a slow-down in the rate of healing, as the wound continues to stay in the inflammation stage to get rid of the bacteria and other associated debris. This extended inflammation period could also lead to further tissue damage to the wound bed. Studies have shown that surgical wound infections can increase the number of days required for hospitalisation, which is a concern both from the patient's perspective, as well as from a health economics perspective (Bowler et al., 2001).

Both acute and chronic wound can be infected. Looking at external factors first, for acute traumatic wounds, the likelihood of infection is higher when

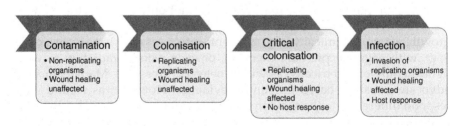

FIGURE 2.3
From contamination to infection (de Leon et al., 2016)

patients do not present for treatment until six or more hours after the injury, or for compression wounds (such as pressure sores and crush injuries) or bite wounds, and/or if there are foreign bodies in the wound (Richardson, 2004). The presence of foreign bodies or devitalised tissue on the wound bed can favour bacterial growth. For both acute (traumatic or surgical) and chronic wounds, infections can also be caused by external contamination or self-contamination due to the wound size and location, through inadequate hygiene or insufficient precautions taken during dressing changes. The risks are heightened especially when the patient is in an uncontrolled environment or when combined with other systemic risk factors. The main recurring health conditions or comorbidities increasing the susceptibility to infections are poor circulation leading to insufficient oxygen at the wound sites, diabetes, obesity, compromised immune system, decreased mobility and nutritional deficiencies.

In recent years, a bigger focus has been put on the presence of biofilms and their role in the tenaciousness of chronic wounds (Rhoads et al., 2008). A biofilm is a multi-species community of bacteria, held together by a slimy extracellular polymeric substance, which act as a matrix in which the bacteria is encased. The biofilm formation starts with attachment of cells on a surface and the formation of microcolonies. Bacteria then start secreting the extracellular polysaccharide substance, which continues on until they are safely attached into the internal surfaces of a thick biomolecular layer, which presents itself as the mature biofilm structure (Roy et al., 2018). Together, bacteria in a biofilm do not behave like in their free-flowing planktonic state. They are able to withstand more hostile environments, including starvation and desiccation, and they also become more recalcitrant to antimicrobials and the immune system response (Roy et al., 2018). As a community, the microcolony of bacteria in the biofilm has cell-to-cell signalling capabilities, and the organisms within have different roles within the biofilm structure. Together, they are able to have different protein-expressing behaviours that aid the resistance to antimicrobials and the immune response. The deeply embedded species are sheltered from these latter attacks, are less metabolically active, but are also more resistant and able to reconstitute the community.

2.4.1 Treatment of Infected Wounds

Left untreated, wound infections can lead to cross infections, cellulitis, and ultimately bacteraemia and septicaemia, both of which can be fatal. An acute wound is not normally closed up until the infection has been dealt with. An important step in the treatment of the infected wound is to clean and surgically debride the wound bed. This is particularly significant in the case where there are suspected biofilms, as topical or systemic treatments alone are unlikely to have a measurable outcome on the biofilms. Debriding the wound has the additional benefit of ensuring that the wound bed is rid of devitalised tissues and other debris, which could create an environment that encourages bacterial proliferation. The more intact host responses may also be exposed following debridement – this can help the body fight the infection.

Alongside debridement, a systemic antibiotic is often prescribed for the management of clinically infected wounds, particularly when the wound infection is deep or when there is clinical evidence that the infection is systemic. These have high specificity to inhibit or kill certain microorganisms. However, there are concerns over the excessive use of antibiotics and the development of bacterial resistance to them. Topical antimicrobials such as antiseptic ointments or creams, or antimicrobial wound dressings are also used in infection management. They normally have a broader range of antibacterial activity, but some can be harmful to healthy wound healing cells. As the majority of wounds have a polymicrobial aerobic-anaerobic microflora, broad-spectrum antimicrobial agents are more likely to have a positive effect in the management of infected wounds (Bowler et al., 2001). More details on various types of anti-infective ingredients are discussed in Chapter 6.

Notes

1 Allografts here are skin transplants from another donor, generally cadaver.
2 Xenografts here are skin transplants from another species, generally porcine.

References

Berenguer Pérez, M., López-Casanova, P., Sarabia Lavín, R., González de la Torre, H., & Verdú-Soriano, J. (2019). Epidemiology of Venous Leg Ulcers in Primary Health Care: Incidence and Prevalence in a Health Centre – A Time Series Study (2010–2014). *International Wound Journal, 16*(1), 256.

Bowler, P. G., Duerden, B. I., & Armstrong, D. G. (2001, April). Wound Microbiology and Associated Approaches to Wound Management. *Clinical Microbiology Reviews, 14*(2), 244.

Chiu, T., & Burd, A. (2005, July–August). "Xenograft" Dressing in the Treatment of Burns. *Clinical Dermatology, 23*(4), 419.

Collaborative GS. (2017). Determining the Worldwide Epidemiology of Surgical Site Infections after Gastrointestinal Infection Surgery: Protocol for a Multicentre, International, Prospective Cohort Study (GlobalSurg 2). *BMJ Open, 7*, 1.

Collier, M. (2004, January). *Recognition and Management of Wound Infections* (Version 1.0). Retrieved April 16, 2020, from http://www.worldwidewounds.com/2004/january/Collier/Management-of-Wound-infections.html

de Leon, J., Bohn, G. A., DiDomenico, L., Fearmonti, R., Gottlieb, H. D., Lincoln, K., Sha, J. B., Shaw, M., Taveau, H. S., Thibodeaux, K., Thomas, J. D., Treadwell, T. A. (2016, October). Critical Thinking and Treatment Strategies for Wounds. *Wounds: A Compendium of Clinical Research and Practice (Supplement)*, 1. Retrieved September 3, 2020, from https://pdfs.semanticscholar.org/56e3/16d13683d103b00773250a98e be85390d8e4.pdf?_ga=2.79766551.184915936.1599127334-148716857.1586709410

DeSanti, L. (2005, July–August). Pathophysiology and Current Management of Burn Injury. *Advances in Skin & Wound Care, 18*(6), 323.

EWMA. (2004). *Position Document: Wound Bed Preparation in Practice*. London: MEP Ltd. Retrieved from https://ewma.org/fileadmin/user_upload/EWMA.org/ Position_documents_2002-2008/pos_doc_English_final_04.pdf

Guo, S., & DiPietro, L. (2010). Factors Affecting Wound Healing. *Journal of Dental Research, 89*(3), 219.

Heyman, H., Van De Looverbosch, D. E., Meijer, E. P., & Schols, J. M. (2008). Benefits of an Oral Nutritional Supplement on Pressure Ulcer Healing in Long-Term Care Residents. *Journal of Wound Care, 17*, 476.

Moffatt, C., Morison, M. J., & Pina, E. (2004). Wound Bed Preparation for Venous Leg Ulcers. In *European Wound Management Association (EWMA). Position Document: Wound Bed Preparation in Practice*. London: MEP Ltd.

Rhoads, D. D., Wolcott, R., & Percival, S. (2008, November). Biofilms in Wounds: Management Strategies. *Journal of Wound Care, 17*(11), 502.

Richardson, M. (2004, January 27). Acute Wounds: An Overview of the Physiological Healing Process. *Nursing Times, 100*(4), 50.

Roy, R., Tiwari, M., Donelli, G., & Tiwari, V. (2018). Strategies for Combating Bacterial Biofilms: A Focus on Anti-Biofilm Agents and Their Mechanisms of Action. *Virulence, 9*(1), 522. doi:10.1080/21505594.2017.1313372

Sawyer, R., & Evans, H. (2018, May 1). Surgical Site Infection – The Next Frontier in Global Surgery. *The Lancet Infectious Diseases, 18*(5), 477.

Vorstenbosch, J., & Buchel, E. (2019, September 16). *Thermal Burns*. Retrieved April 3, 2020, from Medscape: https://emedicine.medscape.com/article/ 1278244-overview

Woo, K. Y. (2012). Exploring the Effects of Pain and Stress on Wound Healing. *Advances in Skin & Wound Care, 25*(1), 38.

World Health Organization. (2018a). *Global Guidelines for the Prevention of Surgical Site Infection*. Geneva: World Health Organization. Retrieved April 2, 2020, from https://apps.who.int/iris/bitstream/handle/10665/277399/9789241550475-eng.pdf?ua=1

World Health Organization. (2018b). *Protocol for Surgical Site Infection Surveillance with a Focus on Settings with Limited Resources*. Geneva: World Health Organization.

Wound Care Center. (2014, March 24). *How Diabetes Affects Wound Healing* (IB Internet Brands). Retrieved April 8, 2020, from Wound Care Center: https://www.woundcarecenters.org/article/living-with-wounds/ how-diabetes-affects-wound-healing

Wound Source. (2019, April). *Why Won't This Wound Heal? Addressing Common Factors That Impact Wound Healing*. Retrieved April 9, 2020, from Wound Care Center: https://pages.woundsource.com/addressing-common-factors-that-impact-wound-healing/

3

The Requirements for Advanced Wound Care

3.1 General Wound Requirements

The body is designed to deal with minor and moderate breakdown in tissue, but sometimes needs a little extra help in order to make sure that healing occurs in a healthy and predictable manner, or does not get unnecessarily delayed. For large or very deep wounds, or those that involve major organs, significant help is required in order to help it manage not only the localised trauma but also the systemic reactions throughout the body. The main routes of external intervention to help the body to heal are first aid actions, surgical procedures, pharmacological treatment, medical device assistance, wound dressings and nursing care.

The key requirements of a wound and the wound bed are shown in Figure 3.1. The prevention of excessive blood loss and having a clean micro-environment are important starting points for healing. For minor wounds, the body does this automatically by the first and second stages of wound healing involving blood clotting and temporary local inflammation. For larger open wounds, contaminated ones or those that contain slough and other devital-ised tissues, external assistance in the form of application of pressure, surgi-cal procedures, debridement and cleansing of the wound and application of appropriate dressings and/or skin substitutes are important actions required to control blood loss and create a clean environment for the wound to heal.

Another step that generally needs external intervention is protection of the wound from environmental contaminants, bacteria, further physical dam-age, and heat and moisture loss. As the skin barrier properties and normal functions are compromised by the wound, contaminations and infections are more likely. A replacement barrier layer, generally in the form of a dressing or bandage or even skin substitutes in some cases, can be essential. It can serve as protecting layer against contaminants of all sorts, and in some cases, can also provide a degree of cushioning to prevent further tissue damage caused by accidental bumps on the wound site. Wounds are also known to be a pathway for loss of heat and moisture through evaporative loss, and a protecting layer which minimises this loss will help the wound stay on track.

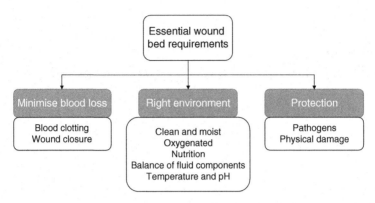

FIGURE 3.1
Key wound bed requirements

Considering the physiological processes, in order for the body to be able to successfully activate and manage all the healing activities, the wound site needs to be healthily perfused, with good access to oxygen and nutrients. A lack of either is a well-accepted cause of wound healing delay. As well as good vascularisation to the wound site, for the wound bed to have a regular supply of oxygen and nutrients, the wound area must also not be under unnecessary physical pressure which may restrict blood flow, or cause any reperfusion injury.

The balance of healing mediators is absolutely important at each stage of wound healing. In reperfusion injury for example, when the cycle of restored blood flow following ischemia is repeated several times, a pro-inflammatory state is induced. When reperfusion occurs, there is an excess of leukocytes and neutrophils, which leads to more cytokines and ROS, and a reduced level of the antioxidant nitric oxide (Zhao et al., 2016). Altogether this fluid composition leads to tissue damage and injury. Imbalances in the microenvironment typically seen in chronic wounds are increased levels of neutrophils, macrophages, proteases, inflammatory cytokines, ROS, and reduced availability of growth factors. The outcome is a prolonged state of inflammation or an inability for the proliferation stage to fully develop due to cellular matrix being destroyed too quickly. The wound fluid composition in chronic wounds, which has been found to be more basic in pH, is reported to block cellular proliferation and angiogenesis when there is an excess of exudate. By contrast, wound fluid from acute wounds, which is more acidic, has been reported to stimulate proliferation of fibroblasts, keratinocytes and endothelial cells, at least *in vitro* (Falanga, 2004).

The modern concept of moist wound healing has been developed from the understanding of acute wounds, and the positive effect of acute wound fluids relates seamlessly to the concept. Despite the negative connotation of chronic wound exudate, the total desiccation of the wound area is not advised either.

TABLE 3.1

Benefits of moist wound healing

Positive impact on wound progression	Positive outcomes
Less intense and less prolonged inflammation	Earlier full-thickness wound contraction
Increased collagen synthesis	Reduced pain
Faster re-epithelialisation rates	Improved cosmesis
Earlier and less prolonged angiogenesis	Reduced infection
Earlier differentiation of keratinocytes to restore the skin barrier function	Reduced overall health care costs
Faster keratinocyte and fibroblast proliferation and migration	

Source: Sharman (2003) and Ovington (2007).

Therefore, moist wound healing is still preferred even for chronic wounds. Moist wound healing is a long-established practice of ensuring that the wound bed has an optimum level of hydration and does not dry out during wound care. The benefits of this principle have been thoroughly explored over the last few decades, particularly in acute wounds. Summed up, it has been shown to accelerate wound healing and is associated with the benefits shown in Table 3.1.

Moist wound healing is all about moisture balance, and making sure that there is no excessive exudate either – which could damage the wound bed (as in chronic wounds), or even the peripheral still-healthy tissues. For a healthy wound, exudate production is normal and facilitates the delivery of essential healing mediators and nutrients. It normally decreases as the wound heals, but for some chronic wounds, e.g., venous leg ulcers, or some acute wounds, e.g., burns and donor sites, the exudate level is excessive and needs to be managed in order to assure the comfort of the patient, or to prevent damage that can occur due to imbalanced, cell-damaging exudate. Left unmanaged, excessive exudate can lead to odour, discomfort, infection, and wound maceration, leaving it and the adjacent skin at risk of further moisture-related or enzyme-related damage, or even infections. In short, in an ideal situation, the wound needs to remain moist but not soggy, and for those with significant exudate, moisture management is essential.

3.2 Patient Needs

In the pursuit of wound healing and closure, it is not difficult to forget that behind the injury is a person. Each individual has his or her own preferences, priorities and sensitivities in dealing with their wound and in managing their quality of life. In some cases, such priorities may necessitate a different approach to the care given, in order to ensure a better chance of compliance to the treatment and therefore a better chance of a positive outcome. Improving the patient experience has been a focus of many healthcare services in developed countries. Patient needs such as the wish for a personalised, individualised approach, for greater control over their health and healthcare decisions, greater dignity and respect, and the right to access to a range of treatments are at the forefront of improving patient experience in the UK for example (Department of Health, 2008). Very similar requirements are likely also applicable in many other countries.

The presence of an injury, whether acute or chronic, or an infection can elicit many different emotions, including fear, stress, anxiety and worry. When the wound is chronic and an infection is long-lasting, other emotions develop too, such as frustration, embarrassment, anger, feeling depressed and not wanting to socialise. Many of these emotions, particularly those that lead to anxiety and stress, eventually have a negative impact on wound healing and even on the perception of the wound and pain.

Pain, which is very much a patient-centred and multidimensional symptom, leads to a cascade of issues. When experienced during movement, pain can lead to the patient becoming less and less mobile and more isolated. At dressing changes, it leads to fear and anxiety in anticipation of dressing changes, and stress during the change. As a result, pain can lead to patients not adhering to a treatment, having a reduced quality of life, experiencing heightened levels of stress or distress and having difficulties in maintaining social relationships (Woo, 2012). The link between pain and stress is a tight and bidirectional one. It is known that stressing about and anticipating pain can make its perception higher. Vice versa, pain can lead to more stress, and the cycle continues. There have been a number of studies demonstrating how stress impacts wound healing, including reducing the immune response, the potential for cell proliferation, resistance against infection and skin barrier recovery (Woo, 2012).

For patients experiencing heavily exuding wounds, the excessive fluids can seriously affect their quality of life. Discomfort, pain, embarrassment, constantly soiled clothing and bedding, frequent dressing changes and healing delays are some of the issues they may have to deal with on a day-to-day basis. Odour can also arise from excessive exudate levels, as well as from infection. Altogether, the effect of excessive exudate and malodour can impact on patients' mental wellbeing and lead to depression, low self-esteem, stress, anxiety, sleep problems, reduced mobility, and even social isolation. An important aspect of the management of wounds and exudate levels therefore is the need to ensure that the quality of life is improved or at the very least is not worsened by the treatment.

For some patients, the ability to continue with their day-to-day activities is very important both for their mental health, self-esteem, dignity, and perhaps

TABLE 3.2

Wound symptoms and patient needs

Wound symptoms	Patient concerns	Treatment needs
Open wounds	Fear, worry, anxiety, stress, embarrassment, inability to do the things that they normally do	Cover and protect the wound, e.g., with a dressing; if required, discreet dressing profile
Pain	Anxiety at dressing changes, worry about mobility, or ability to continue with their day-to-day activities, reduced quality of life and reduced wish to socialise	Low adhering dressings, gentle adhesives, pain management strategies, including pain-relieving dressings
High exudate levels	Embarrassment, discomfort, worry about frequent dressing changes, inconvenience	Absorbent and superabsorbent dressings or systems
Infection	Pain and its associated effects, worry, embarrassment, frustration at healing delay	Antimicrobial treatments or dressings
Odour	Embarrassment, worry, reduce wish to socialise	Debridement, odour control dressings, infection control strategies, including using antibacterial dressings
Non-healing wound	Frustration, anger, embarrassment, depression	Treatments and dressings that can stimulate wound healing and/or re-balance the wound bed

for their financial situation or because others are dependent on them. This needs to be taken into account, for example, with the use of dressings that can withstand the day-to-day activities that the wearer can perform, as well as minimise hindering due to inflexibility or bulk.

For a positive and holistic approach to wound healing, all of the above must be taken into consideration and the treatment and dressings chosen with the right balance of wound healing, reassurance to the patient and management of their emotions (Table 3.2).

3.3 The Role of Wound Dressings

Some of the wound requirements discussed above are managed systemically, surgically or through nursing care. Others, such as providing protection and a moist environment at the wound bed, can be delivered using a dressing, in combination with the appropriate treatment. Dressings have always been used in the care of wounds, and in the last few decades, there has been an acceleration in the development of new flexible materials for use as dressing materials. The basic role of wound dressings used to be as a protective layer against the environment and against further aggression to the wound, and to absorb any fluids. Nowadays advanced wound care entails the use of dressings that perform other functions than being a protective layer. The role of the modern wound dressing is to assist in accelerating wound healing, in conjunction with other care and treatment protocols devised for a patient. How this is achieved depends on the type of wound, the status of the wound and the patient.

3.3.1 Wound Dressing Requirements

From what is known about acute and chronic wounds, and about patient concerns and requirements, there are a number of essential design features for wound dressings that need to be considered. They are grouped into subcategories or levels, illustrated in Figure 3.2. Two requirements that are applicable to all dressings are safety and ease of application and use. All wound dressings must demonstrate safety during and after use, for the patient, the care provider, and towards the environment when disposed of. Ideally, they must all be easy to remove from their packaging, easy to handle, easy to apply and easy to remove. The next level is the protective role of the dressing against external aggressors and contamination. This can be achieved with or without a passive or active management of the wound environment (i.e., fluid management, bioburden management and enzymatic balance). The ultimate level of advanced wound dressing is to actively assist in speeding up healing, e.g., by encouraging it to move through the various stages

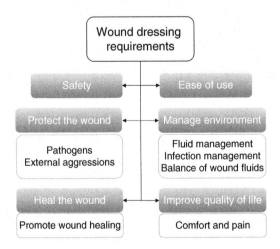

FIGURE 3.2
General wound dressing requirements

of wound healing, and also to assist in improving the quality of life of the patient, such as providing comfort, reducing pain and decreasing stress.

Dressings are a powerful tool in the treatment of wounds and the right choice can positively influence how the wound heals. On the other hand, choosing the wrong dressing can inadvertently make matters worse for the patient and the clinician alike. The choice of a wound dressing depends on the symptoms that the wound presents (e.g., excess exudate, presence of infection, and so on), the underlying issues that need to be managed, on the size and location of the wound and the patient's health, skin health, mobility and lifestyle. As a starting point, some dressing properties to be taken into considerations for specific wounds are given below.

3.3.1.1 Superficial Wounds

For wounds that only concern the upper layer of the skin, which are predicted to heal within a few days with minimal exudate, the purpose of the dressing is to protect the damaged area and if desired, to provide a moist wound healing environment. It is more than likely that for such wounds, unless a large body area is affected, the patient is able to continue with most of their day-to-day activities, including basic requirements for having a wash and a shower. A dressing which is thin, flexible and a good barrier, and which will stay in place (e.g., with a reasonably strong adhesive) is a practical solution to protect the wound from contaminants. Waterproofness is desirable if the wound is likely to get wet. If the dressing is able to occlude or semi-occlude the wound area, the moist environment may help with wound healing. However, if the wound is likely to have an amount of exudate, then an absorbing layer is required.

3.3.1.2 Bleeding Wounds

Very minor bleeding wounds should respond positively with the manual application of pressure, which reduces the blood loss. Within a few minutes of applying pressure on the wound, the wound's coagulating cascade would have started and blood flow should stop. For the lightest wounds, an occlusive dressing is sufficient to provide the pressure and contain any blood. If the wound is a little deeper, an absorbent dressing may be required to be placed on the wound while pressure is applied, with more layers added should the bleeding continue. In other cases, for example, severe acute traumatic wounds, where large arteries and veins have been affected, bleeding does not stop easily and the situation can soon become life threatening. Also, the position of the wound in some cases does not allow adequate pressure to be applied. It is reported that up to 40% of mortality after a traumatic injury is caused by massive haemorrhage (Smith et al., 2013). Under these circumstances, haemostatic dressings can help prevent excessive blood loss

TABLE 3.3

Ideal haemostatic dressing for tactical applications

Patient requirements	Caregiver requirements	Other requirements
Stops severe bleeding fast	Poses no risk to medics	Safe for the patient, carer and environment
Causes no pain	Ready to use	Inexpensive and cost-effective
Causes no thermal injury	Requires little or no training	Biodegradable
Flexible and conformable	Durable and lightweight	Bioabsorbable
Easily removed	Practical	
Does not leave residues	Easy to use in austere conditions	
No toxicity	Stable at extreme temperatures	
No side effects	Long shelf life	

by chemically or physically helping the blood to coagulate. Ideally, these dressings should work fast (within minutes), should be easy to apply, be easily conformed to the wound area and also be able to manage blood that is already on the wound bed. A more comprehensive list of requirements was developed for military applications (Kheirabadi, 2011), and has been adapted in Table 3.3. A number of haemostatic materials are available commercially and, it is important to balance the absolute haemostatic efficiency versus side effects and other complications that may be incurred, or indeed other wound aspects that may take priority. Some of technologies are used as base materials for dressings, and discussed in Chapter 4; others are additives, discussed in Chapter 6.

Some wounds may present with minor bleeding but also with other significant aspects to manage, such as excessive exudate. For example, donor sites, ulcers and other partial or full-thickness wounds may have minor concurrent bleeding, which could benefit from being managed using a dressing that has both good fluid handling capabilities and some haemostatic properties. The decision on whether haemostatic properties are required in a dressing would depend upon the overall wound situation.

3.3.1.3 Wounds with Exudate

Fluids from wounds, especially when in excessive quantities, need to be managed in order to prevent further damage to the wound bed, to the peri-wound area, and to allow the patient to have a good quality of life. Wounds that require 1–2 dressing changes a day are considered mild to moderate; those that need 2–3 dressing changes a day are deemed moderate and more than 3 changes daily are considered heavy (Dabiri et al., 2016). Exuding wounds need to be dressed with materials that take away the exudate from the wound

TABLE 3.4

Ideal properties of dressings for highly exuding wounds

Fluid handling properties	Other desirable properties
High absorption capacity	Can be used under compression
No strikethrough	Minimal trauma and pain on removal
No sideways spreading of fluids	Comfortable, flexible, conformable
Locking in of fluids (no leakages and no maceration or excoriation)	Stays intact and can be left in place for long duration
	Protection from contaminants and infection
	Cost-effective

Source: Gardner (2012).

bed. This means that it should be able to absorb the fluid, prevent it from spreading outside of the wound area, retain fluid in its structure so that it does not squeeze back onto the wound or through the dressing outer layer or clothing (especially if venous compression therapy is used alongside), and/ or evaporate the excess. A summary of ideal properties for dressings used in the management of highly exuding wound is given in Table 3.4. A large number of materials have been developed for light to heavy exuding wounds. The decision on the appropriate one for each wound is based on the amount of exudate, the type of wound, its position, the cost and how often the dressing can be changed. Where dressing change is a concern, dressings that can hold more fluid for longer can reduce the frequency of the changes. When the amount of fluid is extremely high, a supporting medical device to get rid of the fluid (such as NPWT) may have to be used in combination with a dressing.

It is important to highlight at this point that many dressings used for exudate management are simply there to deal with the fluids and possibly to prevent additional damage. When the presence of excessive damaging fluids is the cause of delayed healing, managing the exudate levels could kick start the healing process. However, for many cases, unless the dressings contain other actives or are part of a combination treatment, they are unlikely to address the underlying causes of the wound. Therefore, it is important that while the fluid is being managed for the patient's comfort and to prevent further damage to the wound, other treatment avenues are also considered to treat the underlying cause or contributory factors.

3.3.1.4 Granulating and Epithelialising Wounds

Wounds that start to show some granulation tissue at the base can still be exuding, although generally to a lesser amount. Dressings that can manage the fluids and protect the wound are still indicated, however, care must be taken with regards to not damaging new cells, nor creating an environment that could lead to over-granulation. As new capillaries are formed, followed by new epithelium, it is important not to overly disrupt or destroy them and cause unnecessary trauma with dressing changes. Materials with low adherence to the wound bed, and which can maintain a moist environment are ideal. The use of some highly evaporative dressings, which could have been used to manage a heavily exuding stage, may dehydrate the wound bed and cause cells to stick to the wound dressing. This can lead to damage and pain upon dressing changes.

3.3.1.5 Dry Wounds or Wounds with Eschar

Wounds that do not produce much exudate can be dehydrated and under such conditions, cell growth is hampered and the healing mediators are unable to spread and participate optimally in the healing process. Allowed to remain dry for long, the wound may eventually result in the formation of eschar, a thick, dry dark scab of dead tissue on the surface of the wound. To prevent wounds from over-drying, and reaching that stage, a moisture-donating dressing, preferably with an occlusive layer may be helpful. Such dressings normally have a high water content, which acts as a reservoir for the wound, keeping it moist, not wet. An occlusive layer will prevent moisture from unnecessarily evaporating from the dressing or wound bed.

When eschar is present, it needs to be removed in order to allow the wound to continue healing. This procedure is conducted either surgically, or using an enzymatic treatment or a moisture-donating dressing that softens the hard tissue first and subsequently enables the body to deal with the eschar itself (autolytic debridement). In the latter case, a high water content dressing slowly helps to restore moisture to the wound bed and softens the hardened layer at the same time. With moisture level at the wound bed becoming more balanced, the body's own phagocytes and enzymes can gradually get back to work and start to get rid of the dead tissue. Although significantly slower than other debridement methods, this is normally conducted when the size of the eschar is not significant or if other treatments are contraindicated. In the case where enzymatic debridement is chosen as the preferred treatment of choice, the dressing applied on top should protect the wound and maintain a moist environment, enabling the proteolytic enzyme preparation to digest the necrotic tissues at its own pace.

3.3.1.6 Sloughy, Fibrinous Wound Beds

Slough on the surface of the wound bed consists of devitalised tissue mixed with fibrins, degraded extracellular matrix proteins, exudate, white blood cells and bacteria, and presents itself as a tan-yellow coloured layer, sometimes securely adhered to granulation tissue (Dabiri et al., 2016). Its presence hampers the wound from properly granulating and epithelialising, and puts the wound at higher risk of infection. Debridement is necessary to remove the slough, and as mentioned above, can be done surgically, or using enzymatic preparations or dressings that facilitate autolytic debridement.

The cause of the excessive slough is an over-activity of proteases, which breaks down newly formed granulation tissue as well as other biologically active proteins on the wound bed such as growth factors and cytokines (Dabiri et al., 2016). Exudate from chronic wounds has been found to contain excessive amounts of proteases. Dressings may be able to address this issue – by locking away excess fluids from the wound bed, and/or by the delivery of active ingredients that can moderate the proteolytic degradation.

3.3.1.7 Infected Wounds

In Chapter 2, antimicrobial dressings were highlighted as one of three main pillars of the treatment of infected wounds – the other two being debridement and cleansing of the wound bed and systemic medication. There are a substantial number of antimicrobial dressings commercially available and there is no single dressing that is universally suitable for all types of infected wounds. At the base, one of the key requirements for dressing such wounds should be to help reduce the bacterial load without being cytotoxic to the freshly growing tissues. In order to do so, there are a number of properties that come into play such as how efficacious the dressing is when in use (for example as measured by the amount of bacteria killed), how long this efficacy lasts, what type of bacteria can the dressing deal with, and whether the efficacy is consistent over the wear time of the product (Table 3.5).

The clinician needs to consider other aspects of the wound and the patient's requirements before being able to make the correct decision. Infected wounds also present with other complications such as an increased exudate level, pain, swelling and odour, which should also be considered in the dressing choice.

TABLE 3.5

Properties to consider for antimicrobial dressings

Antimicrobial properties	Other dressing requirements
Bactericidal efficacy	Safe, non-allergenic, non-cytotoxic to cells
Sustained antimicrobial effect	Maintains a moist healing environment
Consistency over time	Provides exudate management if necessary
Consistency over the whole wound area	Pain-free and atraumatic removal
Broad-spectrum activity	Odour control
Speed of antimicrobial activity	Easy to use and apply
Protection from cross-contamination	

3.3.1.8 Sensitive Skin or Painful Wounds

Low adherence to the wound bed is a desired characteristic for any wound dressing. Where wound bed adherence is high (such as with traditional cotton gauze or a simple cotton dressing pad), ingrowth of tissue cells into the dressing can lead to trauma and pain upon its removal, and a risk of increasing the wound size or unnecessarily delaying healing. For sensitive skin and for wounds that are painful, dressings that will not cause trauma or contact allergies to the wound or to the peri-wound skin during wear or upon removal are essential. This applies not only to the wound-contact layer of the dressing, but also to any adhesives that would be in contact with the surrounding skin. For example, the frequency of contact allergy is high in patients with venous leg ulcers, and the skin around the ulcers is often fragilised. Dressings that are non-adherent on the wound bed, that provide atraumatic removal, have a low risk of allergic reactions, and that contain gentle adhesives if they are to be used, are recommended (Rippon et al., 2007).

3.3.1.9 Surgical Wounds

For clean surgical wounds, the primary concern of a dressing is to protect the wound from external contamination and surgical site infection and manage exudate levels, if any. An effective occlusive or semi-occlusive dressing with or without an absorbent layer is perfect for this purpose. When other aspects of the nursing care are taken into consideration, other dressing properties may become necessary too. Mobility is essential for example, in the case where the patient is quickly required to start physiotherapy and exercising, or where the surgery is at or near a joint. A dressing that is more flexible, conformable and even stretchable can facilitate movement. For surgical sites that are painful, dressings that can contribute to the overall pain management – including gentle cushioning or atraumatic removal during dressing changes, will lead to a better patient experience and quality of life.

3.3.1.10 Anatomical Locations

The majority of dressings are available as square or rectangular shapes. For anatomically challenging locations such as the heel, hands, face, digits or the sacral area, some practitioners may find it difficult or very time consuming to utilise these basic shapes and achieve good dressing-to-wound contact, or seal the edges efficiently. If the dressing gapes, is incorrectly placed, and is not in contact fully with the wound bed, there is the risk of leakage of fluids, contamination and infection. For an exuding wound, fluids can pool in the gaps and lead to maceration, excoriation and damage of the wound bed, or of other contacting areas including the peri-wound skin.

For the practitioner, using a dressing designed for a specific position speeds up the dressing application and change time. However, not all dressings are available in anatomical shapes, and it may be then required to cut and shape a product to optimise the close contact of the dressing surface to the wound surface, as demonstrated by Fletcher (2007). The cuttability of a dressing – without it losing its integrity or becoming too difficult to handle – is essential in order to enable clinicians to perform this procedure. The mass production of dressings means that under most business models, it is unfortunately not possible for shaped dressings to be made in all anatomically challenging positions due to their low volume requirements. Practitioners have to show creativity and skill in the cutting of standard shaped dressings, while still adhering to their best local practice for avoiding contaminations and risk of infections when the sterile package is open.

3.3.1.11 Deep Tunnelling Wounds

Some wounds tunnel deep or across under the surface of the skin, with minimal breakdown of the epidermis. The risk for such wounds is that the small area of broken skin on the surface may appear healed and closed up, but the underneath cavity remains unhealed and even infected. The path of the tunnelling wound may be difficult to visualise because the majority of the wound is underneath what seems to be healthy skin. If not dressed properly, an exuding tunnelling wound will experience fluid pooling and its related issues. The cavity needs to be packed with an appropriate dressing material. Ideally, this needs to be flexible and strong enough to be pushed through small apertures, be able to closely contact the wound bed, and be easily removed without falling apart. Once properly packed inside the cavity, the dressing is then able to manage exudate, ensure a moist wound healing environment, and help in the cleansing of the wound. Typically, such materials are in ribbon forms, which are narrower in shape to more easily get in and can be pulled out when the dressing needs changing.

3.3.1.12 Burns

Wounds from burns have quite specific challenges, some of which are immediate, and others medium and long term. From the start in the burns care process, the prevention of infection, particularly for larger wounds is critical, as the body's immune response may be compromised. Due to this, antimicrobial treatments, including dressings are the norm in certain countries. Dressings are used as a source of antimicrobial actives, and a way to protect the burnt area from external contamination as well as from loss of heat and dehydration. For partial-thickness burns, appropriate exudate management is necessary to deal with the potentially large amounts of fluids released.

TABLE 3.6

Desired dressing's characteristics for small burns wounds

Characteristics	Deemed essential	Deemed desirable
Lack of adhesion to the wound bed	45.8%	41.7%
Pain-free dressing	55.4%	44.6%
Absorbency	34.2%	53.5%
Ease of removal	64.5%	33.9%
Antimicrobial activity	43.0%	40.5%

Source: Selig et al. (2012).

Where there is a copious amount of exudate, a highly absorbent dressing is preferred so as not to have to change the dressing too frequently.

Ideally, dressing changes should be minimised, to lower the chances of contamination, reduce disruption of the healing process, particularly growth of new cells, and also minimise pain and discomfort for the patient during the changes. A global survey of burns specialists, on the topic of treatment of small burns (<20% TBSA), revealed that nearly half the respondents (49.6%) deemed the most important dressing characteristic to be a 'non-adherent, non-traumatic wound interface', which stresses that removal of the dressing for dressing changes is an area of concern (Selig et al., 2012). Most of the clinicians surveyed would rather not to have to change the dressing daily, preferring instead twice weekly changes (36.4%), alternate days (29.6%) or even weekly (24.6%). Some of the desired characteristics for the ideal dressings, as surveyed, are summarised in Table 3.6.

As shown above, pain is a concern for clinicians and of course for patients, particularly in the case of partial-thickness burns, where the nerve endings are exposed and tender. Pain increases the anxiety and stress levels of the patients and may contribute to reduce compliance to the care recommendations, such as physiotherapy and dressing changes. Dressings that are pain-free upon wear and removal, but also those that can help soothe or provide comfort during wear are appealing in some cases.

The characteristics summarised in Table 3.6 address mainly the immediate needs to manage the wound and the patient's comfort. Looking further, ideally, advanced burn dressings should be able to help the patient recover with the best outcome possible, not just heal the wound per se. Often, and understandably so, the longer term outcomes can be neglected in favour of the immediate survival requirements. Where possible, medium to longer term outcomes need to be taken into consideration such as the ability to maintain a sufficient range of motion and movement, and the aesthetic aspect of the scarring tissue.

Hypertrophic scarring is a typical skin complication that can occur following severe burns. The skin becomes raised, with different pigmentation, vascularity, thickness and hardness. As well as aesthetically undesirable, if the scar is close to a joint, scar contracture can lead to reduced movement at the joint, particularly in the absence of adequate physiotherapy. Burns or post-burns dressings that can help reduce scarring or skin contraction are important to consider, particularly in aesthetically or functionally important locations such as the face, joints, fingers, etc. Similarly, and particularly in these positions, dressings should ideally be fully conformable to the wound bed, and yet enable some movement particularly in the later days of healing where some physiotherapy may be required.

A final small point worth noting with regards to dressings for burns is the availability of different dressing sizes. Burns are one of the few wounds where in some cases, large areas may be affected. For major burn injuries (e.g., >25% TBSA of partial-thickness burn in an adult), dressing application and changes can be facilitated with the availability of large dressings that can be used for areas such as the torso, back and legs.

3.4 Skin Substitutes

Dressings are typically used for wounds where there is sufficient viable skin tissue for the body to self-regenerate over time. In certain cases, such as in severe burns or severe chronic wounds, the wound is too deep or too slow to heal and may require skin grafting from donor or cadaver sites, or tissue-engineered skin substitutes to help. The demarcation between advanced dressing and skin substitutes is not totally clear, and there is an overlap in certain cases. Skin substitutes are used to replace the epidermis, or both the epidermis and dermal layer, with or without a primary and a secondary dressing. Like dressings, they are intended to perform some of the functions of the skin – at the least, those functions related to being a protective barrier, to preventing fluid loss and microbial contamination. They can be applied on a temporary basis, similar to dressings, or typically longer term, or even permanently in certain cases. They are normally used when traditional and advanced wound care dressings are not deemed to be sufficient for the required outcome on the wound being treated, typically on burns, donor sites and some chronic wounds.

Skin substitutes can be fully synthetic, or they can contain natural biomaterials and/or cultured live cell suspensions with or without a supporting matrix. Skin substitutes that do not contain live cells (acellular) provide a temporary scaffold or template that encourages the growth of fibroblasts, blood vessels and epithelial cells in patients where the wound healing cascade is not fully compromised. Typically, they contain biomaterials such as collagen and hyaluronic acid, which inherently promote the activity of viable cells in the wound. The source of the bioactive material used in commercial acellular skin substitutes ranges from animal to human cadaveric. A structural support material may be incorporated to provide some stability, and an outer layer to act as a barrier layer. Where present, the latter prevents evaporative water loss, heat loss, and protects against bacterial contamination to some extent too. In general, acellular skin substitutes only provide temporary coverage to open wounds, and need to be replaced by a split skin graft or re-grafted, except in small wounds where re-epithelialisation can occur (Vig et al., 2017).

Skin substitutes with live cells are defined as being cellular. The cells can be grown onto a matrix, membrane or mesh that also act as a scaffold for further growth. The scaffold is made of a material that needs to be physically removed or that can be bioresorbed by the body. Cellular skin substitutes are allogeneic or autologous. Those that are autologous use cells from the same patient harvested during a biopsy from the epidermis and/or dermis, or from the patient's follicles, which are then grown over a few weeks onto a substrate (Vig et al., 2017). While the main benefit of this route is that there is a low risk of rejection, the downside is that it takes time for the cells to be cultured. Substitutes with allogeneic cells are seeded with cultured human neonatal foreskin fibroblasts and are therefore available faster when needed. However, as with any transplants from another donor, disease transmission is a small risk. Also, the allogeneic cells do not survive for a long time, so therefore only offer a temporary solution in some cases. Whether autologous or allogeneic, live cells enhances the chance of speeding up the wound healing process, including in chronic wounds. When placed on the wound, the new cells can proliferate and produce growth factors and extracellular matrix components (Vig et al., 2017). However, vascularisation is difficult and the type of cells that can be transferred is typically limited to keratinocytes and fibroblasts, which limits the regeneration of the skin structure. The base substrate, if there is one, needs to be removed after a certain time, unless it is made from a short-term biodegradable material.

3.5 The Clinician's Perspective

In the final section of this chapter on the requirements for advanced wound care, it is important to briefly raise the perspective of the caregivers, particularly in the context of modern healthcare. A patient-centred approach to healthcare is essential; however, the challenges of clinicians and practitioners must not be overlooked, in order to ensure that the patient's experience is optimised. Like many professions, wound care specialists are faced with the challenges linked to lack of time, bottom-line costs and risk mitigation. In parallel, the socio-demographical and population health aspects, which are big drivers for the advanced wound care market, bring on their specific challenges that clinicians are faced with. Dressing design for advanced wound care must take all of this into consideration.

Taking the example of time: where possible, features and design characteristics that enable the clinician to perform dressing applications and dressing changes faster (without compromising on the quality of the procedure) are desirable. Packaging must be easy to open, the dressing must be easy to remove from the packaging, as well as easy to handle, apply and remove during dressing changes. Dressings that can be kept on safely for longer while still being efficacious are time savers too, by default of reducing the number of dressing changes. With an increasing number of overweight and obese patients, larger dressings can save the wound care practitioner the time of unpacking and overlapping several smaller dressings in the case of treating large wounds.

In recent years, there has been an increasing need for some patients to be cared for in the community instead of at a hospital. While in their home setting, patients need to feel that their dressings will be able to stay securely and comfortably in place for the whole time that they will be without nursing assistance. It is also important that the dressing is and remains an effective protection against infections. Compared to a hospital, the home environment is uncontrolled from a cleaning and space / set-up perspective, as this responsibility is that of the home owner or renter, who may be the patient himself or herself and find it physically or mentally difficult to prepare and maintain the right environment. where the dressing changes will take place may therefore be sub-optimal, or even contaminated with a range of microorganisms. The nurse practitioner has the extra challenge of having to complete dressing changes as aseptically as practically possible in an environment that may not be fit for purpose. Requirements of dressings used in a home setting must thus be to have packaging that enables aseptic changes, to be easy to open and apply, without the need for specialist equipment and ideally for the changes to be rapid and pain-free. A better understanding of the activities performed by nurses and other caregivers can help with the development of dressings optimised for home care. More about useability and designing to facilitate the clinician's task will be discussed in Chapter 7.

References

Dabiri, G., Damstetter, E., & Phillips, T. (2016). Choosing a Wound Dressing Based on Common Wound Characteristics. *Advances in Wound Care*, 5(1), 32.

Department of Health. (2008). *High Quality Care for All*. The Stationery Office. Retrieved August 9, 2020, from http://webarchive.nationalarchives.gov.uk/20130107105354/http://www.dh.gov.uk/prod_consum_dh/groups/dh_digitalassets/@dh/@en/documents/digitalasset/dh_085828.pdf

Falanga, V. (2004). Wound Bed Preparation: Science Applied to Practice. In *European Wound Management Association (EWMA) Position Document: Wound Bed Preparation in Practice*. London: MEP Ltd. Retrieved from file:///C:/Users/user/Downloads/pos_doc_English_final_04.pdf

Fletcher, J. (2007, May). *World Wide Wounds*. Retrieved April 30, 2020, from Dressings: Cutting and Application Guide: http://www.worldwidewounds.com/2007/may/Fletcher/Fletcher-Dressings-Cutting-Guide.html

Gardner, S. (2012). Managing High Exudate Wounds. *Wound Essentials, 7*(1), 1–3.

Kheirabadi, B. (2011, April–June). Evaluation of Topical Hemostatic Agents for Combat Wound Treatment. *US Army Medical Department Journal, 2*, 25.

Ovington, L. (2007). Advances in Wound Dressings. *Clinics in Dermatology, 25*, 33.

Rippon, M., White, R., & Davies, P. (2007). Skin Adhesives and Their Role in Wound Dressings. *Wounds UK, 3*(4), 76.

Selig, H. F., Lumenta, D. B., Giretzlehner, M., Jeschke, M. G., Upton, D., & Kamolz, L. P. (2012). The Properties of an "Ideal" Burn Wound Dressing – What do we Need in Daily Clinical Practice? Results of a Worldwide Online Survey Among Burn Care Specialists. *Burns, 38*, 960.

Sharman, D. (2003). Moist Wound Healing: A Review of Evidence, Application and Outcome. *The Diabetic Foot, 6*(3), 112.

Smith, A., Laird, C., Porter, K., & Bloch, M. (2013). Haemostatic Dressings in Prehospital Care. *Emergency Medicine Journal, 30*, 784.

Vig, K., Chaudhari, A., Tripathi, S., Dixit, S., Sahu, R., Pillai, S., Dennis, V. A., Singh, S. R. (2017, April). Advances in Skin Regeneration Using Tissue Engineering. *International Journal of Molecular Science, 18*(4), 789. doi:10.3390/ijms18040789

Woo, K. Y. (2012). Exploring the Effects of Pain and Stress on Wound Healing. *Advances in Skin & Wound Care, 25*(1), 38.

Zhao, R., Liang, H., Clarke, E., Jackson, C., & Xue, M. (2016, December 11). Inflammation in Chronic Wounds. *International Journal of Molecular Science, 17*(12), 2085.

4

Base Materials for Wound Dressings

4.1 Natural Materials and Their Derivatives

Raw materials used for the manufacture of wound dressings can be broadly split into two categories: (1) natural polymers and their derivatives and (2) synthetic polymers. In the first group to be discussed in this section, the materials are produced using a naturally available source directly, or as raw materials which are then chemically modified. The sources are typically vegetal or animal, and to a lesser extent microbial. The benefits of using a natural resource are that if managed properly, it could be sustainable in the long run, and the waste material is more likely to be environmentally friendly and biodegradable. On the flip side of the coin, natural resources suffer from the challenge of variability, which in some cases can be quite high from batch to batch.

4.1.1 Celluloses

One of the most widely available sources of raw materials is cellulose, which is a polysaccharide that can be obtained from plants and trees, and also on a smaller scale, from certain species of bacteria (bacterial cellulose). Cellulose-based materials are deemed to be biocompatible and generally do not cause an inflammatory response in the body. The most well-known and simplest of cellulosic dressings are the humble cotton gauze and pads, which are often referred to as 'traditional' wound dressings. Cotton was widely used before the development of modern wound dressings, due to its easy availability, low cost, high wet and dry strength, and good absorbency. However, while traditional cotton dressings can provide a small degree of protection and reasonable absorbency for the wound, as soon as fluids strike through the material, the wound becomes at risk of infection. Cotton fibres are in addition notorious for sticking to a wound as it starts to dry out, making the removal and changing of the dressing difficult, damaging and painful. A solution to this problem has been to impregnate gauze dressings with a non-adherent substance such as petrolatum. This forms the basis of many modern advanced wound dressings, utilising different base materials impregnated with active ingredients, a topic covered in Chapter 6.

Throughout textile history, there have been several developments in utilising other abundant sources of cellulose, such as processed wood pulp, to make new higher purity cellulosic fibres and powders, with less variability. Some of these have been subsequently successfully used in the medical industry, for example, viscose rayon fibres and sodium carboxymethyl cellulose (CMC) fibre, both used as textile structures. Other examples of cellulose derivatives that are film-forming or fibre-forming and have been explored as potential medical components or dressings include methyl cellulose, hydroxypropyl cellulose, hydroxyethyl cellulose, cellulose acetate and CMC sulphate. Modifications to the glucose units making up the long linear cellulose polymer, and to how they are packed together result in materials with different physical and bioactive properties, that can be processed in a range of forms, from sheets films and hydrogels to fibres. For many of the chemical processing routes, it is possible to convert the cellulose in various structural forms, including powder, fibres, slivers, yarns or even fabric rolls.

4.1.1.1 Sodium Carboxymethyl Cellulose

CMC or its sodium salt sodium CMC are common materials used in the food and consumer goods industries due to being non-toxic, hypoallergenic and being able to modify or thicken the viscosity of many food and non-food formulations. It does so by its absorption, swelling and gelling properties. Made primarily from softwood pulp or cotton linters, the process involves derivatising natural cellulose by binding carboxymethyl groups to some of the hydroxyl groups of the glucose units of the cellulose polymer. The number of carboxymethyl groups added determines the degree of substitution. Along with the degree of polymerisation, the number of carboxymethyl groups substituted in turn determines the solubility, viscosity, gel-forming ability, fluid handling capacity and other physical properties of the CMC. CMC in powder form is used in hydrocolloid sheet dressings, in combination with a number of other gel-forming, moisture-retentive agents, which together help maintain a moist wound environment. It has also been used extensively in many other research activities involving the development of new fibrous or flexible sheet materials with potential uses in medical dressings, again due to its gel-forming and fluid handling capabilities. Some examples of its use as powder or fibres are given in Box 4.1.

In fibre form, the physical properties of sodium-CMC textile dressings have been demonstrated to be beneficial for wound healing (Table 4.1). *In vitro*, sodium-CMC dressings have been reported to have greater fluid retention capabilities under compression compared to open-celled foams, better-sustained contact with a simulated wound bed, less lateral spread of fluids, less fibroblast adhesion, to be less detrimental to fibroblast contraction and to cell viability (Walker et al., 2010). The contact between the dressing and the wound bed is normally reinforced with the accumulation of fibrin and fibronectin

TABLE 4.1

Characteristics of sodium CMC fibre dressings

Physical properties	Wound healing benefits
High and rapid absorption of fluids	Wound exudate management Less frequent dressing changes required, less disruption to the healing process
Rapidly gels when in contact with fluids	Locks in harmful exudate components Protects surrounding skin by retaining fluid even under compression and preventing the spread of exudate to the peri-wound areas Less pain and trauma upon removal of the gelled dressing
Fibres swell when in contact with fluids	Prevents micro-concentration of exudates in micro-pools by contouring very closely to the irregular wound bed surface and maintaining the close contact

Source: Walker and Parsons (2010).

between the two layers, which act as temporary adherents while preventing ingrowth of cells into the dressing (Richters et al., 2004; Richetta et al., 2011).

The sodium-CMC fibres are produced from highly refined reformed cellulose fibres made from wood pulp. The regenerated cellulose fibres are treated chemically to add carboxymethyl groups, the component that confers the gel-forming ability. A specifically controlled degree of substitution is targeted in order to create a fibre with just enough carboxymethyl groups to be able to absorb high amounts of fluids, swell and transform into a gel when hydrated, but still retain some form of structural integrity and strength to enable it be handled when wet. Too much carboxymethyl groups will lead to the fibres being easily disintegrated when gelled, and too little will result in insufficient gelling and absorption. CMC fibres are reported to be able to absorb up to 25 times their own weight (Uzun, 2018).

The ability to absorb fluid and the rapid gelation of the fibrous mass are linked to several wound healing benefits such as an effective absorption and retention of exudate, the ability to lock in fluids and bacteria, and conformity of the dressing to the topology of the wound bed (Walker & Parsons,

2010). The retention property of the material is of particular interest as this means that fluid does not easily squeeze out or spread out. Up to 90% of fluid absorbed in CMC fibre dressings can be retained even under mild compression (Walker et al., 2010). This retention also indicates that wound exudate components are also 'locked' into the gelled network. Interestingly, it was also found that other than fluids and bacteria, sodium-CMC fibres are also able to draw in and retain inflammatory cells such as neutrophils (Hoekstra et al., 2002; Richters et al., 2004). The outcome of this is a better micro-environment at the wound bed, enabling better growth of keratynocytes and faster reepithelialisation. The modulation of proteases such as MMPs in the gelled fibres has also been observed *in vitro* (Krejner & Grzela, 2015). An unexplained mechanism to reduce MMP activity aside to the physical gel-blocking route was also observed in the latter study.

4.1.1.2 Oxidised Cellulose

Another derivative of cellulose, oxidised cellulose is characterised by its haemostatic and bioabsorbable properties, which means that after a number of weeks, it is naturally degraded and absorbed by the body. Made from a plant raw material such as cotton, the derivatisation is conducted through controlled oxidisation by nitrogen dioxide or dinitrogen tetroxide to create polyuronic acid (Kunio & Schreiber, 2013; Lewis et al., 2013). The hydroxyl groups of the cellulose polymer are oxidised into carboxylic acid groups, and like with other derivatisation processes, the properties of the finished product depend on the number of hydroxyl groups that have been oxidised, and on the nature of the starting raw materials. The process can also be conducted using regenerated cellulose fibres such as viscose or lyocell as the starting point, instead of native cellulose, in which case the material is then termed oxidised regenerated cellulose. The oxidisation can be performed on a range of flexible structural forms suitable for dressings, including mesh, gauze, fibrillar tufts and sponges and this makes it available in easy-to-handle forms. Some commercialised examples are given in Box 4.2.

BOX 4.2   EXAMPLES OF COMMERCIALISED OXIDISED CELLULOSE

	Unique Selling Points
• Surgicel® range of dressings (Ethicon) • BloodSTOP gauze (Curad) • Promogran™ range and family of dressings (Acelity) (with collagen) • m.doc® used in gels and films (Tricol Biomedical) • Resorba® Cell range (Advanced Medical Solutions)	Haemostatic Bioresorbable Antibacterial

Oxidised cellulosics have been used successfully where clinicians have not been able to control bleeding (Hazarika, 1985; Lagman et al., 2002), and have also been demonstrated to lead to faster healing compared to standard dressings (Cagri et al., 2006). The mechanism of action of oxidised cellulose and oxidised regenerated cellulose is not fully understood but it is believed to be a physical effect only, and therefore only works with patients with an intact coagulation cascade. Upon being in contact with blood, the material swells and gels, coagulating with haemoglobin and forming a matrix that activates the clotting pathway and the formation of fibrin (Hazarika, 1985; Chiara et al., 2018). It has been found that oxidised cellulose has superior haemostatic properties compared to the regenerated cellulose version, and this could be linked to the fibrous structure, which creates more exposed surface area (Lewis et al., 2013). Both types have a low pH, which can help to maintain an environment unsuitable for bacteria, making it antimicrobial to a broad range or organisms. This has some advantages for use where infection prevention and haemostatic control are both needed, e.g., in certain donor site and burns cases.

4.1.1.3 Bacterial Cellulose

Bacterial or microbial cellulose is synthesised by bacteria such as *Gluconacetobacter xylinus* (formerly *Acetobacter xylinum*), and secreted outside the cells through pores. The pure, natural cellulose is formed in a gelatinous membrane, with a structure consisting of an ultrafine network of cellulose nanofibers organised into sub-fibrils, micro-fibrils, and bundles of micro-fibrils (Hoenich, 2006). The cellulosic purity means that no chemical treatments are required to remove non-cellulosic components such as lignin and hemicelluloses, as in the case with plant-based cellulose products. The fibres, which have a high degree of crystallinity, are oriented in the same direction, resulting in a material of high mechanical strength. They also possess a high fluid handling capacity and should be able to absorb and retain exudate while keeping the wound moist. However, if the bacterial cellulose is dried first, rehydration is poor due to the high crystallinity of the fibres and the closing of all micellar spaces when dry.

A summary of the key inherent properties of bacterial cellulose is provided in Table 4.2. As with many fibre-forming processes, the physical properties of the material vary with the manufacturing and processing conditions. For example, parameters such as the pore size and the total fibre surface area affect the fluid handling capacities, while the crystallinity influences the strength and fluid handling properties. Culture growth conditions, culture media components, the presence of specific additives in the synthesis, and starting and finishing processes can affect the structural characteristics and subsequently the physical properties.

While the inherent properties of bacterial cellulose are of interest for the wound care market, and while there are reports of improved healing (Portela

TABLE 4.2

Properties of bacterial cellulose

Safety	Physical properties	Other benefits
Non-toxic	Higher surface area per fibre	Versatility in manufacture
Biocompatible	Flexible, conformable	Additional properties can be built in
Non-carcinogenic	Absorbs and retains moisture*	Potential for pain relief
High purity	High mechanical strength	Autolytic debridement
Biodegradable	Variable porosity	

Source: Portela et al. (2019).
* When not dried out.

et al., 2019), there has been limited commercial success to date. The potential of the material is the process versatility, including the ability to 3D print the cellulose, and the ability to combine it with other compounds or actives to create bioactive or other multifunctional properties on a biofriendly base. A range of additives have been explored for the manufacture of composite bacterial celluloses with different properties. Examples are hydroxypropyl methyl cellulose, CMC, chitosan, alginates, *aloe vera*, glycerine, acrylic acid, poly(vinyl alcohol), silver nanoparticles, hyaluronan, zinc oxide, arginine, stem cells, etc. (Portela et al., 2019). With these modifications and additions, other properties can be engineered, including those related to the wound healing process, such as increased collagen synthesis, improved tissue regeneration and granulation, enhanced epithelialisation and fibroblast proliferation and drug-delivery properties.

4.1.2 Alginates

Alginate (or alginic acid) is the most widely available marine biopolymer and is obtained from sea algae, chemically processed and typically then transformed into pellets. In the making of alginate fibres, the pellets are then turned into an aqueous sodium alginate solution and wet spun into a calcium chloride coagulation bath to form calcium alginate fibres. There is an interesting degree of versatility in the fibre-forming process, which enables various versions of alginate fibres to be easily manufactured. Altering the coagulation bath, for example, is a way to create different salts of the alginate fibres, such as sodium-calcium alginates (with faster gelling characteristics), or zinc alginates (with better haemostatic characteristics), or to form fibres incorporating antibiotics (Hampton, 2004; Rajendran et al., 2016; Schoukens, 2019). Fibres are also not the only form in which alginates are available. Sponges, films, gels and hydrogels can be manufactured, and the powder version is also used in the making of many other medical polymeric composites. Its use in the medical industry is encouraged by its high biocompatibility, low toxicity and biodegradability.

The key properties of interest with alginates in the context of wound care are the high fluid uptake, the ability of the fibres to gel and the mild haemostatic effect, all of which have a positive wound healing outcome. The fibres are able to absorb up to about 20 times their own weight, which makes them suitable for medium to heavily exuding wounds, reducing the necessity for frequent dressing changes (Dabiri et al., 2016). As the fibres absorb fluid, they form a gel, which helps to maintain a moist wound healing environment, facilitate autolytic debridement and prevent traumatic removal during dressing changes. The gelling and fluid uptake characteristics are influenced by the proportion and arrangement of d-mannuronic acid and l-guluronic acid, which make up the linear polysaccharide. High guluronic alginates have higher wet strength. Alginates with high mannuronic acid units have higher fluid uptake and faster swelling speed, because the calcium ions in the mannuronic units are more easily replaced by sodium ions from wound fluids (Qin, 2016; Uzun, 2018). This ion interchange occurs when the dressing becomes in contact with sodium-rich exudate or plasma. As the sodium ions bind to the polymer backbone and re-form sodium alginate or calcium-sodium alginate, the solubility and gelation of the fibres increase, but the balance of guluronic units contributes to maintaining the wet integrity.

As with CMC fibres, the gelation of a dressing helps it maintain a moist wound healing environment, manage exudate and its components and reduce pain at dressing changes. *In vitro* studies have shown that alginate can bind elastase, lower the amount of pro-inflammatory cytokines and reduce free radical formation (Wiegand et al., 2009). Alginate fibres have been demonstrated to result in faster pressure ulcers size reduction and to faster healing and comfort of donor sites compared to traditional practice (Attwood, 1989; Sayag et al., 1996; O'Donoghue et al., 1997). They have also been found to result in less blisters, less pain upon removal and to be easier to remove than other basic dressings used (Dawson et al., 1992; Ravnskog et al., 2011).

The calcium ions released from the calcium alginate fibres are understood to assist the body's own blood coagulation cascade, imparting mild haemostatic properties to the dressing. Calcium ions are required throughout the coagulation process and are particularly required in the formation of fibrin polymers. In a study comparing alginate swabs and standard surgical gauze, it was found that less blood loss was observed with the alginate group, and a reduced operating time was achieved as well (Blair et al., 1990). Caution is however advised on its use as a haemostat dressing on a dry wound, as leaving blood clots to dry can cause the dressing to adhere to the wound. If this occurs, care must be taken to remove the dressing with minimal tissue damage and pain. Similarly, as for any highly absorbing dressing, alginates should not be used on dry wounds due to the risk of dehydration damage to the wound bed, and adherence to granulation tissue which could lead to pain and damage upon removal. The various properties of alginate fibres make them appropriate for use in a range of exuding wound types, chronic

BOX 4.3   EXAMPLES OF COMMERCIAL USES OF ALGINATES IN WOUND DRESSINGS

• Tegaderm® Alginate (3M) • ActivHeal® Alginate (Advanced Medical Solutions) • ActivHeal® Aquafiber® (Advanced Medical Solutions) • Kaltostat® Alginate (Convatec) • Biatain® Alginate (Coloplast) (also containing CMC) • Algisite* M (Smith + Nephew) • CalciCare™ and Restore™ ranges (Hollister) • NU-DERM™ (Acelity) (with CMC fibres)	**Unique Selling Points** Gel forming Fluid handling Mild haemostatic

or acute, superficial or tunnelling. For example, granulating wounds in ulcers tend to be moist, as can some wet tunnelling wounds, making alginates a good choice; however, some epithelialising wounds have very low exudate amounts, making alginates not appropriate (Sharman, 2003). A wide number of alginate dressings are commercially available worldwide. Generally, they are available as fibrous dressings or pads, which require a secondary dressing or bandage to hold it in place. Some examples are given in Box 4.3.

4.1.3 Chitin and Chitosan

Chitin is yet another abundant source of natural polysaccharide that can be processed into various derivatives and forms. As a waste product of the seafood industry, it can be widely and cheaply found in the shells of common crustacea such as shrimps and crabs. It is also found in the exoskeleton of other arthropods, some molluscs and in the cell walls of fungi. Chitosan is a common chitin derivative, a deacetylated version made of linear arrangements of D-glucosamine and N-acetyl-D-glucosamine units, which make it soluble in aqueous solutions. The chitosan amino and hydroxyl groups can be chemically modified into various chitosan derivatives. The degree of deacetylation, combined with the molecular weight of the polymer, determines its chemical, physical and biological properties. Its solubility in weak organic acids makes it easy to process into multiple forms, including films, hydrated membranes, hydrogels, sponges, scaffolds, fibres and powder. Chitosan has been successfully used to coat other materials such as textiles, particularly cotton gauze. Its versatility in its structural form and in its range of chemical derivatives has made it a polymer of interest to researchers in the medical textiles field, particularly since it is known to be biocompatible, biodegradable and of low toxicity, and reported to have antimicrobial and haemostatic properties.

The mild antimicrobial properties of chitosan are explained by several proposed mechanisms of action. The disruption of the cell membrane or cell wall has been cited as one of the mechanisms; interaction with microbial DNA, chelation of essential metals and of nutrients, and the physical blocking of nutrients to inhibit microbial growth have also suggested to be other potential mechanisms (Matica et al., 2019). Cell wall disruption occurs due to the electrostatic interactions between the positively charged polymer (at a pH of around 6 and under) and the negatively charged cell membranes of bacteria and fungi. Low molecular weight chitosan can further go through the disrupted cell membrane and interact with DNA, inhibiting the synthesis of proteins in the microorganism. The antibacterial efficacy is dependent on the polymer's molecular weight, its degree of acetylation, the pH, the original source of the chitin and the type of microorganism present. Like its haemostatic effect, it improves when the degree of acetylation goes up, increasing its solubility and charge. The antimicrobial aspect of chitosan has not been fully commercially exploited in the medical field. While complexing or incorporation of chitosan with other antimicrobial actives has been explored to increase the antimicrobial efficacy, most commercialised chitosan-based products concentrate their claims on its haemostatic properties instead. Some of these examples are given in Box 4.4.

The ability of chitosan and its derivatives to help in haemostasis is speculated to be also linked to the positive charge of the material. Red blood cells are negatively charged and the electrostatic adhesion of the polymer to the blood cells physically agglomerates the latter together to start the clotting process (Matica et al., 2019). In turn, the platelets are encouraged to adhere to the polymer too, to activate and to aggregate. Chitosan has been described as a mucoadhesive agent in the context of its mechanism of action, due to the fact that it works by physically sealing bleeding wounds (Granville-Chapman et al., 2011). *In vitro*, chitosan and its derivatives have been shown to increase platelet adhesion and induce the increased expression of certain platelet receptors, to reach the required levels for platelet aggregation and haemostasis (Chou et al., 2003; Periayah et al., 2004). A number of *in vivo* studies have shown the ability of chitosan dressings and granules to reduce the total amount of blood loss (Kozen et al., 2008; Gegel et al., 2010).

BOX 4.4   EXAMPLES OF COMMERCIAL USES OF CHITOSAN IN WOUND DRESSINGS

	Unique Selling Points
• Celox Rapid (Celox)	Haemostatic
• HemCon® PRO range (Tricol Biomedical)	Antimicrobial
• ChitoFlex® PRO range (Tricol Biomedical)	
• Opticell (Medline) (alginate with chitosan)	

Clinically, chitosan dressings have also been found to help stop bleeding in uncontrolled external haemorrhages when other standard measures (typically the use of gauze and pressure) have not been successful, and to bring on a faster haemostasis and reduced blood loss compared to standard treatment (Wedmore et al., 2006; Brown et al., 2009; Granville-Chapman et al., 2011; Hatamabadi et al., 2015). One of the major areas of use for commercial haemostatic chitosan dressings, e.g., those mentioned in Box 4.4, are by the military for pre-hospital casualty care. Milder haemostatic products are indicated for use on minor bleeding wounds, including chronic ones.

4.1.4 Collagen and Gelatine

Collagen is a major natural structural protein, produced by fibroblasts to form and strengthen the extracellular matrix. It is heavily involved in the wound healing process due to its chemotactic role. Starting from participating in the haemostasis phase, it has an important function in the inflammatory phase and the proliferative phase – stimulating various cellular migration and contributing to new tissue development. Disturbances in the wound healing cascade have an impact on the development and deposition of new collagen in a wound, leading to delayed healing. For example, in chronic wounds, the recruitment of fibroblasts can be retarded, the expression of the collagen gene in fibroblasts can be suppressed, and an elevated amount of proteolytic enzymes, which destroy new and existing collagens and elastin, may be present in wound exudate (Fleck & Simman, 2010). When introduced in wound care, collagen can support the body's own healing process, encourage the deposition and organisation of newly formed collagen and stimulate, recruit and help the migration of specific cells such as macrophages and fibroblasts (Fleck & Simman, 2010; Smith + Nephew, 2020). In addition, it can also reduce the activity of proteolytic enzymes by acting as a sacrificial element and rebalancing the wound bed environment positively. For these reasons, it is used in temporary skin substitutes and bioactive dressings, some examples shown in Box 4.5.

Collagen is generally obtained from animal (bovine, porcine, avian, equine or piscean) sources and can be reformed into gels, sheets, membranes, fibres, powder, sponges and foam. Processing it to make it into a form suitable for use, and purifying to make it antigenic, can cause collagen to become denatured – whereby the triple-helical basic structure is disrupted. The denatured collagen essentially becomes gelatine. Gelatine itself is able to help in the wound healing process, e.g., by being a readily available source of amino acids necessary for tissue reconstructions, by being an accessible source of sacrificial proteins to neutralise certain excess proteases and by attracting fibroblasts and endothelial cells responsible for forming granulation tissue (Matthews, 2011; Hochstein, 2014). It has been found that denatured collagen successfully increased fibroblast and keratinocyte proliferation and sped up

---

BOX 4.5   EXAMPLES OF COMMERCIALISED COLLAGEN DRESSINGS AND SKIN SUBSTITUTES

• Oasis® Matrix range (Smith + Nephew) (porcine collagen) • Promogran™ range and family of dressings (Acelity) (with oxidised cellulose) • Fibracol™ (Acelity) (collagen with alginate) • Neuskin-F™ (Medira) (piscean collagen) • PURACOL® (Medline Industries) • Matriderm® (Medskin Solutions) (bovine collagen with elastin) • Biobrane^ (Smith + Nephew) – collagen peptides with nylon and silicone • Apligraf® (Organogenesis) – fibroblasts and keratinocytes on collagen matrix	**Unique Selling Points** Bioactive wound healing Scaffold for cell growth

---

wound healing *in vitro*, more so than the non-denatured version (Egles et al., 2008). The non-denatured version of collagen, with its higher proportion of the original triple helical structure, is said to be a more natural 3D structure for fibroblasts, to bind better with elastin, to conserve elastin better, to maintain its wet structural integrity for longer on the wound bed and as a result provide collagen for longer on site (Hochstein, 2014; Medline Industries Inc., 2018). Higher quantities of non-denatured, native collagen can be achieved with newer and gentler extraction and purification processes. It is worth noting that aside to differences in the type of collagen, the source of the collagen, its macro structure and porosity, the percentage of collagen content in the dressing, and most likely other factors too, affect the properties and efficacy as a wound healing material. A morphological study of different collagen products concluded that if the collagen substructure is too large or too small, it may not be suitable for sustaining cell movement and that if the fibrils are too thin or too thick, they may influence the persistence and integrity of the product and the collagen accessibility on the wound bed (Karr et al., 2011).

Some Clinical studies on chronic wounds and donor sites comparing the use of a collagen dressing versus other standard treatments, or adjunct to another treatment have shown that speed to healing is higher with the collagen dressings (Mostow et al., 2005; Romanelli et al., 2010; Brown-Etris et al., 2019; Carvalho et al., 2011). However, not all reports demonstrate the superiority of collagen over other more conventional treatments. In a study comparing collagen dressings versus other standard treatments on burns and chronic wounds, it was found that although healthy granulation tissue appeared earlier over collagen-dressed wounds, no significant difference in the completeness of healing over the study period was observed (Singh et al., 2011). In another study comparing collagen with hydrocolloids, no significant difference was observed in healing outcomes or rates between the two dressing types (Graumlich et al., 2003). A systematic review of studies on collagen-based wound dressings for treating diabetic foot ulcers concluded that although there are some benefits of using the collagen dressings, there is no evidence that they should replace current gold standards of care (Holmes et al., 2013). There was also no evidence to prove the superiority of any particular collagen type.

4.1.5 Hyaluronic Acid and Its Derivatives

Hyaluronic acid, also known as hyaluronan, is a naturally occurring linear polysaccharide widely found in the connective tissue and vitreous and synovial fluids of mammals. Its highly hygroscopic behaviour, unusual viscoelastic properties, good biocompatibility and non-antigenic characteristics have made it a material of interest in the development of cosmetics and advanced wound care products. There has been a number of reports of its potential role in wound healing. Notably, hyaluronic acid is thought to be linked to scar-less healing in foetuses, and *in vitro* has been shown to promote collagen and other protein synthesis and cell division, and enhance keratinocyte proliferation (Mast et al., 1993; Greco et al., 1998; Price et al., 2007). The effect and role of hyaluronic acid on tissue vary significantly based on its molecular weight (Stern et al., 2006). Large hyaluran polymers are space-filling, anti-angiogenic, immunosuppressive and impede differentiation. Medium-sized versions protect the integrity of the epithelial layer and are involved in wound repair and regeneration. Smaller sized fragments are inflammatory, immuno-stimulatory and angiogenic. Hyaluronic acid-based products may therefore have different effects on a wound if they vary widely in their molecular weight.

Hyaluronic acid is extracted from natural sources such as rooster combs, or produced on a large and controllable scale by microbial fermentation. The high hygroscopicity of the polymer, whilst less of a problem for creams and pastes in the cosmetic industry, makes it difficult to be used as a dressing, as it tends to liquefy easily upon contact with a small amount of water. The derivatisation of hyaluronic acid is now conducted in order to improve the polymer's structural stability, while still maintaining the biological efficacy. One example is the esterification of the free carboxylic group, which increases the hydrophobic components of the polymer and enables it to be processed into different forms.

As wound care products, derivatised hyaluronic acids can be processed in a range of formats, including sheets or mesh, impregnated dressings, fibrous dressings, sponges, hydrogels and creams. It is used as topical treatments and dressings, as well as scaffolds for tissue engineering and for transplanting

**BOX 4.6 EXAMPLES OF COMMERCIALISED TECHNOLO-
GIES AND DRESSINGS WITH HYALURONIC ACID
DERIVATIVES**

	Unique Selling Points
• HYAFF® technology (Haemo Pharma) • Hyalofill®, Hyalomatrix® and Hyalosafe® (Anika Therapeutics) (with HYAFF®) • Sorelex® (Contipro) (with octenidine)	Bioactive wound healing Scaffold for cell growth

autologous cells onto deeper tissue wounds. Box 4.6 gives some commercial examples.

A number of studies have been conducted demonstrating the ability of hyaluronic acid to heal acute and chronic wounds when used as a topical care (Vazquez et al., 2003; Voinchet et al., 2006; Barrois et al., 2007). Hyaluronic acid gauze was found to perform better than standard hydrocolloid dressings in the treatment of various chronic leg ulcers (Dereure et al., 2012). In a review of nine studies on the use of hyaluronic acid derivatives, the conclusion was that in most cases, they significantly improved the healing of chronic and acute wounds (Voigt & Driver, 2012). Used as a carrier to transplant autologous human keratinocytes onto recalcitrant diabetic foot ulcers or trauma wounds, it was found to give positive outcomes in pilot studies (Hollander et al., 2001; Lobmann et al., 2003). However, a further review of the use of hyaluronic acid on chronic wounds found the evidence still limited, despite an indication of certain benefits (Shaharudin & Aziz, 2016). More recently, it was found that although hyaluronic acid-based products were effective for treating chronic wounds, patients with sclerodermic (inflammatory) ulcers experienced a worsening of their ulcers – due to the fact that hyaluronic acid, particularly the lower molecular weight version, can produce a pro-inflammatory effect (Gualdi et al., 2019).

4.1.6 Other Natural Polymers

Natural polymers have always been attractive for use in the medical field due to their wide availability, biodegradability, safety, non-toxicity and potential for biocompatibility. The previous sections covered mostly well-explored materials, but the following are worth a mention due to various reports on their potential for accelerating wound healing.

4.1.6.1 Dextran

Dextran is a bacterial branched exopolysaccharide consisting of repeating glucose molecules, and synthesised from sucrose by certain lactic-acid bacteria. As a medicine, it is used intravenously as a blood plasma volume expander. It is also used in the food industry as a thickener. More recently, dextran has been used in the development of advanced wound care scaffolds, as it is easily formed into hydrogels or electrospun fibrous mats, often with other polymers or actives. Being highly hydrophilic, dextran is able to bring in properties such as softness, swelling ability, water vapour transmission, elasticity, porosity and in some cases protein absorption capabilities (Hwang et al., 2010). It is also a good carrier for many protein biomolecules, can be biodegradable *in situ* and with proper modifications and formulation, it has been shown to be customisable to have specific functionalities, many of which suitable for scaffolds for drug delivery and tissue engineering (Sun & Mao, 2012).

On its own, dextran hydrogel has been shown *in vivo* to promote neovascularisation and skin regeneration after a week from a burn wound (Sun et al., 2011). The hydrogel scaffold was found to facilitate early inflammatory and endothelial cell infiltration, leading to greater blood flow compared to otherwise treated and untreated controls. Of note, the higher-ratio dextran hydrogel (with polyethylene glycol diacrylate) was found to facilitate accelerated cell infiltration compared to the low-ratio version. It also degraded faster *in situ*, due to a more efficient neutrophil penetration.

Dextran hydrogels have been combined with other materials to improve the physical or bioactive properties of such materials. For example, oxidised dextran has been used to modify silk fibroin nanofibres in order to improve its hydrophilicity (Kim et al., 2014). The dextran-modified silk was found to have faster water absorption and a higher swelling ratio than the untreated silk fibroin nanofibre mats, which enabled it to manage a moist wound healing environment better, hence leading to better wound healing.

Some other dextran-based potential advanced wound care materials have included chitosan and growth factors (Ribeiro et al., 2013), polyvinyl alcohol and gentamicin (Hwang et al., 2010) and bacterial cellulose (Lin et al., 2017). In each of the above reports, faster or improved wound healing was observed *in vivo*, compared to a control or conventional product. Other reported *in vitro* and *in vivo* observations that contribute to the re-establishment of skin architecture and function are as follows: enhanced re-epithelialisation rates, higher fibroblast cell growth rates, more collagen tissues, and less inflammatory cells. In some cases, the effect of the addition of dextran in the composition of the material on wound healing is clearly seen, for example, when combined with bacterial cellulose and compared with bacterial cellulose alone (Lin et al., 2017). In other cases, the dextran component is present to create the right physico-chemical structure, for example, when it is used for controlled release of actives such as growth factors or medicines. Its versatility in processing and its biodegradability also make it a useful component of electrospinning solutions, where it has been mixed with a number of other polymers and actives to create nanofibrous membranes and scaffolds with potential for slow release of ingredients at the wound site.

4.1.6.2 Elastin

Elastin is a major component of the skin's extracellular matrix, providing elasticity to the different layers and underlying tissues. Elastin is highly insoluble, which limits its applications, but the soluble derivatives such as elastin peptides, tropoelastin and digested elastins are more versatile to be used in material processing and have been integrated with other structures, or formed into hydrogels, electrospun scaffolds, and coatings for other materials. Tropoelastin in particular has been of interest and is reported to release peptides that are chemotactic for monocytes, macrophages, neutrophils, endothelial cells, keratinocytes and fibroblasts (Machula et al., 2014). A study where tropoelastin was incorporated into a synthetic commercial dermal regeneration template showed that angiogenesis was increased, indicating a potential to improve wound healing where slow blood vessel ingrowth is a problem (Wang et al., 2015). Electrospun tropoelastin scaffolds have been used as a delivery system for stem cells, demonstrating faster wound closure and better epithelial thickness *in vivo* compared to a control (Machula et al., 2014). Similarly, another *in vivo* study using fibroin-elastin crosslinked scaffolds also showed that the scaffolds with the higher levels of elastin had the most beneficial effect on wound healing, accelerating re-epithelialisation and wound closure (Vasconcelos et al., 2012). When compared with commercialised hydrogels and a control, a fibroin-elastin hydrogel demonstrated a higher epithelialisation rate in a mice full-thickness wound model, but did not lead to a larger newly formed granulation area (Kawabata et al., 2018). However, in their guinea pig model, which had a thicker dermis, the silk-elastin hydrogel showed a higher wound healing capacity than a standard hydrocolloid paste, and this was attributed to an accumulation of fibroblasts in the gel, subsequently producing collagen.

The incorporation of elastin in dermal substitutes and wound dressings may be associated with an increase in elasticity in the repaired or regenerated skin. A pilot clinical study comparing the treatment of severe burns with split-thickness skin grafting with and without a commercially available collagen-elastin dermal substitute concluded that using the collagen-elastin matrix resulted in better skin elasticity (Ryssel et al., 2008). Further studies of the matrix (Matriderm®) demonstrated a reduction in wound contraction, improvement in elasticity and quality of scar tissue and its potential in the treatment of skin injuries where there are high strains and high risk of scar contracture and poor skin quality, such as hand burns (Haslik et al., 2007, 2010; Cervelli et al., 2011).

4.1.6.3 Silk Fibroin and Sericin

Silk is typically extruded naturally by the larvae *Bombyx mori* (or other silk-spinning arthropods), and consists of two major protein components: fibrillar fibroin and glue-like sericin. The two are separated in the silk production process by a process called degumming; with fibroin being the main component used in the silk industry and sericin ending up as a waste by-product. Both components have been of interest in the biomedical field, due to their biocompatibility, biodegradability, biological and physical characteristics. Both have been explored significantly, in various structural and morphological forms, on their own and incorporating other bioactive components.

Electrospinning has been one of the processing techniques of choice for silk fibroin in the last couple of decades, producing nanofibre sheets of varying porosity and offering the possibility of incorporating various other components within the structure. Electrospun silk fibroin has been studied *in vivo* on a burn wound model and found to speed up wound healing, epithelialisation, collagen production, and to modulate the pro-inflammatory cytokines involved in wound healing (Ju et al., 2016). Fibroin was also processed with chitosan, elastin, epidermal growth factors (EGF), honey and gelatine, with positive outcomes with respect to *in vitro* fibroblast cell attachment and proliferation, epithelialisation, collagen formation and/or speed of wound closure (Schneider et al., 2009; Cai et al., 2010; Kanokpanont et al., 2012; Vasconcelos et al., 2012; Yang et al., 2017). Other actives or composite components found in the fibroin literature include silver nanoparticles, hydroxyapatite, insulin, alginate, polylactic acid, and many more. The ability to combine fibroin with other materials increases its versatility as a raw material. In addition, an interesting feature of processed fibroin as opposed to natural silk is that it can be engineered to degrade at a slow rate without causing an inflammatory reaction or interfering with the healing process (Schneider et al., 2009). Both of these processing features make it a material of potential for scaffolds or the delivery of actives to a wound site.

Sericin, the glue component keeping the fibroin together as it is being spun, is a largely unutilised by-product of the silk industry, which has led to much research into its potential in the medical industry. The effect of sericin on inflammatory mediators has been investigated *in vitro* and *in vivo*, concluding that sericin promotes the wound healing process without causing inflammation (Aramwit et al., 2009). Clinically, the wound healing properties of sericin have been demonstrated in the treatment of burn wounds in a randomised clinical trial using silver zinc sulfadiazine cream with and without added sericin cream (Aramwit et al., 2013). In this small trial, the sericin group was found to heal faster than the control group, without any severe reaction in any wounds. In dressing form, sericin has been incorporated into polyvinyl alcohol (PVA) scaffolds or nanofibrous structures, with positive wound healing observations. *In vitro*, the incorporation of sericin was found to endow the PVA dressing with free radical scavenging capacity, antibacterial activity, the ability to encourage higher cell proliferation, to have greater antioxidant potential and help with faster healing (Gilotra et al., 2018). In a clinical study on split-thickness donor site wounds, PVA/sericin was found to be less adhesive, to lead to faster healing and to reduce pain better than a standard commercial dressing (Siritientong et al., 2014). Other than PVA, the incorporation of sericin with other carrier materials has been explored to create more bioactive combinations. Some examples in the literature include collagen, gelatine, chitosan, CMC and bacterial cellulose. The formation of sericin-only gel films, sponges and hydrogels is also possible, by cross-linking or ethanol precipitation (Teramoto et al., 2008; Lamboni et al., 2015).

4.2 Synthetic Polymers

Manufactured by polymerising raw material components in a precise and controlled process, synthetic polymers are artificially created and have the advantage of not being as variable as polymers produced naturally by plants, bacteria or animals. The processing route into a number of shapes and morphologies is also more direct, yet more versatile, without complex requirements to pre-treat or modify the polymer before turning it into a processable form. Chemically, synthetic polymers have the advantage that their mechanical and degradation kinetics can be manipulated more reliably and precisely, and they can also be designed with chemical functional groups to assist in wound management. One of their long-term limitations is that most are manufactured from hydrocarbons derived from crude oil – which is widely agreed to be limited in long-term supply. The first synthetic polymers commercialised on a large scale also had the disadvantages of being non-biodegradable and therefore a source of microplastic pollution. However, over time, this has changed and biodegradable synthetic polymers are now commonly manufactured. The level of biodegradability varies from short term, i.e., in the case of a dressing or scaffold, over the duration of the wound healing timescale, to long term, whereby the polymer degrades naturally over time when disposed of.

4.2.1 Nylon (PA)

Nylon is a polyamide (PA) which is commonly used in many other industries, including the fashion industry and as packaging films in the food industry, due to its mechanical properties, stability, inertness and low cost. Typically, it is made by a condensation polymerisation reaction using an amine and a carboxylic acid, with variations in the monomers creating different types of nylon (two common ones being nylon 66 and nylon 6). Despite not being hydrophilic, nylon has been used in wound care under various forms because of its strength and low reaction to tissues. It is used as removable sutures, dressing material and support for skin substitutes. Typically, nylon is manufactured in smooth continuous filaments. This, with their thermoplastic characteristic, makes it ideal to use for the formation of fine filament

---

BOX 4.7   EXAMPLES OF DRESSINGS AND SKIN SUBSTITUTE WHERE NYLON IS USED

- Mepitel® (Mölnlycke Health Care) – silicone-coated polyamide mesh
- Atrauman® Ag (Hartmann) – silver-coated polyamide mesh
- Biobrane^ (Smith + Nephew) – silicone membrane with collagen and nylon mesh
- Silverlon® range (Argentum Medical) – silver-coated nylon fabric
- Actisorb™ range (Acelity) – activated charcoal in nonwoven nylon fabric
- Silvercel™ range (Acelity) – silver-coated nylon fibres with alginate and CMC

---

nonwovens, knits, mesh and nets, used to support or contain other materials. The smoothness of the fibres helps in minimising adherence of bacteria and tissue cells to the surfaces. However, being fairly non-reactive to tissue and fluids, nylon itself does not contribute to wound healing; it mainly serves as a support for other more active materials. Some examples of where traditional nylon is used commercially in wound dressings and skin substitutes are given in Box 4.7.

Newer applications of nylon in advanced wound care research include using it as a main polymer in electrospinning with another active. Some examples from the research literature include gelatine (Panthi et al., 2013), silver nanoparticles (Pant et al., 2012), antibacterial violacein pigment (Osman & Setu, 2018), soybean (Dias et al., 2019), chitosan (Nirmala et al., 2011) and chitosan/polyethylene oxide for antimicrobial effects (Keirouz et al., 2020).

4.2.2 Polyester (PET)

Another low-cost and readily available polymer, polyester is a category of polymers containing the ester functional group in their chain. The most common type of polyester is polyethylene terephthalate (PET), widely used in the fashion, home interior, packaging and plastic-related industries. Like nylon, polyester is cheap, easy and versatile to manufacture and has excellent mechanical properties and stability. Like nylon, polyester in the wound care industry is used in different shapes and forms, and primarily to provide a low-cost structural support or backing material. The melt-extruded fibres can be easily turned into knits, nonwoven mats, meshes and nets and the resulting textiles are readily impregnated, coated or otherwise combined with other materials to provide wound healing benefits. A large number of commercially available dressings have a polyester component included within the structure; some examples are provided in Box 4.8. In the case of Dermabond® Prineo®, a glue is applied on top of a polyester mesh and polymerised. While it is the glue component that holds the skin together, and provides the protective barrier function, the polyester mesh, as with many other wound dressings, provides the necessary strength, support and stability to the glue. This

---

BOX 4.8 EXAMPLES OF DRESSINGS WITH POLYESTER COMPONENTS

- Mepore® (Mölnlycke Health Care) – nonwoven polyester backing layer
- ActivHeal® Silicone Wound Contact Layer (Advanced Medical Solutions) – silicone-coated knitted polyester
- Silflex (Advancis Medical) – silicone-coated polyester mesh
- Atrauman® (Hartmann) – ointment impregnated polyester tulle
- Physiotulle® range (Coloplast) – hydrocolloid impregnated knitted polyester net
- UrgoTul (Urgo Medical) – hydrocolloid impregnated polyester mesh
- Dermabond® Prineo® – (J&J) – skin glue with polyester mesh
- Acticoat◊ range (Smith + Nephew) – polyester with nanocrystalline silver

---

combination used after hip arthroplasty was compared with a regularly used dressing, and showed to result in less post-operative complications, despite the glue having a higher rate of skin reaction (Herndon et al., 2020).

Adding bioactive functionality to polyester has been of interest for a number of years. This can be achieved via many processing techniques, including coating, surface deposition, surface modification, plasma modification and polymerisation, electrospinning, polymer grafting, and so on. Physically, the formation of PET nanofibrous mats by electrospinning creates structures that mimic the extracellular matrix and can act as potential scaffolds (Gustafsson et al., 2012). Chemically and biologically, the goal of imparting antimicrobial properties to polyester or polyester blends has been explored using multiple routes, including the addition of nanocrystalline silver (Fong & Wood, 2006), silver nanoparticles coating (Radulescu et al., 2016), silver-loaded chitosan nanoparticles (Ali et al., 2011), chitosan and honey (Arslan et al., 2014), magnetite nanoparticles with essential oils (Anghel et al., 2013), herb extracts on plasma-modified fibres (Shu et al., 2017) and plasma-polymerised polyester (Peršin et al., 2012). Adding hydrogels to the surface of polyester films and textiles enables them to gain other functionalities such as low wound bed adhesion, antibacterial or controlled release drug delivery (Ning et al., 2014; Pour et al., 2015; Norouzi et al., 2019). The versatility of polyester as a base polymer to modify and build onto makes it an interesting material to fuel research and development, however, so far, its commercial uses have mainly been as a supporting or strength providing substrate.

4.2.3 Polyurethane (PU)

Polyurethane is a polymer of alternating units joined by urethane (or carbamate) links, and typically made by reacting a di- or tri-isocyanate with a polyol. Depending on various manufacturing and raw material variables, PUs can be made with different chemical, physical and biological properties.

**BOX 4.9   EXAMPLES OF COMMERCIALISED USE OF POLYURE-
THANE IN WOUND DRESSINGS**

- ActivHeal® Foam range (Advanced Medical Solutions) – PU foam pad and PU membrane
- Allevyn◊ range (Smith + Nephew) – multilayer PU foam
- Acticoat◊ Moisture Control (Smith + Nephew) – PU foam with other layers
- Biatain® range (Coloplast) – PU foam
- Mepilex® range (Mölnlycke Health Care) – PU foam with silicone
- PolyMem® (Ferris) – PU matrix with added ingredients
- Tielle™ range (Acelity) – PU foam and membrane
- Tegaderm™ Foam (3M) – PU foam with other layers
- Tegaderm™ film (3M) – PU film with adhesive
- Opsite◊ (Smith + Nephew) – PU film with adhesive
- Comfeel® Plus range (Coloplast) – PU film with PU foam or other materials
- Mepore® Film (Mölnlycke Health Care) – PU film

They can be hydrophilic or hydrophobic, have different permeation and degradation profiles, or they can be hard, soft, flexible, elastomeric, or adhesive. The versatility in their properties and manufacturability (they can be formed into films, sponges, foams, adhesive layers, fibres, nanofibres, hydrogels, particles, etc.), and their non-toxic, sterilisable and non-allergenic profile, make them a prime material for use in the medical industry.

PU is already significantly and successfully used in wound dressings, as seen from some examples of commercialised products in Box 4.9. Mostly they are used in the form of absorbent and cushioning hydrophilic foams or thin protective films, the latter either in a multilayer system with other materials or with an adhesive layer only. The soft and elastomeric qualities of some polyurethanes make them comfortable, conformable and gentle to the touch, proving protection and cushioning in the form of foam dressing. The semi-permeability of certain PU films makes them ideal to act as a protective barrier that allows the evaporation of water vapour and the exchange of oxygen and carbon dioxide, but leaves them impermeable to microorganisms and liquids.

The processing and formulation of PU as a foam, one of its main uses in the wound care industry, result in dressings with different wound management capabilities, mostly related to the foam pore characteristics. PU foams can have a range of moisture vapour transmission rate, fluid absorption and fluid retention capabilities, which all affect the moisture management potential (Lee et al., 2016). The pore size may also influence the interactions at the wound-dressing interface, including if and how the dressing adheres to the wound bed as the wound heals. The safety and efficacy of various PU foams and foam/films combinations have been largely demonstrated clinically, with foams being significantly used in chronic wounds and films as cover dressings. The foam market, with PU as polymer of choice, is estimated to take about 30% share of the total global wound care market, with an expected CAGR growth of 33% to 2027 (DataM Intelligence, 2020). PU foams are known to have good absorbency, to satisfactorily manage exudate, to reduce dressing change requirements, to help with wound healing and closure, to reduce pain during wear time and to have painless removal in a range of wounds (Schulze, 2003; Franks et al., 2007; Leonard et al., 2009; Hurd et al., 2009; Lee et al., 2016).

To change the biophysical properties of PU, functional ingredients and actives are added to them, including alginates and hyaluronic acid for improved wound healing, and antimicrobials (Lee et al., 2001). Many different development and manufacturing routes have been reported for antibacterial PU foams, and several are commercially available, e.g., foams impregnated with antimicrobials such as various silver formulations, polyhexamethylene biguanide or povidone-iodine. In *in vivo* studies comparing various commercial antibacterial foams with gauze, the foams were unsurprisingly found to lead to better healing than the gauze, with some showing better angiogenesis and collagen deposition than others (Lee & Song, 2018). Clinically, there is evidence that the wound healing capabilities of different antibacterial PU foams differ from product to product, whether this is due to the base foam or to the antibacterial agent (Jørgensen et al., 2005).

Other than conventional outer layer dressings, PU is also being used in the development of scaffolds for tissue engineering and the nanofibrous mat form has been shown to be suitable to assist in cell attachment and proliferation without any additional coating (Gustafsson et al., 2012; Rottmar et al., 2015). The benefits of using PU as scaffolds lie in its elastomeric properties, which enable it to flex as required where required, and its tailorable biodegradability, which enables control over how long the scaffold should last for. PU scaffolds have also been developed in combination with other bioactive materials such as collagen (Sin et al., 2010), silk-fibroin (Petrini et al., 2001), or electroactive materials such as polyvinylidene fluoride (PVDF) (Guo et al., 2012).

Research on novel materials and combinations continues to involve PU. More recently, more complex combinations of PU with other materials have been investigated for wound dressings. One example is the development of a bilayer PU/propolis and polycaprolactone/gelatine material to create multifunctional aspects within one dressing (Eskandarinia et al., 2020). Another example is the use of PU/siloxane membranes for the electroactive stimulation of wound healing, which leads to an antibacterial and antioxidant effect and stimulation of cell growth and proliferation (Gharibi et al., 2015).

4.2.3.1 Elastane

Elastane, or spandex, is the generic name given to elastomeric textiles such as Lycra®, which are characterised by very high elasticity and high recovery. Typically, such materials can be stretched to over 200% and up to 800%

of their original length before breaking (Senthilkumar et al., 2011; Xiong & Tao, 2018). Also sometimes referred to as copolymers of polyether-polyurea, elastane is made of long-chained polymers of at least 85% segmented polyurethane, with soft and hard segments linked by urethane bonds. The elasticity is principally attributed to the soft segments, whereas the hard segments contribute to stability and strength. The filaments can be made by different techniques but the most common one is by solution dry spinning. The prepolymer is prepared, reacted with diamine acid, diluted, extruded, heated, twisted and finished. Elastane fibres are often blended with other man-made or natural fibres, or made into core-spun structures, where they act as the central core and are wrapped with a sheath of other fibres.

Elastane fibres do not claim to have any wound healing properties and are not normally used in primary wound dressings. However, they are mentioned here because their unique elasticity and rapid recovery are essential in secondary dressings such as compression therapy and pressure garments. They are also included in bandages and other secondary dressings to provide a degree of stretch and comfort during use.

4.2.4 Polyvinyl Alcohol (PVA)

PVA is a water-soluble polymer prepared by the hydrolysis of polyvinyl acetate or other vinyl ester-derived polymers. Its easy film-forming characteristics make it widely used in textiles and coatings. Its biocompatibility, low toxicity and biodegradability have made it another polymer of high interest for the medical industry, including in the manufacture of contact lenses, hydrogels and foams/sponges. The PVA sponge can be used as an analytical tool for assessing the healing process (Deskins et al., 2012). Foams and sponges are also used as dressings. Unlike PU foams, PVA ones are rigid in their dry state and in most cases when used in wound care, need to be premoistened first to restore some softness and flexibility (Sambasivam et al., 2006). Being stiffer, PVA foams can be used where compression or collapse of a dressing is not desirable, e.g., when used on certain locations such as tunnelling wounds, with NPWT devices. The PVA foams are also reported to be less adherent to the wound and to have higher tensile strength for ease of removal from difficult to reach wounds (KCI, 2015). Some examples of PVA-containing foams are provided in Box 4.10.

BOX 4.10   EXAMPLES OF COMMERCIALISED PVA FOAMS

- Hydrofera Blue® (Hydrofera) – PVA and PU foam with antibacterials
- V.A.C.® WHITEFOAM™ dressing (Acelity) – hydrophilic PVA
- Invia White Foam NPWT (Medela) – hydrophilic PVA

PVA foams and sponges have been developed with chitosan and chitosan derivatives. With chitosan, it has been found to have excellent haemostatic performance and lead to enhanced wound healing, with increased re-epithelialisation and decreased granulation tissues (Zhao et al., 2019). PVA-chitooligosaccharides sponges have been found to accelerate the early stages of wound healing (You et al., 2004). A composite of fibroin-chitosan derivative-PVA was reported to improve the formation of blood vessels at the wound bed and promoting tissue regrowth (Li et al., 2014).

The other form in which PVA has been significantly explored in the context of wound dressing research is as a hydrogel. However, because of its inherent stiffness, limited elasticity and limited water absorption properties, PVA has been processed in blends and composites with other polymers, to create combinations with better wound management properties. The role of the PVA component is in some cases to enhance the mechanical and physicochemical properties of the other blended-in polymers. The research literature provides a large number of reports on the development and characterisation of PVA hydrogels mixed with a range of natural materials including alginate, dextran, starch and hydroxyethyl starch, glucan, gelatine, and in particular chitosan and its derivatives (Kamoun et al., 2015, 2017). With the blending of more hydrophilic, bioactive polymers, and even with the addition of a medicinal agent within the hydrogel, a compromise in the mechanical properties may be observed, but this often to the benefit of improved wound healing capabilities as demonstrated *in vivo* (Kim et al., 2008; Hwang et al., 2010; Sung et al., 2010). For example, the addition of chitosan to PVA hydrogels tends to improve swelling capacity, water transmission, antibacterial and antifungal properties (Kamoun et al., 2017).

In addition to blending in natural materials, PVA hydrogels have also been blended with synthetic polymers such as polyethylene glycol (PEG) and polyvinyl pyrrolidone (PVP) to improve on the moisture handling and other physicochemical properties. PVA/PVP hydrogels were found to have a range of water absorption properties depending on the proportions of each component; they were also found to be a good microbial barrier (Razzak et al., 1999). For additional functionalities, other actives such as nanoparticles, clay and natural extracts can also be incorporated with the PVA or PVA blend, to design potential wound dressing materials (Kamoun et al., 2015).

4.2.5 Polyglycolic Acid (PGA) and Polylactic Acid (PLA)

Polyglycolic acid (PGA), or polyglycolide, is an aliphatic polyester, made by polycondensation or ring-opening polymerisation from glycolic acid. It is a high-strength biodegradable and biocompatible polymer, which is used on its own or as a copolymer in bioresorbable sutures and scaffolds. PGA is highly susceptible to hydrolysis, losing strength and mass, leaving glycolic acid as the resulting degradation product (Prieto & Guelcher, 2014). Glycolic acid is a natural metabolite and is gradually disposed of by the body.

Polylactic acid (PLA), like PGA, it is another biodegradable and bioresorbable polyester, but is made by the condensation of lactic acid with a loss of water, or by the ring-opening polymerisation of lactide. PLA is a more sustainable polymer as the starting material is derived from natural sources, by bacterial fermentation of corn, sugarcane, potatoes and other biomass. It is commonly used as a copolymer with PGA, producing poly(lactic-co-glycolic acid) or polyglactin (PLGA), which is also used as a resorbable suture material, orthopaedic repairs and cartilage tissue engineering. Commercially as a wound dressing, PLGA also makes up the bioresorbable mesh scaffold Dermagraft® by Organogenesis, which is supplied with cultured fibroblasts for advanced wound care. A modified version of this technology has been reported in the literature, with web-like collagen microsponges in the mesh's openings, shown to enhance fibroblast cell seedings, improve cell distribution and subsequently facilitate the uniform formation of tissue (Chen et al., 2005).

PLA, PGA and PLGA can be used as carriers for a number of actives because of their biodegradable and bioresorbable properties. They can be made in the form of porous microspheres or nanoparticles or nanofibres, all containing active ingredients, as a form of slow-release system. The small size of the spheres, particles or fibres is associated with a greater surface area to volume ratio, and therefore greater exposure of the actives to the wound bed. Nanoparticles of PLGA have been loaded with a number of actives, such as ciprofloxacin hydrochloride for antibacterial efficacy (Choipang et al., 2018), peptide LL37 and vascular growth factors for enhanced wound healing (Chereddy et al., 2014, 2015). As a carrier for medicinal actives and extracts, PLGA has some benefits as the degradation rate is controllable and tuneable. Nanofibrous PLGA scaffolds have been loaded with pain killer and anti-inflammatory agent ibuprofen, degrading in 6 days following release of the drug over several days (Cantón et al., 2010). Thymoquinone-loaded PLA/cellulose acetate nanofibrous mats exhibited antibacterial effects resulting from the thymoquinone, and the mats were found to also promote wound healing by increasing re-epithelialisation and controlling the formation of granulation tissue *in vivo* (Gomaa et al., 2017). PLA nanofibres loaded with curcumin extract has been found to increase the rate of wound closures compared with PLA nanofibres alone by promoting the attachment and proliferation of cells (Nguyen et al., 2013).

Taking advantage of the fact that porous nanofibrous mats are additionally thought to physically resemble the structure of the skin's extracellular matrix, PLGA nanofibres have been produced with incorporated bioactive materials to try to create composites with improved wound healing properties. In early examples of work, collagen-modified nanofibrous PLGA and PLGA/ gelatine nanofibrous scaffolds have been developed and characterised

(Khorsand-Ghayeni et al., 2016; Vázquez et al., 2019). Vázquez et al. (2019) demonstrated that a ratio of 7:3 of PGLA:gelatine led to higher cell proliferation and degraded completely after 4 weeks implantation, with no residual inflammatory reaction.

4.2.6 Poly-ε-Caprolactone (PCL)

Another biodegradable aliphatic polyester, poly-ε-caprolactone (PCL) is made by the ring-opening polymerisation of ε-caprolactone, and has been used in many biomedical applications including drug delivery systems, implants, tissue engineering and absorbable sutures. Its widespread use is due to several of its properties, including its biodegradability, its ability to be hydrolysed by the body, the ease with which it can be processed into many different forms, its melt processability due to its low melting point and high thermal stability, its compatibility to a wide range of other polymers, and the relatively low cost (Azimi et al., 2014).

Although the use of PCL on its own as a wound dressing material has been investigated and found to be positive *in vivo* (Ng et al., 2007; Buzgo et al., 2019), most reported development work involves the use of PCL in combination with other polymers and/or actives. As with PGA and PLA, the biodegradation of PCL is one of the driving characteristics for its use in the biomedical field. The polymer makes an ideal carrier for actives and pharmaceuticals that need to be delivered at an injury site. The biodegradation of PCL is slower than that of PLA, which in the context of being used as a drug release bioresorbable polymer, makes it suitable for long-term uses. For slow-release dressings, or other shorter-term solutions, PCL nanofibre mats and scaffolds made by electrospinning, due to their higher surface area ratio, are able to release their cargo over a period of hours and days rather than months. One example is curcumin-loaded PCL nanofibres, which have been developed and investigated for use on diabetic wounds. The fibres were found to release their active component over a 3-day period and *in vivo*, to reduce inflammatory induction and increase the rate of wound closure (Merrell et al., 2009). Another example is curcumin-loaded PCL/chitosan films, reinforced with clay, which showed release of the curcumin over a period of several days, with a faster rate over the first 12-hour period, and with the addition of the clay (Huang et al., 2019). Other reported actives or pharmaceuticals loaded onto PCL and PCL containing structures for slow release include heparin, diclofenac, ampicillin, silver nanoparticles, iodine, carvacrol, thymol, chamomile, nitric oxide, among others.

PCL has been used as a strength-providing substrate and polymer base for bioactive materials such as hyaluronic acid, chitosan and collagen. It can also be used to improve the processability of other polymers – for example, it was added to cellulose acetate to make it easier to electrospin (Suteris et al., 2020). Ultra-thin PCL membranes, surface-modified with hyaluronic acid, were found to give comparable *in vivo* wound healing outcomes to a commercially available polyamide-silicone dressing (Cai et al., 2014). The lightweight and thin PCL membrane conforms better to the contours of the wound bed, and like the silicone control, was non-adherent, hence minimising trauma upon removal. Electrospun PCL and PCL with collagen have both been found to support keratinocyte cell attachment and growth, with the addition of collagen increasing the hydrophilicity of the nanofibres (Zeybek et al., 2014).

4.2.7 Polyacrylic Acid (PAA)

Polyacrylic acid (PAA) is a high molecular weight water-soluble polymer made from the polymerisation of acrylic acid. Its water solubility makes it an easy material to electrospin from, and it is also commonly made into hydrogels, with or without other polymers. The hydrogels are characterised by a high swelling capability in moist conditions, which is an attractive characteristic in wound care, particularly in the context of moist wound healing. PAA is also differentiated by being pH-responsive, due to the presence of carboxylic acid, which makes it interesting as a polymer for reactive drug release dressings. At higher pH, PAA and its blends demonstrate a higher release rate of incorporated actives than at lower pH.

In work using electrospun PAA/PVA with antimicrobial peptides, it was found that, as well as having a 2-week-long antibacterial effect, sustained release was observed in acidic environments, and a rapid release at higher pH values (Amariei et al., 2018). A similar increased release was observed in a bacterial cellulose/PAA hydrogel dressing material, loaded with an antibiotic. The hydrogel was found to have an increase in its swelling capacity and faster release of the active agent at a pH of 8 when a chronic wound is more prone to bacterial growth and biofilm formation (Chuah et al., 2018). A prior but different study demonstrated *in vivo* that acrylic acid and bacterial cellulose hydrogels were non-cytotoxic, and that the right combination would induce re-epithelialisation, fibroblast proliferation, collagen deposition, and could accelerate wound healing (Mohamad et al., 2014).

In other hydrogel formulations, PAA has been used as a polymer base or copolymer base for various hydrogel wound dressing development, including: with PEG (Bialik-Wąs et al., 2013), with chitosan and polyhydroxyethyl methacrylate (Yao et al., 2019), with citraconyl-chitosan (Rusu et al., 2015) and with chitin (Sangjun et al., 2003). The latter chitin-PAA hydrogel was studied *in vivo* and found to lead to more epithelialisation, faster wound closure and less scarring than a control dressing. Additional wound dressing developments include PAA grafted with carboxymethyl chitosan to produce a porous superabsorbent polymer (Chen et al., 2016), regenerated cellulose/PAA films (Bajpai et al., 2014) and electrospun PVA/PAA with ciprofloxacin hydrochloride and *aloe vera* (Serinçay et al., 2013).

4.2.8 Polyethylene Glycol (PEG)/Polyethylene Oxide (PEO)

Polyethylene glycol (PEG), also known as polyethylene oxide (PEO) or poly-oxyethylene (POE) depending on the molecular weight, is a hydrophilic, bio-compatible, flexible, non-toxic and non-immunogenic ether-based material. It is synthesised by the polymerisation of ethylene oxide or ethylene glycol. The polymer can be linear or branched, and the hydroxyl end groups can be converted into symmetrical or asymmetrical functional groups, which make it an extremely versatile polymer to be used in making hydrogels. PEG hydrogels are used as adhesives for wound closures, controlled release substrates and base materials for dressings.

As a sealant, biodegradable PEG hydrogel was compared with a standard skin sealant *in vitro* and *in vivo* (Chen et al., 2018). It was found that incision closure was enhanced in the flexible PEG hydrogel group, which also exhibited a higher level of collagen at the wound site compared to the control. Haemostatic hydrogel tissue adhesives were developed using a chitosan backbone grafted with PEG modified with tyramine (Lih et al., 2012). The resulting curable hydrogels were found to have better adhesiveness than commercial fibrin glue. In addition to the significant stopping of bleeding due to both the adhesiveness and haemostatic characteristics of the chitosan component, *in vivo* results demonstrated superior healing effects when compared to suture, fibrin blue and cyanoacrylate glue.

As with most hydrogels, which are characterised by having a high water content, PEG hydrogels as dressings should be able to help maintain a moist wound environment, favourable for wound healing. For this reason, PEG can be added to other materials to improve their absorptive and moisture-retaining abilities, and their suitability to be used for wound healing. For example, a supramolecular elastomer based on silicone and PEG has been developed, improving on the absorption rate, adhesive ability and water vapour permeability of the starting silicone (Deng et al., 2016). To increase absorbency, CMC-PEG hydrogels have been produced as a potential for wound dressings, with a degree of swelling that is tailorable between 100 and 500% (Capanema et al., 2018). Several *in vivo* studies have shown the potential benefits of including PEG in wound dressings, in combination with other materials. A PEG-protein hydrogel dressing has been shown to promote fast re-epithelialisation by creating a moist environment that encourages keratinocytes proliferation (Shingel et al., 2006).

PEG is also suitable as a material to carry and slowly release drugs over time due to its controllable degradation profile. Chitosan-PEG-(polyvinyl pyrrolidone) loaded with tetracycline hydrochloride and coated onto a substrate was shown to result in good antimicrobial efficacy, with fast healing and minimum scarring (Anjum et al., 2016). In another complex formulation, hyaluronic acid with PEG hydrogel encapsulates nanogels containing chlorohexidine to create multiple wound healing benefits (Zhu et al., 2018). The release of the chlorohexidine and the antimicrobial properties were shown to be prolonged over a period of 240 hours, while the dressing itself was shown *in vivo* to have rapid haemostatic capacity and lead to accelerated wound healing.

A large body of research has been conducted on the development of numerous hydrogels that include PEG, PEO and POE; the above examples are only a small fraction. Due to its versatility in modification, its biocompatibility, safety and inertness, PEG hydrogels will continue to be a material of interest in the development of biomedical polymers.

4.2.9 Polyvinyl Pyrrolidone (PVP)

Polyvinyl pyrrolidone (PVP), or also called polyvidone or povidone is a linear polymer widely used in the biomedical, cosmetic, pharmaceutical and food industries, and manufactured by the free-radical polymerisation of the monomer N-vinylpyrrolidone. Its ability to complex with iodine has resulted in commercial antibacterial PVP-iodine solution and powder, commonly used in the medical setting. A small number of wound dressing containing PVP-iodine compositions are available commercially (Box 4.11). Studies comparing Betafoam® with silver-based foams have found the PVP-iodine dressings to have comparable (if not more rapid) *in vitro* antibacterial efficacy to the silver ones, to have lower cytotoxicity to fibroblasts, and to be similar in wound healing efficacy in the management of partial-thickness burns (Jung et al., 2017; Jeong et al., 2019). This effect is due to the active ingredient iodine, discussed further in Chapter 6; but the enabling complexing agent is the PVP. Electrospun PVP-iodine and PVP-iodine with other polymers have also been a topic of interest for many researchers, including the concept of *in situ* electrospinning onto a wound bed (Liu et al., 2018).

From a wound dressing polymer perspective, the film- and fibre-forming properties of PVP and its hygroscopic nature have made it a useful polymer to explore with electrospinning and hydrogels. Crosslinked PVP hydrogel has excellent transparency, biocompatibility and impermeability to bacteria. *In vivo* tests of PVP hydrogels showed that they exhibited faster wound recovery and less discolouration compared to the topical antibiotic and control (Varzaneh et al., 2015).

BOX 4.11   EXAMPLES OF PVP-IODINE CONTAINING WOUND DRESSINGS

- INADINE™ (PVP-I) (Acelity) – knitted mesh impregnated with PEG/PVP-iodine
- Povitulle® (CD Medical) – gauze with PVP-iodine
- Betafoam® (Genewel) – PU foam with PVP-iodine

Like most of the man-made polymers discussed above, PVP is also often blended with other materials to improve its mechanical and biophysical properties, or to impart moisture handling properties to another polymer. Irradiated PVP with PEG and agar exhibited good elasticity, transparency, flexibility, water absorption capacity as well as impermeability to bacteria (Himly et al., 1993). PVP/CMC hydrogels were found to have better gel strength, flexibility and transparency than hydrogels made of only individual components (Wang et al., 2007). It was also found that the gel fraction and swelling rate can be optimised based on the proportions of the individual components. PVP with alginate and silver nanoparticles were found to have excellent absorption capacity and moisture permeability, with the silver contributing to a strong antimicrobial effect (Singh & Singh, 2012). PVP/PEG hydrogels were reported to have some antibacterial and antifungal properties, compared to a hydrocolloid control and to be biocompatible, as tested *in vitro* (Biazar et al., 2012). PVP incorporating silica nano-aggregates in the form of hydrogel and fibrous dressings resulted in good wound contraction and increased re-epithelialisation (Öri et al., 2017). A PVP with chitosan and titanium dioxide composite demonstrated improved strength with the addition of the titanium dioxide, excellent antibacterial activity with the chitosan, and overall accelerated healing *in vivo* compared with gauze, chitosan dressings and an antibiotic cream (Archana et al., 2013). A similar antibacterial and wound healing outcome was reported with chitosan-PVP-silver oxide films (Archana et al., 2015).

The water solubility of the polymer also makes it an interesting candidate for the gradual release of pharmaceuticals or other actives – in contact with wound fluid, non-crosslinked PVP is dissolved and easily removed. A number of pharmaceuticals have been incorporated in PVP and PVP-blends, including neomycin, indomethacin, bleomycin and ciproflaxin. When ciprofloxacin was incorporated into PVP-based foils and nanofibre mats, the nanofibres released their maximum load after 6 hours while the foils rapidly achieved their maximum and maintained it over 24 hours, even proving to be effective as an anti-biofilm (Rancan et al., 2019). Similarly, electrospun micro- and nanofibre mats with propolis and silver nanoparticles were found to have a fast release of the actives, depending on the polymer concentration and solvent (Adomavičiūtė et al., 2016).

4.2.10 Superabsorbent Polymers (SAP)

There are various references to superabsorbent polymers (SAPs), both from synthetic and natural sources (Zohuriaan-Mehr & Kabiri, 2008). However, the most commonly referred to SAPs are polyacrylate polymers, which are high molecular weight polyelectrolytes typically made from acrylic acid or acrylamides and a crosslinker by solution or suspension polymerisation. Due to their ability to absorb several times their own weight of fluids, and their ability to gel, they are intensively used as absorbent materials for sanitary consumer goods such as nappies, adult incontinence products, feminine hygiene products and the like. SAPs are mostly used in granules or particle form, but are also available in fibrous form. The level and rate of absorption vary according to the degree of crosslinking and the morphology of the SAP. The granules, particles or fibres can swell significantly upon contact with fluids, gelling with the moisture and retaining the fluids under compression. In wound dressings, as in personal consumer goods, SAP granules or particles need to be bagged or enclosed to make the product easier to handle, wear and remove. This is typically done with a nonwoven contact layer and outer layer. In this format, the dressing cannot be cut to size without spilling its contents. Some examples of polyacrylate-containing dressings are provided in Box 4.12.

Polyacrylates have an ionic charge which has been linked to the fluid handling properties and also to protein binding capabilities. Absorption is understood to occur through osmotic pressure caused by the concentration gradient of electrolytes inside and outside the particles, followed by expansion of the macromolecular chains due to electrostatic repulsion, and entrapment of the fluid and its components in the porous structure (Zohuriaan-Mehr & Kabiri, 2008; Wiegand & Hipler, 2013; Rogers & Rippon, 2017). Studies have shown that SAPs can inhibit MMPs activity *in vitro* and *in vivo* and also bind collagenases, elastases and inhibit free radical formation *in vitro* (Eming et al., 2008; Wiegand et al., 2011; Wiegand & Hipler, 2013). The mechanism of inhibition of MMPs is by directly binding to the proteinase and through the ionic charge, binding with calcium and zinc ions. The latter are necessary for enzymatic activity. In a retrospective study on chronic wounds, it was found that SAP dressings could be an effective, atraumatic and easy-to-use method of debriding wounds, by their strong ability to attract proteins and bacteria into the dressing, while keeping the wound bed moist (Paustian & Stegman, 2003). When compared with an enzymatic treatment, no significant

---

BOX 4.12   EXAMPLES OF DRESSINGS CONTAINING SUPER-ABSORBENT POLYMERS

	Unique Selling Points
• Cutimed® Sorbion® Sachet S (BSN Medical) – enclosed cellulose fibres and polyacrylate particles • Mextra® (Mölnlycke) – enclosed particles • HydroClean® (Hartmann) – enclosed particles, activated with Ringer's solution • UrgoClean (Urgo) – nonwoven polyacrylate fibres with acrylic core • Vliwasorb® Pro (Lohmann & Rauscher) – enclosed particles • Tegaderm™ Superabsorber (3M) – enclosed particles	Super absorbing Protein binding Debriding properties

difference was found between a superabsorbent-containing dressing and enzyme-containing ointment (König et al., 2005). This suggests that it could be a suitable alternative to autologous debridement when more aggressive methods are not recommended.

4.2.11 Silicone

Silicones or polysiloxanes are polymers made up of siloxane units. Typically, they are rubber-like in mechanical properties, but they can be made in different consistencies, from liquids to semi-solids and solids. They are chemically inert, do not facilitate bacterial growth, do not cause skin reactions or systemic toxicity and cannot be absorbed by the body. Silicones are widely used in many consumer, healthcare and industrial goods, including as sealants, adhesives, insulation, utensils, etc. In the medical field, due to their inertness, silicones of various composition and physical characteristics have been used as implants, contact lenses, epidermal substitute components, scar treatment sheets, and as contact layer and adhesive coatings for wound dressings.

In skin substitutes or regeneration templates, a silicone layer is used as the epidermal layer to protect the wound from heat and moisture loss, as well as from infection. The thin silicone layer can be porous (semi-permeable) or non-porous, and is typically the outer layer of the dermal substitute. This layer is then combined with a scaffolding structure containing a biomaterial such as collagen or viable cells. The matrix form of the bioactive contact layers provides a template for the patient's fibroblasts to migrate and grow, and for effective revascularisation. Examples of skin substitutes with a silicone layer are given in Box 4.13. Of those, Integra® and Biobrane^ are two of the most popular in academic research, and have been used with positive outcomes for burns, scar contraction surgery, and chronic wounds.

Silicones on their own have been used as a treatment for hypertrophic scarring and keloid management. These are conditions where the collagen formation upon healing is excessive and results in a raised scar. While the mechanism of action of silicone therapy on scars is not fully determined, it is believed that it could involve a localised rise in temperature, occlusion of the scar and hydration of the upper layer of the skin, increased oxygen tension,

---

BOX 4.13   EXAMPLES OF SILICONE-CONTAINING SKIN SUBSTITUTES

- Biobrane^ (Smith + Nephew) – collagen peptides with nylon mesh and silicone
- Integra® (Integra Lifesciences) – collagen-choidrontin fibrous matrix and silicone
- Hyalomatrix® (Haemo Pharma) – hyaluronic acid ester fibrous matrix on silicone
- Pelnac™ (Eurosurgical) – atelocollagen sponge with silicone

BOX 4.14   EXAMPLES OF SILICONE GEL SHEETS FOR SCAR MANAGEMENT

- CICA-CARE◊ (Smith + Nephew)
- Mepiform® (Mölnlycke) – soft silicone laminate
- MediClear™ Scar (Covalon) – PU film coated with soft silicone
- Epi-Derm range (Biodermis) – with or without soft fabric backing

direct action of the silicone oil and polarisation of scar tissue (Berman et al., 2007; Mustoe, 2008). Silicone sheets or topical gels are used both for the prevention and reduction of scar formation. Typically, they must be used for extended periods of time, e.g., in a study where improvements in tissue elasticity and scar volume were observed, the silicone dressing was used for a minimum of 12 hours a day and up to 2 months (Ahn et al., 1991).

Some examples of silicone gel sheets for scar management are given in Box 4.14. Most tend to be self-adhesive and cuttable to cover the scar. However, one of the disadvantages of sheets compared to gel is that they can be limited in terms of how well they can conform and intimately contact the scar in difficult or delicate anatomical locations. Larger (or longer) scars are also more difficult to cover properly. Silicone gels and creams have subsequently become part of the scar management toolkit. Creams containing silicone oil are thought to only be effective when used in conjunction with an occlusive dressing, whereas self-drying silicone gels are believed to be as efficacious as the sheets in the improvement of scars (Mustoe, 2008). However, while there is some evidence on the ability of silicone to improve the colour and volume of already-formed scars (Berman et al., 2007; Mustoe, 2008), a prevention study using silicone sheet and gels post-surgery found that the silicone-based products investigated were not able to prevent the formation of hypertrophic scars, but on the contrary, seemed to develop more excessive scarring (Niessen et al., 1998).

Soft silicone is a family of solid silicones, which is soft, conformable and tacky, and used in wound dressings as an atraumatic adhesive layer. As an inert material, it does not have an intrinsic effect on the wound healing processes per se, but in combination with other materials or dressings, is able to contribute to the care of wounds, principally by offering a solution to provide adherence without damage to the wound or surrounding skin. Handling of wound fluids in these cases is dealt with by a secondary dressing, or absorbing layer within the dressing. Some examples of atraumatic adhesive dressings are given in Box 4.15.

A number of laboratory and clinical studies have demonstrated the atraumatic benefits of soft silicones particularly when they are compared with the

BOX 4.15 EXAMPLES OF SOFT SILICONE WOUND DRESSINGS FOR MINIMAL TRAUMA

- Safetac® technology (Mölnlycke) – soft silicone layer used on the Mepitel® contact layer range with polyamide mesh, Mepilex® PU foam range and Mepitac® fixation range
- Biatain® silicone (Coloplast) – PU foam with soft silicone contact layer
- Activheal® Silicone range (Advanced Medical Solutions) – foam or knit with soft silicone layers
- ADAPTIC TOUCH™ (Acelity) – silicone wound contact layer
- Atrauman® Silicone (Hartmann) – two-sided soft silicone gel on polyester mesh
- Silflex (Advancis Medical) – polyester mesh with soft silicone
- Dermatac™ Drape (Acelity) – silicone/acrylic adhesive

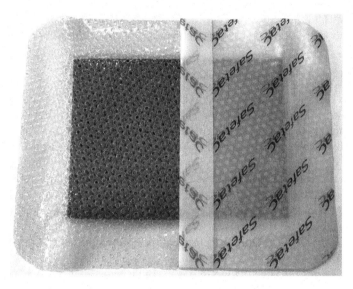

FIGURE 4.1
An example of a dressing with a soft atraumatic apertured silicone adhesive, shown here partly covered with the release layer

stronger and more aggressive adhesives such as acrylic ones (White, 2005; Rippon et al., 2007; Meuleneire & Rücknagel, 2013). It is understood that the silicone adhesives are able to gently adhere to dry skin, but not to the moist wound bed, instead allowing fluids to pass through apertures in the silicone layer (seen in Figure 4.1). Also, due to their microfluidity, they are able to conform intimately to the contours of the skin, ensuring a more secure seal. The soft adhesion to surrounding skin does not increase over time and is in itself not damaging upon removal.

Studies of different adhesive dressings on healthy volunteers showed that dressings with soft silicone adhesive were among those that removed the least stratum corneum from healthy skin (Dykes et al., 2001; Matsumara et al., 2014). Comparing a silicone adhesive dressing, non-silicone one, despite demonstrating no significant difference in the peel force required to remove the dressing, the silicone dressing was found to have a lower amount of skin cells and proteins on its surface (Warring et al., 2008). Clinically, the combination of a non-adhering moist area and gentle dry skin adhesion with minimal disruption of skin cells translates to less pain upon dressing changes and also during wear time. This has been demonstrated in several studies in paediatric patients (Morris et al., 2009), burns patients (Silverstein et al., 2011), on split-thickness grafts (Patton et al., 2013), and in a large multinational survey including both chronic and acute wounds (White, 2008). The benefits of soft silicone-containing dressings have therefore been widely demonstrated as a gentle adhesive; however, they have a high cost, require a minimum thickness layer to be effective, and cannot be sterilised by gamma irradiation without affecting the performance of the silicone layer.

4.2.12 Other Adhesives for Dressings

Several types of adhesives have been on the market for wound dressings, used either as a full-contact layer or border layer (for so-called island dressings) or on tapes used to secure other dressings. The purpose of an adhesive is normally to keep the dressing in place during wear and give the patient the ability to continue with their day-to-day activities, including moving about, showering where a waterproof backing layer is present, and even sleeping with the reassurance that the dressing will not move out of position. While doing so, they need to keep the skin as healthy as possible, and not negatively interfere with the wound healing process.

Adhesives for dressings need a fine balance of properties and performance. On the one hand, the bond between the dressing and the adhesive needs to be strong enough to be fit for purpose. This means keeping the dressing in place, protecting the wound from external contamination, and protecting the environment from wound contamination too. On the other hand, if it is too strong, or if the bond is formed on the wound bed, it risks damaging the healthy and healing tissue when the dressing is being removed. This results in pain and disruption of the healing process, and potentially unnecessary delayed healing. Adhesion strength is further complicated by skin variability, including skin health, sebum levels, moisture and hair levels, and even the presence of topical residues such as creams and other ointments. In general, it is possible to modify the properties and performance of the adhesives chemically (e.g., by varying the amount of tackifiers and resins) and by controlling the adhesive pattern on to the substrate. As a simplistic example, where more moisture vapour transmission is required, the adhesive may be applied in a dot pattern or reverse dot pattern instead of all over.

Traditional adhesives in wound dressings are acrylic based – e.g., methacrylates and epoxy diacrylates. These tend to be widely available and cost-effective (particularly compared to soft silicones, which command a higher premium), and applied as a border adhesive surrounding a central pad, or on the whole contact surface, e.g., of a transparent PU film. Acrylic adhesives are normally permeable to water vapour, the degree of which is influenced by the thickness of the adhesive and its formulation. The bond between acrylic adhesives and the skin can be quite strong, however, unlike some other more modern adhesive materials, they do not 'flow' to contour the microscopic topography of the skin (Neil, 2016). As a result, the seal may become imperfect and can lead to leakages or maceration of surrounding areas. The disadvantages of traditional acrylic adhesives are their tendency to cause skin stripping and irritation and to leave residues on the skin (Dykes et al., 2001; Rippon et al., 2007). When compared with a silicone adhesive, for example, an acrylic adhesive foam dressing was found to be more painful to remove, in correlation with a finding of higher levels of protein and cellular material on the acrylic adhesive (Warring et al., 2008).

Some clinicians recommend avoiding the use of traditional adhesive dressings on venous leg ulcers due to the high frequency of contact allergy and fragile nature of the skin (Rippon et al., 2007). More recently, to counter the issues of skin trauma, low trauma acrylic adhesives have been developed with the benefits of good adhesion, conformity, gentle removal with no residue, the ability to be repositioned, and at lower costs than silicones. Acrylic adhesives can now be modified to have different tack and adhesion properties by altering the formulation and with the addition of tackifiers.

Other alternative adhesives to acrylic and silicones are zinc oxide (used on plasters and tapes), PU and synthetic rubber-based adhesives. Rubber adhesives are strong but not breathable and likely to leave residues when removed. They are not recommended for long wear time, repeated applications or sensitive skin (Tebrake, 2014). Like acrylics, PU and zinc oxide adhesives have been reported to lead to skin stripping and are therefore not recommended for sensitive skin (Cutting, 2008).

Two wound dressing materials that can also double up as adhesives are hydrocolloids and hydrogels. As these are structural combinations of multiple base raw materials, they are discussed more in detail in Chapter 5. In the context of wound dressing adhesives, despite being able to intimately conform to the skin, they suffer from losing their adhesiveness when in contact with exudate. In addition, hydrocolloids have also been linked to trauma and pain upon removal (Cutting, 2008).

A study on the effect of various types of adhesives on the upper layer of the skin found that the worst offenders were dressings with acrylic adhesives and hydrocolloids (Matsumara et al., 2014). The ones which disrupted the least number of cells in the stratum corneum were found to be soft silicone-based ones and self-adhesive PU foam. Normally, when dressings are removed with skin cells attached to the adhesive, they lose their stickiness. Adhesives to which skin cells do not adhere to are re-positionable, which can be a benefit upon application, particularly for wounds that are difficult to dress.

4.3 About Sustainability and Waste Management

To end this chapter, this short section is intended to increase awareness of the sustainability and disposal aspect of dressings and other medical devices for advanced wound care. The base materials used for the dressings are one of the influencing factors in determining the sustainability and waste impact of the dressing. In the earlier subsections, some reference was made to the availability of resources for the manufacture of the various materials described. Some are produced from petrochemicals, which makes them dependent on fossil fuel extraction and the environmental impacts associated. Others are manufactured from widely available natural and renewable materials, but this may still generate a negative environmental impact. For example, cotton is biodegradable in landfills (unlike PET and PA), but a life cycle assessment from cradle to grave concluded that the environmental burden of cotton textiles is higher than that of PET and PA (van der Velden et al., 2014).

The concept of sustainable healthcare involves aspects of efficiency and responsibility from the beginning to the end. From the advanced wound care perspective, throughout the whole lifecycle of the product and care, the bottom-line impact on the environment, the patient and carer and on costs should be considered. Raw material supplies, the manufacture of the product, packaging and transporting, the use of the product, and its disposal must be managed to minimise waste and any negative impact on the environment wherever possible. Existing positive steps include, for example, utilising managed forests of fast-growing trees for the manufacture of man-made or modified cellulosics, use of waste materials and by-products from other industries as raw materials (e.g., as with chitosan), the use of recyclable or biodegradable packaging materials, optimisation of product designs and sizes for minimal waste, human factors, and so on.

Waste is a significant aspect in the healthcare industry, consisting of both general, non-hazardous waste and hazardous or contaminated waste. The latter is estimated to be about 15% of the amount of waste generated by the industry, with high-income countries generating on average about 0.5 kg of hazardous waste per bed per day, and low-income countries about 0.2 kg (WHO, 2018). This proportion is likely to vary considerably given that the segregation of hazardous and non-hazardous waste can be done differently in different countries, regions, or even care settings. For example, a 2015/2016 survey in the National Health Service in England indicated that 33% of bagged waste was deemed infectious and hazardous, higher than the WHO estimate (Royal College of Nursing, 2018). The total amount of waste produced by the healthcare industry also varies greatly from country to country, being correlated to the gross domestic product (GDP), accessibility of healthcare and other socio-economic factors (Minoglou et al., 2017). The USA and Canada have the highest levels of total waste per bed per day (more than 8 kg/bed/day), by contrast, lower income countries such as Morocco, Nepal and Mauritius have less than 1 kg/bed/day of healthcare waste. Waste in Europe and Asia fall somewhere in between these two extremes.

Waste disposal in the advanced wound care industry is constrained by the contamination of used products. Uncontaminated parts of the products, including primary packaging (which is the sterile barrier), secondary and tertiary packaging, and instructions for use can be recycled where possible. Unused, clean waste dressings are normally not recycled – they are more likely treated as general waste, which is disposed of in landfills. Dressings that have been in contact with wound fluids including blood and exudate are classed as contaminated, clinical, infectious or hazardous. Due to the risks they may pose to others, they are normally separated from other non-contaminated waste and need to be decontaminated first.

Previously, incineration used to be the method of choice for disposing of hazardous healthcare waste; however, it is now recognised that aside from the pollution, incineration of certain materials may release carcinogens and therefore require specialised gas cleaning equipment to comply with emission standards. For certain types of healthcare waste, such as infectious ones, incineration is still required at a specialist facility. Other methods of treating hazardous wastes can be used such as autoclaving, microwaving, steam treatment with internal mixing and chemical treatment. The latter can also lead to the release of harmful chemical substances in the environment if the appropriate handling, storage and disposal measures are not in place. Decontaminated hazardous waste can be subsequently disposed of in landfills, unless classified as too hazardous to do so.

The base material or polymer used in advanced wound care has a significant contribution to the impact of the product on the environment, not only from a manufacturing perspective, but also in terms of waste. However, other factors also contribute, including actives and additives (Chapter 6), the product design, how it used and how often it needs to be changed, whether devices are single-use disposable or can be repurposed, and how it is packaged. In the development of advanced wound care materials and the selection of materials to be used, the balance of clinical benefits that a material can provide versus environment and cost is an important one. The stronger the evidence for clinical efficacy, the more acceptable the premiums become.

References

Adomavičiūtė, E., Stanys, S., Žilius, M., Juškaitė, V., Pavilonis, A., & Briedis, V. (2016). Formation and Biopharmaceutical Characterization of Electrospun PVP Mats with Propolis and Silver Nanoparticles for Fast Releasing Wound Dressing. *BioMed Research International*, 4648287. doi:10.1155/2016/4648287

Ahn, S. T., Monafo, W. W., & Mustoe, T. A. (1991, April). Topical Silicone Gel for the Prevention and Treatment of Hypertrophic Scar. *Archives of Surgery, 126*(4), 499. doi:10.1001/archsurg.1991.01410280103016

Ali, S. W., Rajendran, S., & Joshi, M. (2011, January 10). Synthesis and Characterization of Chitosan and Silver Loaded Chitosan Nanoparticles for Bioactive Polyester. *Carbohydrate Polymers, 83*(2), 438. doi:10.1016/j.carbpol.2010.08.004

Amariei, G., Kokol, V., Boltes, K., Letón, P., & Rosal, R. (2018). Incorporation of Antimicrobial Peptides on Electrospun Nanofibres for Biomedical Applications. *RSC Advances, 49*, 28013. doi:10.1039/c8ra03861a

Anghel, I., Holban, A. M., Andronescu, E., Grumezescu, A. M., & Chifiriuc, M. C. (2013, April). Efficient Surface Functionalization of Wound Dressings by a Phytoactive Nanocoating Refractory to Candida Albicans Biofilm Development. *Biointerphases, 8*, 12. doi:10.1186/1559-4106-8-12

Anjum, S., Arora, A., Alam, M. S., & Gupta, B. (2016, July 11). Development of Antimicrobial and Scar Preventive Chitosan Hydrogel Wound Dressings. *International Journal of Pharmaceutics, 508*(1–2), 92. doi:10.1016/j.ijpharm.2016.05.013

Aramwit, P., Kanokpanont, S., De-Eknamkul, W., & Srichana, T. (2009, May). Monitoring of Inflammatory Mediators Induced by Silk Sericin. *Journal of Bioscience and Engineering, 107*(5), 556. doi:10.1016/j.jbiosc.2008.12.012

Aramwit, P., Palapinyo, S., Srichana, T., Chottanapund, S., & Muangman, P. (2013). Silk Sericin Ameliorates Wound Healing and Its Clinical Efficacy in Burn Wounds. *Archinves of Dermatological Research, 305*, 585. doi:10.1007/s00403-013-1371-4

Archana, D., Singh, B. K., Dutta, J., & Dutta, P. K. (2013, June 5). In Vivo Evaluation of Chitosan–PVP–Titanium Dioxide Nanocomposite as Wound Dressing Material. *Carbohydrate Polymers, 95*(1), 530. doi:10.1016/j.carbpol.2013.03.034

Archana, D., Singh, B. K., Dutta, J., & Dutta, P. K. (2015, February). Chitosan-PVP-Nano Silver Oxide Wound Dressing: In Vitro and In Vivo Evaluation. *International Journal of Biological Macromolecules, 73*, 49. doi:10.1016/j.ijbiomac.2014.10.055

Arslan, A., Şimşek, M., Aldemir, S. D., Kazaroğlu, N. M., & Gümüşderelioğlu, M. (2014). Honey-Based PET or PET/Chitosan Fibrous Wound Dressings: Effect of Honey on Electrospinning Process. *Journal of Biomaterials Science, Polymer Edition, 25*(10), 999. doi:10.1080/09205063.2014.918455

Attwood, A. (1989). Calcium Alginate Dressing Accelerates Split Skin Graft Donor Site Healing. *Brirish Journal of Plasric Surgery, 42*, 373.

Azimi, B., Nourpana, P., Rabiee, M., & Arbab, S. (2014). Poly (ε-Caprolactone) Fiber: An Overview. *Journal of Engineered Fibers and Fabrics, 9*(3), 74.

Bajpai, M., Bajpai, S. K., & Gautam, D. (2014). Investigation of Regenerated Cellulose/Poly(Acrylic Acid) Composite Films for Potential Wound Healing Applications: A Preliminary Study. *Journal of Applied Chemistry*, 1. doi:10.1155/2014/325627

Barrois, B., Carles, M., Rumeau, M., Tell, L., Toussaint, J.-F., Bonnefoy, M., & de Vathaire, F. (2007). Efficacy and Tolerability of Hyaluronan (Ialuset) in the Treatment of Pressure Ulcers: A Multicentre, Non-Randomised, Pilot Study. *Drugs R&D, 8*(5), 267. doi:10.2165/00126839-200708050-00001

Berman, B., Perez, O. A., Konda, S., Kohut, B. E., Viera, M. H., Delgado, S., Zell, D., & Li, Q. (2007). A Review of the Biologic Effects, Clinical Efficacy, and Safety of Silicone Elastomer Sheeting for Hypertrophic and Keloid Scar Treatment and Management. *Dermatologic Surgery, 33*, 1291. doi:10.1111/j.1524-4725.2007.33280

Bialik-Wąs, K., Tyliszczak, B., & Pielichowski, K. (2013). Preparation of Innovative Hydrogel Wound Dressings Based on Poly(Acrylic Acid). *Chemik Science-Technique-Market, 67*(2), 99. Retrieved from https://www.researchgate.net/publication/283016718_Preparation_of_innovative_hydrogel_wound_dressings_based_on_polyacrylic_acid

Biazar, E., Roveimiab, Z., Shahhosseini, G., Khataminezhad, M., Zafari, M., & Mjadi, A. (2012). Biocompatibility Evaluation of a New Hydrogel Dressing Based on Polyvinylpyrrolidone/Polyethylene Glycol. *BioMed Research International, 343989*. doi:10.1155/2012/343989

Blair, S., Jarvis, P., Salmon, M., & McCollum, C. (1990). Clinical Trial of Calcium Alginate Haemostatic Swabs. *BJS Society, 17*(5), 568.

Brown, M. A., Daya, M., & Worley, J. (2009). Experience with Chitosan Dressings in a Civilian EMS System. *Journal of Emergency Medicine, 37*(1), 1.

Brown-Etris, M., Milne, C. T., & Hodde, J. P. (2019, February). An Extracellular Matrix Graft (Oasis® Wound Matrix) for Treating Full-Thickness Pressure Ulcers: A Randomized Clinical Trial. *Journal of Tissue Viability, 28*(1), 21. doi:10.1016/j.jtv.2018.11.001

Buzgo, M., Plencner, M., Rampichova, M., Litvinec, A., Prosecka, E., Staffa, A., Kralovic, M.; Filova, E.; Doupnik, M.; Lukasova, V.; Vocetkova, K.; Anderova, J.; Kubikova, T.; Zajicek, R.; Lopot, F.; Jelen, K.; Tonar, Z.; Amler, E.; Divin, R.; & Fiori, F. (2019, May). Poly-ε-Caprolactone and Polyvinyl Alcohol Electrospun Wound Dressings: Adhesion Properties and Wound Management of Skin Defects in Rabbits. *Regenerative Medicine, 14*(5), 423. doi:10.2217/rme-2018-0072

Cagri, U. A., Sahin, A. M., Hakan, O., & Omer, S. (2006). An Alternative Dressing Material for the Split-Thickness Skin Graft Donor Site: Oxidized Regenerated Cellulose. *Annals of Plastic Surgery, 57*(1), 60.

Cai, E. Z., Lee, J., & Wen, F. (2014, November). Bio-Conjugated Polycaprolactone Membranes: A Novel Wound Dressing. *Archives of Plastic Surgery, 41*(6), 638. doi:10.5999/aps.2014.41.6.638

Cai, Z.-X., Mo, X.-M., Zhang, K.-H., Fan, L.-P., Yin, A.-L., He, C.-L., & Wang, H.-S. (2010). Fabrication of Chitosan/Silk Fibroin Composite Nanofibers for Wound-Dressing Applications. *International Journal of Molecular Sciences, 11*, 3529. doi:10.3390/ijms11093529

Cantón, I., Mckean, R., Charnley, M., Blackwood, K. A., Fiorica, C., Ryan, A. J., & MacNeil, S. (2010, February 1). Development of an Ibuprofen-Releasing Biodegradable PLA/PGA Electrospun Scaffold for Tissue Regeneration. *Biotechnology and Bioengineering, 105*(2), 396. doi:10.1002/bit.22530

Capanema, N. S., Mansur, A. A., de Jesus, A. C., Carvalho, S. M., de Oliveira, L. C., & Mansur, H. S. (2018, January). Superabsorbent Crosslinked Carboxymethyl Cellulose-PEG Hydrogels for Potential Wound Dressing Applications.

International Journal of Biological Macromolecules, *106*, 1218. doi:10.1016/j.ijbiomac.2017.08.124

Carvalho, V. F., Paggiaro, A. O., Isaac, C., Gringlas, J., & Ferreira, M. C. (2011). Clinical Trial Comparing 3 Different Wound Dressings for the Management of Partial-Thickness Skin Graft Donor Sites. *Journal of Wound Ostomy and Continence Nursing*, *38*(6), 643.

Cervelli, V., Brinci, L., Spallone, D., Tati, E., Palla, L., Lucarini, L., & De Angelis, B. (2011, August). The Use of MatriDerm® and Skin Grafting in Post-Traumatic Wounds. *International Wound Journal*, *8*(4), 400. doi:10.1111/j.1742-481X.2011.00806.x

Chen, G., Sato, T., Ohgushi, H., Ushida, T., Tateishi, T., & Tanaka, J. (2005, May). Culturing of Skin Fibroblasts in a Thin PLGA-Collagen Hybrid Mesh. *Biomaterials*, *26*(15), 2559. doi:10.1016/j.biomaterials.2004.07.034

Chen, S.-L., Fu, R.-H., Liao, S.-F., Liu, S.-P., Lin, S.-Z., & Wang, Y.-C. (2018, February). A PEG-Based Hydrogel for Effective Wound Care Management. *Cell Transplantation*, *27*(2), 275. doi:10.1177/0963689717749032

Chen, Y., Zhang, Y., Wang, F., Meng, W., Yang, X., Li, P., Jiang, J., Tan, H., & Zheng, Y. (2016, June 1). Preparation of Porous Carboxymethyl Chitosan Grafted Poly(Acrylic Acid) Superabsorbent by Solvent Precipitation and Its Application as a Hemostatic Wound Dressing. *Materials Science and Engineering: C*, *63*, 18. doi:10.1016/j.msec.2016.02.048

Chereddy, K. K., Her, C.-H., Comune, M., Moia, C., Lopes, A., Porporato, P. E., Vanacker, J., Lam, M. C., Steinstraesser, L., Sonveaux, P., Zhu, H., Ferreira, L. S., Vandermeulen, G., & Préat, V. (2014, November). PLGA Nanoparticles Loaded with Host Defense Peptide LL37 Promote Wound Healing. *Journal of Control Release*, *47*, 138. doi:10.1016/j.jconrel.2014.08.016

Chereddy, K. K., Lopes, A., Koussoroplis, S., Payen, V., Moia, C., Zhu, H., Sonveaux, P., Carmeliet, P., des Rieux, A., Vandermeulen, G., Préat, V. (2015, November). Combined Effects of PLGA and Vascular Endothelial Growth Factor Promote the Healing of Non-Diabetic and Diabetic Wounds. *Nanomedicine*, *11*(8), 1975. doi:10.1016/j.nano.2015.07.006

Chiara, O., Cimbanassi, S., Bellanova, G., Chiarugi, M., Mingoli, A., Olivero, G., Ribaldi, S., Tugnoli, G., Basilico, S., Bindi, F., Briani, L., Renzi, F., Chirletti, P., Di Grezia, G., Martino, A., Marzaioli, R., Noschese, G., Portolani, N., Ruscelli, P., Zago, M., Sgardello, S., Stagnitti, F., & Miniello, S. (2018, August 29). A Systematic Review on the Use of Topical Hemostats in Trauma and Emergency Surgery. *BMC Surgery*, *18*, 68.

Choipang, C., Chuysinuan, P., Suwantong, O., Ekabutr, P., & Supathol, P. (2018, October). Hydrogel Wound Dressings Loaded with PLGA/Ciprofloxacin Hydrochloride Nanoparticles for Use on Pressure Ulcers. *Journal of Drug Delivery Science and Technology*, *47*, 106. doi:10.1016/j.jddst.2018.06.025

Chou, T., Fu, E., Wu, C., & Yeh, J. (2003, March 14). Chitosan Enhances Platelet Adhersion and Aggregation. *Biochemical and Biophysical Research Communications*, *302*(3), 480.

Chuah, C., Wang, J., Tavakoli, J., & Tang, Y. (2018, December). Novel Bacterial Cellulose-Poly (Acrylic Acid) Hybrid Hydrogels with Controllable Antimicrobial Ability as Dressings for Chronic Wounds. *Polymers (Basel)*, *10*(12), 1323. doi:10.3390/polym10121323

Cutting, K. (2008, May). Impact of Adhesive Surgical Tape and Wound Dressings on the Skin, with Reference to Skin Stripping. *Journal of Wound Care, 17*(4), 157. doi:10.12968/jowc.2008.17.4.28836

Dabiri, G., Damstetter, E., & Philips, T. (2016, January 1). Choosing a Wound Dressing Based on Common Wound Characteristics. *Advances in Wound Care, 5*(1), 32.

DataM Intelligence. (2020, October 8). *Foam Dressings Market, Size, Share, Opportunities and Forecast, 2020–2027.* Hyderabad: DataM Intelligence.

Dawson, C., Armstrong, M., Fulford, S., Faruqi, R., & Galland, R. (1992). Use of Calcium Alginate to Pack Abscess Cavities: A Controlled Clinical Trial. *Journal of the Royal College of Surgeons of Edinburgh, 37*(3), 177.

Deng, W., Lei, Y., Zhou, S., Zhang, A., & Lin, Y. (2016). Absorptive Supramolecular Elastomer Wound Dressing Based on Polydimethylsiloxane–(Polyethylene Glycol)–Polydimethylsiloxane Copolymer: Preparation and Characterization. *RSC Advances, 57*(6), 51694. doi:10.1039/C6RA07146E

Dereure, O., Mikosinki, J., Zegota, Z., & Allaert, F. A. (2012, November). RCT to Evaluate a Hyaluronic Acid Containing Gauze Pad in Leg Ulcers of Venous or Mixed Aetiology. *Journal of Wound Care, 21*(11), 539. doi:10.12968/jowc.2012.21.11.539

Deskins, D. L., Ardestani, S., & Young, P. P. (2012, April 18). The Polyvinyl Alcohol Sponge Model Implantation. *Journal of Visualized Experiments, 62*, 3885. doi:10.3791/3885

Dias, F. T., Ingracio, A. R., Nicoletti, N. F., Menezes, F. C., Agnol, L. D., Marinowic, D. R., Soares, R. M. D., da Costa, J. C., Falavigna, A., & Bianchi, O. (2019, June). Soybean-Modified Polyamide-6 Mats as a Long-Term Cutaneous Wound Covering. *Materials Science and Engineering: C, 99*, 957. doi:10.1016/j.msec.2019.02.019

Dykes, P. J., Heggie, R., & Hill, S. A. (2001, February 1). Effects of Adhesive Dressings on the Stratum Corneum of the Skin. *Journal of Wound Care, 10*(2), 7. doi:10.12968/jowc.2001.10.2.26054

Egles, C. E., Shamis, Y., Mauney, J. R., Volloch, V., Kaplan, D. L., & Garlick, J. A. (2008, July). Denatured Collagen Modulates the Phenotype of Normal and Wounded Human Skin Equivalents. *Journal of Investigative Dermatology, 128*(7), 1830.

Eming, S., Smola, H., Hartmann, B., Malchau, G., Wegner, R., Krieg, T., & Smola-Hess, S. (2008, July). The Inhibition of Matrix Metalloproteinase Activity in Chronic Wounds by a Polyacrylate Superabsorber. *Biomaterials, 29*(19), 2932. doi:10.1016/j.biomaterials.2008.03.029

Eskandarinia, A., Kefayat, A., Agheb, M., Rafienia, M., Baghbadorani, M. A., Navid, S., Ebrahimpour, K., Khodabakhshi, D., & Ghahremani, F. (2020). A Novel Bilayer Wound Dressing Composed of a Dense Polyurethane/Propolis Membrane and a Biodegradable Polycaprolactone/Gelatin Nanofibrous Scaffold. *Scientific Reports, 10*, 3063. doi:10.1038/s41598-020-59931-2

Fleck, C., & Simman, R. (2010, September). Modern Collagen Wound Dressings: Function and Purpose. *Journal of the American College of Certified Wound Specialists, 2*(3), 50.

Fong, J., & Wood, F. (2006, December). Nanocrystalline Silver Dressings in Wound Management: A Review. *International Journal of Nanomedicine, 1*(4), 441. doi:10.2147/nano.2006.1.4.441

Franks, P. J., Moody, M., Moffatt, C. J., Hiskett, G., Gatto, P., Davies, C., Furlong, W. T., Barrow, E., & Thomas, H. (2007, March). Randomized Trial of Two Foam

Dressings in the Management of Chronic Venous Ulceration. *Wound Repair and Regeneration*, 15(2), 197. doi:10.1111/j.1524-475X.2007.00205.x

Gegel, B., Burgert, J., Cooley, B., MacGregor, J., Myers, J., Calder, S., Luellen, R., Loughren, M., & Johnson, D. (2010, November). The Effects of BleedArrest, Celox, and TraumaDex on Hemorrhage Control in a Porcine Model. *Journal of Surgical Research*, 164(1), 125.

Gharibi, R., Yeganeh, H., Rezapour-Lactoee, A., & Hassan, Z. M. (2015). Stimulation of Wound Healing by Electroactive, Antibacterial, and Antioxidant Polyurethane/ Siloxane Dressing Membranes: In Vitro and in Vivo Evaluations. *ACS Applied Materials Interfaces*, 7(43), 24296. doi:10.1021/acsami.5b08376

Gilotra, S., Chouhan, D., Bhardwaj, N., Nandi, S. K., & Mandal, B. B. (2018, September 1). Potential of Silk Sericin Based Nanofibrous Mats for Wound Dressing Applications. *Materials Science and Engineering: C*, 90, 420. doi:10.1016/j.msec.2018.04.077

Gomaa, S., Madkour, T. M., Moghannem, S., & El-Sherbiny, I. M. (2017, December). New Polylactic Acid/Cellulose Acetate-Based Antimicrobial Interactive Single Dose Nanofibrous Wound Dressing Mats. *International Journal of Biological Macromolecules*, 105(1), 1148. doi:10.1016/j.ijbiomac.2017.07.145

Granville-Chapman, J., Jacobs, N., & Midwinter, M. (2011, May). Pre-Hospital Haemostatic Dressings: A Systematic Review. *Injury*, 42(5), 447.

Graumlich, J. F., Blough, L. S., McLaughlin, R. G., Milbrandt, J. C., Calderon, C. L., Abbas Agha, S., & Scheibel, L. W. (2003, February). Healing Pressure Ulcers with Collagen or Hydrocolloid: A Randomized, Controlled Trial. *Journal of the American Geriatrics Society*, 51(2), 147.

Greco, R. M., Iocono, J. A., & Ehrlich, H. P. (1998). Hyaluronic Acid Stimulates Human Fibroblast Proliferation within a Collagen Matrix. *Journal of Cellular Physiology*, 177, 465.

Gualdi, G., Monari, P., Cammalleri, D., Pelizzari, L., & Pinton, P. (2019, March). Hyaluronic Acid-Based Products Are Strictly Contraindicated in Scleroderma-Related Skin Ulcers. *Wounds*, 31(3), 81.

Guo, H.-F., Li, Z.-S., Dong, S.-W., Chen, W.-J., Deng, L., Wang, Y.-F., & Ying, D.-J. (2012, August 1). Piezoelectric PU/PVDF Electrospun Scaffolds for Wound Healing Applications. *Colloids and Surfaces B: Biointerfaces*, 96, 29. doi:10.1016/j.colsurfb.2012.03.014

Gustafsson, Y., Haag, J., Jungebluth, P., Lundin, V., Lim, M. L., Baiguera, S., Ajalloueian, F., Del Gaudio, C., Bianco, A., Moll, G., Sjöqvist, S., Lemon, G., Teixeira, A., & Macchiarini, I. P. (2012). Viability and Proliferation of Rat MSCs on Adhesion Protein-Modified PET and PU Scaffolds. *Biomaterials*, 33, 8094. doi:10.1016/j.biomaterials.2012.07.060

Hampton, S. (2004). The Role of Alginate Dressings in Wound Healing. *The Diabetic Foot*, 7(4), 162.

Haslik, W., Kamolz, L.-P., Manna, F., Hladik, M., Rath, T., & Frey, M. (2010, February). Management of Full-Thickness Skin Defects in the Hand and Wrist Region: First Long-Term Experiences with the Dermal Matrix Matriderm®. *Journal of Plastic, Reconstructive & Aesthetic Surgery*, 63(7), 360. doi:10.1016/j.bjps.2008.09.026

Haslik, W., Kamolz, L.-P., Nathschläger, G., Andel, H., Meissl, G., & Frey, M. (2007, May). First Experiences with the Collagen-Elastin Matrix Matriderm® as a Dermal Substitute in Severe Burn Injuries of the Hand. *Burns*, *33*(3), 364. doi:10.1016/j.burns.2006.07.021

Hatamabadi, H. R., Zarchi, F., Kariman, H., Dolatabadi, A., Tabatabaey, A., & Amini, A. (2015, February). Celox-Coated Gauze for the Treatment of Civilian Penetrating Trauma: A Randomized Clinical Trial. *Trauma Monthly*, *20*(1), 23862.

Hazarika, E. Z. (1985). Oxidised Regenerated Cellulose: An Effective Emergency Haemostatic in Burns Surgery. *British Journal of Plastic Surgery*, *38*, 419.

Herndon, C. L., Coury, J. R., Sarpong, N. O., Geller, J. A., Shah, R. P., & Cooper, H. J. (2020, June). Polyester Mesh Dressings Reduce Delayed Wound Healing Rates after Total Hip Arthroplasty Compared with Silver-Impregnated Occlusive Dressings. *Arthorplasty Today*, *6*(2), 158. doi:10.1016/j.artd.2020.01.013

Himly, N., Darwis, D., & Hardiningsih, L. (1993, October–December). Poly(n-Vinylpyrrolidone) Hydrogels: 2. Hydrogel Composites as Wound Dressing for Tropical Environment. *Radiation Physics and Chemistry*, *42*(4–6), 911. doi:10.1016/0969-806X(93)90400-0

Hochstein, A. O. (2014, August). Collagen: Its Role in Wound Healing. *Podiatry Management*, 103.

Hoekstra, M., Hermans, M., Richters, C., & Dutrieux, R. (2002, March). A Histological Comparison of Acute Inflammatory Responses with a Hydrofibre or Tulle Gauze Dressing. *Journal of Wound Care*, *11*(3), 113.

Hoenich, N. (2006). Cellulose for Medical Appliations: Past, Present and Future. *BioResources*, *1*(2), 270.

Hollander, D. A., Soranzo, C., Falk, S., & Windolf, J. (2001, June). Extensive Traumatic Soft Tissue Loss: Reconstruction in Severely Injured Patients Using Cultured Hyaluronan-Based Three-Dimensional Dermal and Epidermal Autografts. *The Journal of Trauma: Injury, Infection, and Critical Care*, *50*(6), 1125. doi:10.1097/00005373-200106000-00024

Holmes, C., Wrobel, J. S., MacEachern, M. P., & Boles, B. R. (2013, January 17). Collagen-Based Wound Dressings for the Treatment of Diabetes-Related Foot Ulcers: A Systematic Review. *Diabetes, Metabolic Syndrome and Obesity: Targets and Therapies*, *6*, 17. doi:10.2147/DMSO.S36024

Huang, Y., Dan, N., Dan, W., & Zhao, W. (2019, December 19). Reinforcement of Polycaprolactone/Chitosan with Nanoclay and Controlled Release of Curcumin for Wound Dressing. *ACS Omega*, *4*, 22292. doi:10.1021/acsomega.9b02217aww3

Hurd, T., Gregory, L., Jones, A., & Brown, S. (2009). A Multi-Centre In-Market Evaluation of ALLEVYN◊ Gentle Border. *Wounds UK*, *5*(3), 32.

Hwang, M.-R., Kim, J. O., Lee, J. H., Kim, Y. I., Kim, J. H., Chang, S. W., Jin, S. G., Kim, J. A., Lyoo, W. S., Han, S. S., Ku, S. K., Yong, C. S., & Choi, H.-G. (2010, September). Gentamicin-Loaded Wound Dressing with Polyvinyl Alcohol/Dextran Hydrogel: Gel Characterization and In Vivo Healing Evaluation. *AAPS PharmSciTech*, *11*(3), 1092. doi:10.1208/s12249-010-9474-0

Jeong, C. S., Kwak, K., Hur, J., & Kym, D. (2019, January). A Pilot Study to Compare the Efficacy and Safety of Betafoam® and Allevyn® Ag in the Management of Acute Partial Thickness Burns. *Burns Open*, *3*(1), 1. doi:10.1016/j.burnso.2018.12.001

Jørgensen, B., Price, P., Andersen, K. E., Gottrup, F., Bech-Thomsen, N., Scanlon, E., Kirsner, R., Rheinen, H., Roed-Petersen, J., Romanelli, M., Jemec, G., Leaper, D. J., Neumann, M. H., Veraart, J., Coerper, S., Agerslev, R. H., Bendz, S. H., Larsen, J. R., & Sibbald, R. G. (2005, March). The Silver-Releasing Foam Dressing,

Contreet Foam, Promotes Faster Healing of Critically Colonised Venous Leg Ulcers: A Randomised, Controlled Trial. *International Wound Journal, 2*(1), 64. doi:10.1111/j.1742-4801.2005.00084.x

Ju, H. W., Lee, O. J., Lee, J. M., Moon, B. M., Park, H. J., Park, Y. R., Lee, M. C., Kim, S. Y., Chao, J. R., Ki, C. S., & Park, C. H. (2016). Wound Healing Effect of Electrospun Silk Fibroin Nanomatrix in Burn-Model. *International Journal of Biological Macromolecules, 85*, 29. doi:10.1016/j.ijbiomac.2015.12.055

Jung, J.-A., Han, S.-K., Jeong, S.-H., Dhong, E.-S., Park, K.-G., & Kim, W.-K. (2017, June). In Vitro Evaluation of Betafoam, a New Polyurethane Foam Dressing. *Advances in Skin & Wound Care: The Journal for Prevention and Healing, 30*(6), 262.

Kamoun, E. A., Chen, X., Eldin, M. S., & Kenawy, E.-R. S. (2015). Crosslinked Poly(Vinyl Alcohol) Hydrogels for Wound Dressing Applications: A Review of Remarkably Blended Polymers. *Arabian Journal of Chemistry, 8*, 1. doi:10.1016/j.arabjc.2014.07.005

Kamoun, E. A., Kenawy, E.-R. S., & Chen, X. (2017, May). A Review on Polymeric Hydrogel Membranes for Wound Dressing Applications: PVA-Based Hydrogel Dressings. *Journal of Advanced Research, 8*(3), 217. doi:10.1016/j.jare.2017.01.005

Kanokpanont, S., Damrongsakkul, S., Ratanavaraporn, J., & Aramwit, P. (2012, October 15). An Innovative Bi-Layered Wound Dressing Made of Silk and Gelatin for Accelerated Wound Healing. *International Journal of Pharmaceutics, 436*(1–2), 141. doi:10.1016/j.ijpharm.2012.06.046

Karr, J. C., Taddei, A. R., Picchietti, S., Gambellini, G., Fausto, A. M., & Giorgi, F. (2011, May). A Morphological and Biochemical Analysis Comparative Study of the Collagen Products Biopad, Promogram, Puracol, and Colactive. *Advances in Skin & Wound Care, 24*(5), 208.

Kawabata, S., Kanda, N., Hirasawa, Y., Noda, K., Matsuura, Y., Suzuki, S., & Kawai, K. (2018, May). The Utility of Silk-Elastin Hydrogel as a New Material for Wound Healing. *Plastic and Reconstructive Surgery – Global Open, 6*(5), e1778. doi:10.1097/GOX.0000000000001778

KCI. (2015). *V.A.C.® Therapy: Clinical Guidelines, A Reference Source for Clinicians.* KCi. Retrieved June 13, 2020, from https://www.acelity.com/-/media/Project/Acelity/Acelity-Base-Sites/shared/PDF/2-b-128h-vac-clinical-guidelines-web.pdf/#EN

Keirouz, A., Radacsi, N., Ren, Q., Dommann, A., Beldi, G., Maniura-Weber, K., Rossi, R. M., & Fortunato, G. (2020). Nylon-6/Chitosan Core/Shell Antimicrobial Nanofibers for the Prevention of Mesh-Associated Surgical Site Infection. *Journal of Nanobiotechnology, 18*, 51. doi:10.1186/s12951-020-00602-9

Khorsand-Ghayeni, M., Sadeghi, A., Nokhasteh, S., & Molavi, M. (2016). *Collagen Modified PLGA Nanofibers as Wound-Dressing.* 6th International Conference on Nanostructures (ICNS6). Kish Island: ICNS6. Retrieved June 14, 2020, from https://www.researchgate.net/profile/Mohammad_Khorsand-Ghayeni2/publication/290427542_Collagen_modified_PLGA_nanofibers_as_wound-dressing/links/572de10d08aeb1c73d129060/Collagen-modified-PLGA-nanofibers-as-wound-dressing.pdf

Kim, J. O., Park, J. K., Kim, J. H., Jin, S. G., Yonga, C. S., Li, D. X., Choi, J. Y., Woo, J. S., Yoo, B. K., Lyoo, W. S., Kim, J. A., & Choi, H. G. (2008, July 9). Development of Polyvinyl Alcohol–Sodium Alginate Gel-Matrix-Based Wound Dressing System Containing Nitrofurazone. *International Journal of Pharmaceutics, 359*(1–2), 79. doi:10.1016/j.ijpharm.2008.03.021

Kim, M. K., Kwak, H. W., Kim, H. H., Kwon, T. R., Kim, S. Y., Kim, B. J., Park, Y. H., & Lee, K. H. (2014). Surface Modification of Silk Fibroin Nanofibrous Mat with Dextran for Wound Dressing. *Fibers and Polymers, 15*(6), 1137. doi:10.1007/s12221-014-1137-2

König, M., Vanscheidt, W., Augustin, M., & Kapp, H. (2005, July). Enzymatic versus Autolytic Debridement of Chronic Leg Ulcers: A Prospective Randomised Trial. *Journal of Wound Care, 14*(7), 320. doi:10.12968/jowc.2005.14.7.26813

Kozen, B. G., Kircher, S., Henao, J., Godinez, F., & Johnson, A. (2008, January 74). An Alternative Hemostatic Dressing: Comparison of CELOX, HemCon, andQuikClot. *Academic Emergency Medicine, 15*(1), 74–81.

Krejner, A., & Grzela, T. (2015, October 15). Modulation of Matrix Metalloproteinases MMP-2 and MMP-9 Activity by Hydrofiber-Foam Hybrid Dressing – Relevant Support in the Treatment of Chronic Wounds. *Central European Journal of Immunology, 40*(3), 391.

Kunio, N. R., & Schreiber, M. A. (2013). Topical Hemostatic Agents. In C. S. Kitchens, C. M. Kessler, & B. A. Konkle (Eds.), *Consultative Hemostasis and Thrombosis* (p. 538). Elsevier.

Lagman, R., Walsh, D., & Day, K. (2002, November 1). Oxidized Cellulose Dressings for Persistent Bleeding from a Superficial Malignant Tumor. *American Journal of Hospice and Palliative Medicine, 19*(6), 417.

Lamboni, L., Gauthier, M., Yang, G., & Wang, Q. (2015, December). Silk Sericin: A Versatile Material for Tissue Engineering and Drug Delivery. *Biotechnology Advances, 33*(8), 1855. doi:10.1016/j.biotechadv.2015.10.014

Lee, J.-S., Cho, Y.-S., Lee, J.-W., Kim, H.-J., Pyun, D.-G., Park, M.-H., Yoon, T. R., Lee, H.-J., & Kuroyanagy, Y. (2001). Preparation of Wound Dressing Using Hydrogel Polyurethane Foam. *Trends in Biomaterials: Artificial Organs, 15*(1), 4.

Lee, J. W., & Song, K. Y. (2018, January). Evaluation of a Polyurethane Foam Dressing Impregnated with 3% Povidone-Iodine (Betafoam) in a Rat Wound Model. *Annals of Surgical Treatment and Research, 94*(1), 1.

Lee, S. M., Park, I. K., Kim, Y. S., Kim, H. J., Moon, H., Mueller, S., & Jeong, Y.-I. (2016). Physical, Morphological, and Wound Healing Properties of a Polyurethane Foam-Film Dressing. *Biomaterial Research, 20*, 15. doi:10.1186/s40824-016-0063-5

Leonard, S., McCluskey, P., Long, S., Butters, V., Winter, R., & Smith, G. (2009). An Evaluation of Allevyn™ Adhesive and Non-Adhesive Foam Dressings. *Wounds UK, 5*(1), 17.

Lewis, K. M., Spazierer, D., Urban, M. D., Lin, L., Redl, H., & Goppelt, A. (2013, July 4). Comparison of Regenerated and Non-Regenerated Oxidized Cellulose Hemostatic Agents. *European Surgery, 45*(4), 213.

Li, X., Li, B., Ma, J., Wang, X., & Zhang, S. (2014, July 1). Development of a Silk Fibroin/HTCC/PVA Sponge for Chronic Wound Dressing. *Journal of Bioactive and Compatible Polymers, 29*(4), 398.

Lih, E., Lee, J. S., Park, K. M., & Park, K. D. (2012, September). Rapidly Curable Chitosan–PEG Hydrogels as Tissue Adhesives for Hemostasis and Wound Healing. *Acta Biomaterialica, 8*(9), 3261. doi:10.1016/j.actbio.2012.05.001

Lin, S.-P., Kung, H.-N., Tsai, Y.-S., Tseng, T.-N., Hsu, K.-D., & Cheng, K.-C. (2017, November). Novel Dextran Modified Bacterial Cellulose Hydrogel Accelerating Cutaneous Wound Healing. *Cellulose, 24*, 4927. doi:10.1007/s10570-017-1448-x

Liu, G.-S., Yan, X., Yan, F.-F., Chen, F.-X., Hao, L.-Y., Chen, S.-J., Lou, T., Ning, X., & Long, Y.-Z. (2018, October). In Situ Electrospinning Iodine-Based Fibrous Meshes for Antibacterial Wound Dressing. *Nanoscale Research Letters, 13,* 309. doi:10.1186/s11671-018-2733-9

Lobmann, R., Pittasch, D., Mühlen, I., & Lehnert, H. (2003, July–August). Autologous Human Keratinocytes Cultured on Membranes Composed of Benzyl Ester of Hyaluronic Acid for Grafting in Nonhealing Diabetic Foot Lesions: A Pilot Study. *Journal of Diabetes and Its Complications, 7*(4), 199. doi:10.1016/S1056-8727(02)00218-0

Machula, H., Ensley, B., & Kellar, R. (2014, May 1). Electrospun Tropoelastin for Delivery of Therapeutic Adipose-Derived Stem Cells to Full-Thickness Dermal Wounds. *Advanced Wound Care, 3*(5), 367. doi:10.1089/wound.2013.0513

Mast, B. A., Diegelmann, R. F., Krummel, T. M., & Cohen, I. K. (1993). Hyaluronic Acid Modulates Proliferation, Collagen and Protein Synthesis of Cultured Fetal Fibroblasts. *Matrix, 13,* 441.

Matica, M., Aachmann, F., Tøndervik, A., Sletta, H., & Ostafe, V. (2019, November 24). Chitosan as a Wound Dressing Starting Material: Antimicrobial Properties and Mode of Action. *International Journal of Molecular Sciences, 20,* 5589.

Matsumara, H., Imai, R., Ahmatjan, N., Ida, Y., Gondo, M., Shibata, D., & Wanatabe, K. (2014, February). Removal of Adhesive Wound Dressing and Its Effects on the Stratum Corneum of the Skin: Comparison of Eight Different Adhesive Wound Dressings. *International Wound Journal, 11*(1), 50. doi:10.1111/j.1742-481X.2012.01061.x

Matthews, K. (2011). Drug Delivery Dressings. In D. Farrar (Ed.), *Advanced Wound Repair Therapy* (p. 361). Woodhead Publishing.

Medline Industries Inc. (2018). *PURACOL®Collagen Wound Dressings.* Retrieved May 26, 2020, from http://www.medline.com/media/catalog/Docs/MKT/LIT385R_BRO_Puracol_1783575.pdf

Merrell, J. G., McLaughlin, S. W., Tie, L., Laurencin, C. T., Chen, A. F., & Nair, L. S. (2009, December). Curcumin Loaded Poly(ε-Caprolactone) Nanofibers: Diabetic Wound Dressing with Antioxidant and Anti-Inflammatory Properties. *Clinical and Experimental Pharmacology and Physiology, 36*(12), 1149. doi:10.1111/j.1440-1681.2009.05216.x

Meuleneire, F., & Rücknagel, H. (2013, May). Soft Silicones Made Easy. *Wounds International,* 1.

Minoglou, M., Gerassimidou, S., & Komilis, D. (2017). Healthcare Waste Generation Worldwide and Its Dependence on Socio-Economic and Environmental Factors. *Sustainability, 9*(2), 220. doi:10.3390/su9020220

Mohamad, N., Amin, M. C., Pandey, M., Ahmad, N., & Rajab, N. F. (2014, December 19). Bacterial Cellulose/Acrylic Acid Hydrogel Synthesized via Electron Beam Irradiation: Accelerated Burn Wound Healing in an Animal Model. *Carbohydrate Polymers, 114,* 312. doi:10.1016/j.carbpol.2014.08.025

Morris, C., Emsley, P., Marland, E., Meuleneire, F., & White, R. (2009, April 27). Use of Wound Dressings with Soft Silicone Adhesive Technology. *Nursing Children & Young People, 21*(3), 38.

Mostow, E. N., Haraway, G. D., Dalsing, M., Hodde, J. P., King, D., & Oasis Venus Ulcer Study Group. (2005, May). Effectiveness of anEextracellular Matrix Graft (OASIS Wound Matrix) in the Treatment of Chronic Leg Glcers: A

Randomized Clinical Trial. *Journal of Vascular Surgery*, 41(5), 837. doi:10.1016/j.jvs.2005.01.042

Mustoe, T. A. (2008). Evolution of Silicone Therapy and Mechanism of Action in Scar Managemen. *Aesthetic Plastic Surgery*, 32, 82. doi:10.1007/s00266-007-9030-9

Neil, A. (2016). *Innovative Non-Silicone Low Trauma Adhesives versus Traditional Silicone Technology: A Review and Comparison*. Lohmann Corporation. Retrieved July 16, 2020, from http://softstickadhesive.com/documents/lohmann-wp-web.pdf

Ng, K. W., Achuth, H. N., Moochhala, S., Lim, T. C., & Hutmacher, D. W. (2007). In Vivo Evaluation of an Ultra-Thin Polycaprolactone Film as a Wound Dressing. *Journal of Biomaterials Science, Polymer Edition*, 18(7), 925. doi:10.1163/156856207781367693

Nguyen, T. T., Ghosh, C., Hwang, S.-G., Tran, L. D., & Park, J. S. (2013). Characteristics of Curcumin-Loaded Poly(Lactic Acid) Nanofibers for Wound Healing. *Journal of Materials Science*, 48, 7125. doi:10.1007/s10853-013-7527-y

Niessen, F. B., Spauwen, P. H., Robinson, P. H., Fidler, V., & Kon, M. (1998, November). The Use of Silicone Occlusive Sheeting (Sil-K) and Silicone Occlusive Gel (Epiderm) in the Prevention of Hypertrophic Scar Formation. *Plastic and Reconstructive Surgery*, 102(6), 1962. doi:10.1097/00006534-199811000-00023

Ning, C., Logsetty, S., Ghughare, S., & Liu, S. (2014, September). Effect of Hydrogel Grafting, Water and Surfactant Wetting on the Adherence of PET Wound Dressings. *Burns*, 40(6), 1164. doi:10.1016/j.burns.2013.12.024

Nirmala, R., Navamathavan, R., Kang, H.-S., El-Newehy, M. H., & Kim, H. Y. (2011, March 1). Preparation of Polyamide-6/Chitosan Composite Nanofibers by a Single Solvent System via Electrospinning for Biomedical Applications. *Colloids and Surfaces B: Biointerfaces*, 83(1), 173. doi:10.1016/j.colsurfb.2010.11.026

Norouzi, M.-R., Ghasemi-Mobarakeh, L., Gharibi, H., Meanmar, R., Ajalloueian, F., & Chronakis, I. S. (2019). Surface Modification of Poly (Ethylene Terephthalate) Fabric by Soy Protein Isolate Hydrogel for Wound Dressing Application. *International Journal of Polymeric Materials and Polymeric Biomaterials*, 68(12). doi: 10.1080/00914037.2018.1493684

O'Donoghue, J., O'Sullivan, S., Beausang, E., Panchal, J., O'Shaughness, M., & O'Connor, T. (1997, January 1). Calcium Alginate Dressings Promote Healing of Split Skin Graft Donor Sites. *Acta Chirurgiae Plasticae*, 39(2), 53.

Öri, F., Dietrich, R., Ganz, C., Dau, M., Wolter, D., Kasten, A., Gerber, T., & Frerich, B. (2017, January). Silicon-Dioxide–Polyvinylpyrrolidone as a Wound Dressing for Skin Defects in a Murine Model. *Journal of Cranio-Maxillofacial Surgery*, 45(1), 99. doi:10.1016/j.jcms.2016.10.002

Osman, S. H., & Setu, S. A. (2018). Fabrication of Nylon-66 Membranes Coated with Violacein Pigment for Wound Dressing Application. *eProceedings Chemistry*, 3(3), 23.

Pant, B., Pant, H. R., Pandeya, D. R., Panthi, G., Nam, K. T., Hong, S. T., Kim, C. S., & Kim, H. Y. (2012). Characterization and Antibacterial Properties of Ag NPs Loaded Nylon-6 Nanocomposite Prepared by One-Step Electrospinning Process. *Colloids and Surfaces A: Physicochemical and Engineering Aspects*, 94. doi:10.1016/j.colsurfa.2011.12.011

Panthi, G., Barakat, N. A., Risal, P., Yousef, A., Pant, B., Unnithan, A. R., & Kim, H. Y. (2013). Preparation and Characterization of Nylon-6/Gelatin Composite

Nanofibers via Electrospinning for Biomedical Applications. *Fibers and Polymers,* *14,* 718. doi:10.1007/s12221-013-0718-y

Patton, M. L., Mullins, R. F., Smith, D., & Korentager, R. (2013, November–December). An Open, Prospective, Randomized Pilot Investigation Evaluating Pain with the Use of a Soft Silicone Wound Contact Layer vs Bridal Veil and Staples on Split Thickness Skin Grafts as a Primary Dressing. *Journal of Burn Care & Research, 34*(6), 674. doi:10.1097/BCR.0b013e3182853cd6

Paustian, C., & Stegman, M. R. (2003, September 1). Preparing the Wound for Healing: The Effect of Activated Polyacrylate Dressing on Debridement. *Ostomy/Wound Management, 49*(9), 34.

Periayah, M. H., Halim, A., Yaacob, N., Saad, A., Hussein, A., Rashid, A., & Ujang, Z. (2004, August 28). Glycoprotein IIb/IIIa and P2Y12 Induction by Oligochitosan Accelerates Platelet Aggregation. *BioMed Research International.*

Peršin, Z., Jesih, A., & Stana-Kleinschek, K. (2012). Depositionof Amino-Containing Film on the Poly(Ethylene Terephthalate) Dressing-Layer for Safe Wound-Healing. *Materials and Technology, 46*(1), 63.

Petrini, P., Parolari, C., & Tanzi, M. C. (2001). Silk Fibroin-Polyurethane Scaffolds for Tissue Engineering. *Journal of Materials Science: Materials in Medicine, 12,* 849. doi:10.1023/A:1012847301850

Portela, R., Leal, C. R., Almeida, P. L., & Sobral, R. G. (2019, July). Bacterial Cellulose: A Versatile Biopolymer for Wound Dressing Applications. *Microbial Biotechnology, 12*(4), 586.

Pour, S. N., Ghugare, S. V., Wiens, R., Gough, K., & Liu, S. (2015, September 15). Controlled In Situ Formation of Polyacrylamide Hydrogel on PET Surface via SI-ARGET-ATRP for Wound Dressings. *Applied Surface Science, 349,* 695. doi:10.1016/j.apsusc.2015.04.181

Price, R. D., Berry, M. G., & Navsaria, H. A. (2007, October). Hyaluronic Acid: The Scientific and Clinical Evidence. *JPRAS An International Journal of Surgical Reconstruction, 60*(10), 1110. doi:10.1016/j.bjps.2007.03.005

Prieto, E. M., & Guelcher, S. A. (2014). Tailoring Properties of Polymeric Biomedical Foams. In P. A. Netti (Ed.), *Biomedical Foams for Tissue Engineering Applications* (p. 129). Woodhead Publishing.

Qin, Y. (2016). *Medical Textiles Materials.* Woodhead Publishing.

Radulescu, M., Andronescu, E., Dolete, G., Popescu, R. C., Fufă, O., Chifiriuc, M. C., … Holban, A. M. (2016, May). Silver Nanocoatings for Reducing the Exogenous Microbial Colonization of Wound Dressings. *Materials (Basel), 9*(5), 345. doi:10.3390/ma9050345

Rajendran, S., Anand, S., & Rigby, A. (2016). Textiles for Healthcare and Medical Applications. In A. R. Horrocks & S. Anand (Eds.), *Handbook of Technical Textiles* (Vol. 2, p. 135). Woodhead Publishing.

Rancan, F., Contardi, M., Jurisch, J., Blume-Peytavi, U., Vogt, A., Bayer, I. S., & Schaudinn, C. (2019). Evaluation of Drug Delivery and Efficacy of Ciprofloxacin-Loaded Povidone Foils and Nanofiber Mats in a Wound-Infection Model Based on Ex Vivo Human Skin. *Pharmaceutics, 11,* 527. doi:10.3390/pharmaceutics11100527

Ravnskog, F.-A., Espehaug, B., & Indrekvam, K. (2011, March). Randomised Clinical Trial Comparing Hydrofiber and Alginate Dressings Post-Hip Replacement. *Journal of Wound Care, 20*(3), 136.

Razzak, M. T., Zainuddin, Erizal, Dewi, S. P., Lely, H., Taty, E., & Sukirno. (1999, June 11). The Characterization of Dressing Component Materials and Radiation Formation of PVA–PVP Hydrogel. *Radiation Physics and Chemistry*, *55*(2), 153. doi:10.1016/S0969-806X(98)00320-X

Ribeiro, M. P., Morgado, P. I., Miguel, S. P., Coutinho, P., & Correia, I. J. (2013, July 1). Dextran-Based Hydrogel Containing Chitosan Microparticles Loaded with Growth Factors to Be Used in Wound Healing. *Materials Science and Engineering: C*, *33*(5), 2958. doi:10.1016/j.msec.2013.03.025

Richetta, A., Cantisani, C., Li, V., Mattozi, C., Melis, L., De Gado, F., Giancristoforo, S., & Calvieri, S. (2011). Hydrofiber Dressing and Wound Repair: Review of the Literature and New Patents. *Recent Patents on Inflammation & Allergy Drug Discovery*, *5*(2), 1.

Richters, C. D., du Pont, J., Mayen, I., Kamperdijk, W., Dutrieux, R., Kreis, R., & Hoekstra, M. (2004, February). Effects of a Hydrofiber Dressing on Inflammatory Cells in Rat Partial-Thickness Wounds. *Wounds*, *16*(2), 63.

Rippon, M., White, R., & Davies, P. (2007). Skin Adhesives and Their Role in Wound Dressings. *Wounds UK*, *3*(4), 76.

Rogers, A. R., & Rippon, M. G. (2017). Describing the Rinsing, Cleansing and Absorbing Actions of Hydrated Superabsorbent Polyacrylate Polymer Dressings. *Wounds UK*, EWMA Special, 48.

Romanelli, M., Dini, V., & Bertone, M. S. (2010, January). Randomized Comparison of OASIS Wound Matrix versus Moist Wound Dressing in the Treatment of Difficult-to-Heal Wounds of Mixed Arterial/Venous Etiology. *Advancees in Skin & Wound Care*, *23*(1), 34.

Rottmar, M., Richter, M., Mäder, X., Grieder, K., Nuss, K., Karol, A., von Rechenberg, B., Zimmermann, E., Buser, S., Dobmann, A., Blume, J., & Bruinink, A. (2015). In Vitro Investigations of a Novel Wound Dressing Concept Based on Biodegradable Polyurethane. *Science and Technology of Advanced Materials*, *16*, 034606. doi:10.1088/1468-6996/16/3/034606

Royal College of Nursing. (2018). *Freedom of Information Follow up Report on Management of Waste in the NHS*. London: Royal College of Nursing.

Rusu, A. G., Tanasa, I. A., Popa, M. I., Butnaru, M., & Verestiuc, L. (2015). *Development of Novel Hydrogels Based on Citraconyl-Chitosan and Poly(Acrylic Acid) as Potential Wound Dressing Materials. 2015 E-Health and Bioengineering Conference (EHB)* (p. 1). Iasi: IEEE. doi:10.1109/EHB.2015.7391527

Ryssel, H., Gazyakan, E., Germann, G., & Öhlbauer, M. (2008, February). The Use of MatriDerm® in Early Excision and Simultaneous Autologous Skin Grafting in Burns – A Pilot Study. *Burns*, *34*(1), 93. doi:10.1016/j.burns.2007.01.018

Sambasivam, M., White, R., & Cutting, K. (2006). Exploring the Role of Polyurethane and Polyvinyl Alcohol Foams in Wound Care. In M. Ågren (Ed.), *Wound Healing Biomaterials* (Vol. 2, p. 251). Woodhead Publishing. doi:10.1016/B978-1-78242-456-7.00012-X

Sangjun, N., Phulsuksombati, D., Pilakasiri, K., Parichatikanond, P., Muensoongnoen, J., Koedpuech, K., Janvikul, W., & Tanodekaew, S. (2003). Animal Study of the Effect of Chitin-PAA and Carboxymethylchitosan Hydrogels on Healing of Deep Thickness Wounds. *Armed Forces Research Institute of Medical Sciences: Annual Progress Report*, 128. Retrieved June 16, 2020, from http://www.afrims.go.th/uploads/report/AR11.pdf

Sayag, J., Meaume, S., & Bohbot, S. (1996). Healing Properties of Calcium Alginate Dressings. *Journal of Wound Care, 5*(8), 357.

Schneider, A., Wang, X. Y., Kaplan, D. L., Garlick, J. A., & Egles, C. (2009, September). Biofunctionalized Electrospun Silk Mats as a Topical Bioactive Dressing for Accelerated Wound Healing. *Acta Biomaterialica, 5*(7), 2570. doi:10.1016/j.actbio.2008.12.013

Schoukens, G. (2019). Bioactive Dressings to Promote Wound Healing. In S. Rajendran (Ed.), *Advanced Textiles for Wound Care* (p. 135). Woodhead Publishing.

Schulze, H.-J. (2003, November 1). Clinical Evaluation of TIELLE* Plus Dressing in the Management of Exuding Chronic Wounds. *British Journal of Community Nursing, 8*(Suppl. 5), S18.

Senthilkumar, M., Anbumani, N., & Hayavadana, J. (2011, September). Elastane Fabrics – A Tool for Stretch Applications in Sports. *Indian Journal of Fibre & Textile Research, 36*, 300.

Serinçay, H., Özkan, S., Yilmaz, N., Koçyiğit, S., Uslu, I., Gürcan, S., & Arisoy, M. (2013). PVA/PAA-Based Antibacterial Wound Dressing Material with Aloe Vera. *Polymer Plastics Technology and Engineering, 52*(13), 1308. doi:10.1080/03602559.2013.814671

Shaharudin, A., & Aziz, Z. (2016, October 2). Effectiveness of Hyaluronic Acid and Its Derivatives on Chronic Wounds: A Systematic Review. *Journal of Wound Care, 25*(10), 585. doi:10.12968/jowc.2016.25.10.585

Sharman, D. (2003). Moist Wound Healing: A Review of Evidence, Application and Outcome. *The Diabetic Foot, 6*(3), 112.

Shingel, K. I., Di Stabile, L., Marty, J.-P., & Faure, M.-P. (2006, December). Inflammatory Inert Poly(Ethylene Glycol)–Protein Wound Dressing Improves Healing Responses in Partial- and Full-Thickness Wounds. *International Wound Journal, 3*(4), 332. doi:10.1111/j.1742-481X.2006.00262.x

Shu, Y.-T., Kao, K.-T., & Weng, C.-S. (2017, August 1). In Vitro Antibacterial and Cytotoxic Activities of Plasma-Modified Polyethylene Terephthalate Nonwoven Dressing with Aqueous Extract of Rhizome Atractylodes Macrocephala. *Materials Science and Engineering: C, 77*, 606. doi:10.1016/j.msec.2017.03.291

Silverstein, P., Heimbach, D., Meites, H., Latenser, B., Mozingo, D., Mullins, F., Garner, W., Turkowski, J., Shupp, J., Glat, P., & Purdue, G. (2011, November–December). An Open, Parallel, Randomized, Comparative, Multicenter Study to Evaluate the Cost-Effectiveness, Performance, Tolerance, and Safety of a Silver-Containing Soft Silicone Foam Dressing (Intervention) vs Silver Sulfadiazine Cream. *Journal of Burn Care & Research, 32*(6), 611. doi:10.1097/BCR.0b013e318236fe31

Sin, D., Miao, S., Liu, G., Fan, W., Chadwick, G., Yan, C., & Friis, T. (2010). Polyurethane (PU) Scaffolds Prepared by Solvent Casting/Particulate Leaching (SCPL) Combined with Centrifugation. *Materials Science and Engineering C: Materials for Biological Applications, 30*(1), 78. doi:10.1016/j.msec.2009.09.002

Singh, O., Singh Gupta, S., Soni, M., Moses, S., Shukla, S., & Mathur, R. (2011, January–April). Collagen Dressing versus Conventional Dressings in Burn and Chronic Wounds: A Retrospective Study. *Journal of Cutaneous and Aesthetic Surgery, 4*(1), 12.

Singh, R., & Singh, D. (2012, November). Radiation Synthesis of PVP/alginate Hydrogel Containing Nanosilver as Wound Dressing. *Journal of Materials Science: Materials in Medicine, 23*(11), 2649. doi:10.1007/s10856-012-4730-3

Siritientong, T., Angspatt, A., Ratanavaraporn, J., & Aramwit, P. (2014). Clinical Potential of a Silk Sericin-Releasing Bioactive Wound Dressing for the Treatment of Split-Thickness Skin Graft Donor Sites. *Pharmaceutical Research, 31,* 104. doi:10.1007/s11095-013-1136-y

Smith + Nephew. (2020, May 23). *Oasis(R) Matrix Products.* Retrieved May 23, 2020, from Smith + Nephew: https://www.smith-nephew.com/key-products/advanced-wound-management/oasis/

Stern, R., Asari, A. A., & Sugahara, K. N. (2006, August 3). Hyaluronan Fragments: An Information-Rich System. *European Journal of Cell Biology, 85*(8), 699. doi:10.1016/j.ejcb.2006.05.009

Sun, G., & Mao, J. J. (2012, November). Engineering Dextran-Based Scaffolds for Drug Delivery and Tissue Repair. *Nanomedicine (London), 7*(11), 1771. doi:10.2217/nnm.12.149

Sun, G., Zhang, X., Shen, Y.-I., Sebastian, R., Dickinson, L. E., Fox-Talbot, K., Reinblatt, M., Steenbergen, C., Harmon, J. W., & Gerecht, S. (2011, December 27). Dextran Hydrogel Scaffolds Enhance Angiogenic Responses and Promote Complete Skin Regeneration during Burn Wound Healing (R. Langer, Ed.). *Proceedings of the National Academy of Sciences of the U.S.A., 108*(52), 20977. doi:10.1073/pnas.1115973108

Sung, J. H., Hwang, M. R., Kim, J. O., Lee, J. H., Kim, Y. I., Sun, J. H., Chang, W., Jin, S. G., Kim, J. A., Lyoo, W. S., Hann, S. S., Ku, S. K., Yong, C. S., & Choi, H. G. (2010, June). Gel Characterization and In Vivo Evaluation of Minocycline-Loaded Wound Dressing with Enhanced Wound Healing Using Polyvinyl Alcohol and Chitosan. *International Journal of Pharmaceutics, 392*(1–2), 232. doi:10.1016/j.ijpharm.2010.03.024

Suteris, N. N., Misnon, I. I., Roslan, R., Zulkifili, F. H., Venugopal, J. R., Yusoff, M. M., & Jose, R. (2020, March). Synthesis and Characterization of Polycaprolactone/Cellulose Acetate by Electrospinning for Wound Dressing Applications. *Materials Science Forum, 981,* 291. doi:10.4028/www.scientific.net/MSF.981.291

Tebrake, M. G. (2014). *Selecting the Right Medical Adhesive Tape: Challenges Facing the Medical Device Designer.* Loughborough, UK: 3M Medical OEM. Retrieved July 18, 2020, from http://multimedia.3m.com/mws/media/1128482O/3m-medical-materials-and-technologies-medical-oem-white-paper

Teramoto, H., Kameda, T., & Tamada, Y. (2008). Preparation of Gel Film from Bombyx Mori Silk Sericin and Its Characterization as a Wound Dressing. *Bioscience, Biotechnology and Biochemistry, 72*(12), 3189. doi:10.1271/bbb.80375

Uzun, M. (2018, January 29). A Review of Wound Management Materials. *Journal of Textile Engineering & Fashion Technology, 4*(1), 53.

van der Velden, N. M., Patel, M. K., & Vogtländer, J. G. (2014, February). LCA Benchmarking Study on Textiles Made of Cotton, Polyester, Nylon, Acryl, or Elastane. *The International Journal of Life Cycle Assessment, 19,* 331. doi:10.1007/s11367-013-0626-9

Varzaneh, R. F., Moshtaghian, J., Talebi, A., & Abedini, F. (2015, January). The Effects of Polyvinyl Pyrrolidone Hydrogel Dressing on Open-Wound Healing in Rats. *Journal of Isfahan Medical School, 32*(313), 2134.

Vasconcelos, A., Gomes, A. C., & Cavaco-Paulo, A. (2012). Novel Silk Fibroin/Elastin Wound Dressings. *Acta Biomaterialia, 8*(8), 3049. doi:10.1016/j.actbio.2012.04.035

Vazquez, J. R., Short, B., Findlow, A. H., Nixon, B. P., Boulton, A. J., & Armstrong, D. G. (2003, February 1). Outcomes of Hyaluronan Therapy in Diabetic Foot Wounds. *Diabetes Research and Clinical Practice, 59*(2), 123. doi:10.1016/S0168-8227(02)00197-3

Vázquez, N., Sánchez-Arévalo, F., Maciel-Cerda, A., Garnica-Palafox, I., Ontiveros-Tlachi, R., Chaires-Rosas, C., Piñón-Zarate, G., Herrera-Enríquez, M., Hautefeuille, M., Vera-Graziano, R., & Castell-Rodríguez, A. (2019, July). Influence of the PLGA/gelatin Ratio on the Physical, Chemical and Biological Properties of Electrospun Scaffolds for Wound Dressings. *Biomedical Materials, 14*(4), 045006. doi:10.1088/1748-605X/ab1741

Voigt, J., & Driver, V. R. (2012, May–June). Hyaluronic Acid Derivatives and Their Healing Effect on Burns, Epithelial Surgical Wounds, and Chronic Wounds: A Systematic Review and Meta-Analysis of Randomized Controlled Trials. *Wound Repair and Regeneration, 20*(3), 317. doi:10.1111/j.1524-475X.2012.00777.x

Voinchet, V., Vasseur, P., & Kern, J. (2006). Efficacy and Safety of Hyaluronic Acid in the Management of Acute Wounds. *American Journal of Clinical Dermatology, 7*, 353.

Walker, M., Lam, S., Pritchard, D., & Cochrane, C. A. (2010). Biophysical Properties of a Hydrofiber(R) Cover Dressing. *Wounds UK, 6*(1), 19.

Walker, M., & Parsons, D. (2010). Hydrofiber(R) Technology: Its Role in Exudate Management. *Wounds UK, 6*(2), 31.

Wang, M., Xu, L., Hu, H., Zhai, M., Peng, J., Nho, Y., Li, J., & Wei, G. (2007, December). Radiation Synthesis of PVP/CMC Hydrogels as Wound Dressings. *Nuclear Instruments and Methods in Physics Research Section B: Beam Interactions with Materials and Atoms, 265*(1), 385. doi:10.1016/j.nimb.2007.09.009

Wang, Y., Mithieux, S. M., Kong, Y., Wang, X.-Q., Chong, C., Fathi, A., Dehghani, F., Panas, E., Kemnitzer, J., Daniels, R., Kimble, R. M., Maitz, P. K., Li, Z., & Weiss, A. S. (2015, March 11). Tropoelastin Incorporation into a Dermal Regeneration Template Promotes Wound Angiogenesis. *Advanced Healthcare Materials, 4*(4), 577. doi:10.1002/adhm.201400571

Warring, M., Rippon, M., Bielfeldt, S., & Brandt, M. (2008, September). Cell Attachment to Adhesive Dressings: Qualitative and Quantitative Analysis. *Wounds UK, 4*(3), 35.

Wedmore, I., McManus, J., Pusateri, A., & Holcomb, J. (2006). A Special Report on the Chitosan-Based Hemostatic Dressing: Experience in Current Combat Operations. *The Journal of TRAUMA(R) Injury, Infection, and Critical Care, 60*(3), 655.

White, R. (2005, November). Evidence for Atraumatic Soft Silicone Wound Dressing Use. *Wounds UK, 1*(3), 104.

White, R. (2008, March 1). A Multinational Survey of the Assessment of Pain When Removing Dressings. *Wounds UK, 4*(1), 14.

WHO. (2018, February 8). *Health-Care Waste.* Retrieved June 23, 2020, from World Health Organization: https://www.who.int/news-room/fact-sheets/detail/health-care-waste

Wiegand, C., Abel, M., Ruth, P., & Hipler, U.-C. (2011, November). Superabsorbent Polymer-Containing Wound Dressings Have a Beneficial Effect on Wound Healing by Reducing PMN Elastase Concentration and Inhibiting Microbial Growth. *Journal of Materials Science: Materials in Medicine*, *22*(11), 2583. doi:10.1007/s10856-011-4423-3

Wiegand, C., Heinze, T., & Hipler, U.-C. (2009, July/August). Comparative In Vitro Study on Cytotoxicity, Antimicrobial Activity, and Binding Capacity for Pathophysiological Factors in Chronic Wounds of Alginate and Silver-Containing Alginate. *Wound Repair and Regeneration*, *17*(4), 511.

Wiegand, C., & Hipler, U.-C. (2013). A Superabsorbent Polymer-Containing Wound Dressing Efficiently Sequesters MMPs and Inhibits Collagenase Activity in Vitro. *Journal of Materials Science: Materials for Medicine*, *24*, 2473. doi:10.1007/s10856-013-4990-6

Xiong, Y., & Tao, X. (2018, June). Compression Garments for Medical Therapy and Sports. *Polymers (Basel)*, *10*(6), 663. doi:10.3390/polym10060663

Yang, X., Fan, L., Ma, L., Wang, Y., Lin, S., Yu, F., Pan, X., Luo, G., Zhang, D., & Wang, H. (2017, April 5). Green Electrospun Manuka Honey/Silk Fibroin Fibrous Matrices as Potential Wound Dressing. *Materials & Design*, *119*, 76. doi:10.1016/j.matdes.2017.01.023

Yao, H.-Y., Lin, H.-R., Sue, G.-P., & Lin, Y.-J. (2019, March 1). Chitosan-Based Hydrogels Prepared by UV Polymerization for Wound Dressing. *Polymers and Polymer Composites*, *27*(3), 155. doi:10.1177/0967391118820477

You, Y., Park, W. H., Ko, B. M., & Min, B.-M. (2004, March). Effects of PVA Sponge Containing Chitooligosaccharide in the Early Stage of Wound Healing. *Journal of Materials Science: Materials in Medicine*, *15*, 297. doi:10.1023/B:JMSM.0000015491.91918.64

Zeybek, B., Duman, M., & Ürkmez, A. Ş. (2014). Electrospinning of Nanofibrous Polycaprolactone (PCL) and Collagen-Blended Polycaprolactone for Wound Dressing and Tissue Engineering. *Usak University Journal of Material Sciences*, *1*, 121. doi:10.12748/uujms.201416506

Zhao, Y.-F., Zhao, J.-Y., Hu, W.-Z., Ma, K., Chao, Y., Sun, P.-J., Fu, X.-B., & Zhang, H. (2019). Synthetic Poly(Vinyl Alcohol)–Chitosan as a New Type of Highly Efficient Hemostatic Sponge with Blood-Triggered Swelling and High Biocompatibility. *Journal of Materials Science: B*, *7*, 1855. doi:10.1039/C8TB03181A

Zhu, J., Li, F., Wang, X., Yu, J., & Wu, D. (2018, April 2). Hyaluronic Acid and Polyethylene Glycol Hybrid Hydrogel Encapsulating Nanogel with Hemostasis and Sustainable Antibacterial Property for Wound Healing. *ACS Applied Materials Interfaces*, *10*(16), 13304. doi:10.1021/acsami.7b18927

Zohuriaan-Mehr, M. J., & Kabiri, K. (2008). Superabsorbent Polymer Materials: A Review. *Iranian Polymer Journal*, *17*(6), 451.

5

Structural Forms and Systems for Dressings

5.1 From Raw Materials to Dressing Structure

The majority of polymeric raw materials discussed in Chapter 4 are versatile enough to be easily manipulated into different forms that can be used in a dressing: fibres, particles, films, foams, etc. Each of these structural forms has its own advantages and disadvantages, making it more or less suited for specific needs. A simplified schematic of some wound dressing requirements, and how structural formats can directly address them is given in Figure 5.1.

In a clinical situation, it is not unusual for dressings of different formats and characteristics to be used in layers and in combination with each other or with devices. As examples, a non-adherent pad needs to be supported with a secondary dressing to keep it in place; an absorbent dressing may have to be used underneath layers of compression bandages; a foam and a cover layer are required in the use of NPWT devices.

Equally, it is quite common for different materials to be layered within a dressing itself, either through lamination, coating, or other type of bonding, to form a multicomponent dressing. Layering enables multiple functionalities to be built in a dressing – for example, an absorbent pad may be given a protective barrier that is impervious to fluids and bacteria, and an adherent border layer for sticking around the wound. Each of these individual layers has its own structural form and properties, and together they form the combined system for the dressing. The challenge of multi-layered dressings is to ensure the structural integrity and stability of the combined layers. Each layer may behave differently during manufacture and use, causing the dressing to distort, delaminate and fall apart prior to or during use. The reaction of the base materials to heat and sterilisation during manufacture, and moisture and stress during wear, for example, may be unequal for each layer, causing uneven shrinkage and eventual delamination of the layers. A good understanding of the physicochemical properties of the base materials is therefore essential for the development of multi-layered dressings.

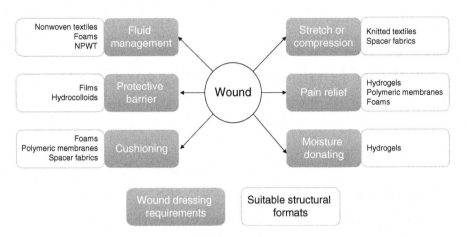

FIGURE 5.1
Examples of wound dressing requirements that structural formats can directly address

5.2 Textiles

Textiles, one of the earliest forms of wound dressings, are now ubiquitous in the wound care industry. Textile materials include all manners of fibrous structures, from randomly distributed fibres to carefully organised structures, from natural fibres to man-made ones, and from regular fibre sizes of a few microns in diameter to nanofibres of less than a micron in diameter. Because textile structures are made of a large number of connected fibres, they can have excellent drapeability, flexibility and conformability to the curves of the human body, which is important when intimate contact is required to the wound bed. The flexibility and conformability depend on the physical properties of the fibres (including their diameter and inherent stiffness), and on how the fibres are connected together. Likewise, other physical properties can be tailored to suit specific needs, by modifying the base material used and the processing parameters. A textile material can be produced with some or all of these processes: fibre formation (or preparation), yarn formation, yarn finishing, fabric formation, fabric finishing and fabric enhancements. At each stage, process variables can be changed to alter the final product's characteristics. One of the basic step determining the properties of the textile sheet is the sheet forming process itself, of which there are three main ways: the nonwoven, woven and knitted processes (Figure 5.2). Each process results in specific physical characteristics making them more suitable for certain uses than others. Wound dressings are made out of all three types of textile structures, and of combinations of.

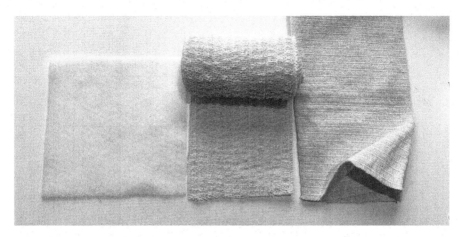

FIGURE 5.2
Textile wound dressings, from left to right: nonwoven, loosely woven and knitted tubular structures

5.2.1 Nonwovens

Nonwoven manufacture is the simplest way of organising fibres together into a mat. Fibres are uniformly but randomly laid as a sheet and are connected by physical entanglements or other bonds such as those achieved using heat or chemicals. The strength of the mat is determined by the number and strength of the bonds between fibres, as well as by the inherent strength of the fibres. There are a number of raw material and manufacturing parameters that can be changed to modify the properties of the resulting mat. By varying the base fibres, the thickness of the nonwoven mat, the density of fibres, the type of inter-fibre bond, and any other finishing treatments, the mechanical properties of the material change. Porosity also changes, which in the context of wound healing, in turn, affects the absorbency, cushioning ability and air permeability.

The nonwoven process is the simplest manufacturing route because there are no intermediate yarns required – a fabric structure is formed directly from fibres, and in some cases directly from the spinneret as the fibres are being spun. As a result of this shortened process, nonwovens are generally very cost-effective and have become widely used in the disposable medical textile sector, for example, as surgical gowns, caps, and other drapes. Globally, 64% of the volume of medical textiles consists of nonwovens (Grand View Research, 2019). In the wound dressing sub-sector, nonwovens are commonly used too. They are used as gauzes, or contact layers in dressings, and in particular, are used for fibrous absorbent pads, for example, of fibres of alginates, CMC and their blends. These pads can be made with or without an adhesive border and film outer layer. Table 5.1 highlights what nonwovens are best and least suited for.

TABLE 5.1

Suitability of nonwovens

Best suited for	Least suited for
Absorbing exudate	Acting as a barrier
Packing tunnelling and deep wounds	
Low-cost disposable wound dressings	

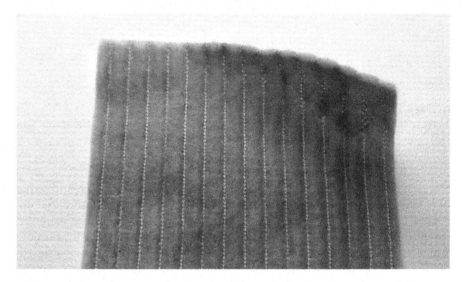

FIGURE 5.3
Nonwoven fabric with reinforcing stitchbonding running vertically

Because of the large amount of interstitial spaces and ability for the fibres to move to accommodate fluid into these spaces, nonwovens are ideal as absorbent structures. They can also be easily cut and packed into deep or tunnelling wounds. However, they do suffer from being generally weaker than other textile structures. To counteract this, there are various ways in which they can be reinforced. For example, additional entanglements and bonds can be created, a secondary backing sheet can be laminated onto the nonwoven or a process called stitchbonding can be performed, whereby rows of stitching are machined through the nonwoven structure to provide extra strength in the direction of the rows. An example nonwoven with reinforcing stitchbonding is illustrated in Figure 5.3.

5.2.2 Woven Fabrics

Woven fabrics are manufactured by the regular and repeating interlacing of yarns (made of twisted fibres), in a general lattice structure. Typically, two sets of yarns are made to weave over and under each other at right angles to each other. The contact points of the interlaced yarns create enough friction to hold the yarns altogether and form the fabric. Woven fabrics tend to be quite strong and stable, with minimal stretch (Table 5.2). They are not ideally suited when a degree of stretch or elasticity is required except when elastic yarns are used. The porosity is controlled by the looseness of the twist in the yarns and the interstitial spaces between the yarns – the more separated the yarns are, the bigger the pores between them, with the most open structures termed woven meshes and nets. Examples of dressings that are woven include some gauzes (including impregnated gauzes to reduce wound adherence, and gauzes made with stretch yarns), meshes and other secondary bandages.

5.2.3 Knitted Fabrics

Knitted structures are made by the inter-looping of yarns and in the simplest of forms of weft knitting, a single yarn is used to inter-loop on itself, one row at a time. More complex knitted structures may have several yarns interlooping in complicated patterns. Like woven fabrics, knitted ones need the extra step of yarn manufacture before the fabric can be formed, so the overall process is lengthier than nonwovens. One of the key benefits of knitted structures is their ability to stretch, in some cases in multi-directions. Stretch occurs as the loops are pulled and straightened, making knitted fabrics both highly extensible and strong. The extension of the fabric depends on the loop structure as well as on the inherent extensibility of the yarn itself. For example, products containing elastane are able to stretch significantly more, as well as recover their original sizes much faster and repeatedly. Warp-knitted structures, in which the yarns interloop with each other vertically tend to result in a less stretchy, more stable material. Another interesting feature of knitted fabrics is that they can also be formed seamlessly and directly in tubular and other three-dimensional forms, as shown in Figure 5.2. Knitted dressings include knitted tubular gauzes, compression bandages for venous leg treatment and for scar treatments. Table 5.3 highlights where knitted structures are best and least useful.

TABLE 5.2

Suitability of woven textiles

Best suited for	Least suited for
Providing strength and stability	When stretch is required
	Heavily exuding wounds

TABLE 5.3

Suitability of knitted materials

Best suited for	Least suited for
When stretch and flexibility is required	When stability is essential
Compression therapy bandages	Acting as a barrier layer
Tubular requirements, e.g., to dress digits	

5.2.4 Spacer Fabrics

Spacer fabrics are three-dimensional textile structures that consist of two lay-ers of fabrics held together by pile fibres or yarns. The latter connect the two layers together and are in the general perpendicular direction to the fab-rics. The pile gives the spacer fabrics their controllable thickness, typically between 1.5 and 10 mm (Ramazan, 2019). They also impart other charac-teristics to the whole structure, such as porosity, density, compression resis-tance, absorbency, uniform pressure distribution, and so on. Typically, the pile fibres can be mono-filaments of synthetic polymers such as PET, which have high modulus and good recovery and therefore give the spacer fabric good resistance to compression. The smoothness of the mono-filaments also makes the spaces within the structure quite large, with good air permeability and circulation. When using other fibres and blends in the pile, a softer, more compressible, but more absorbent version with smaller interstitial spaces can be obtained. The surface properties, extensibility and comfort of the spacer fabrics are determined by the two fabric layers, which can be woven or knit-ted and can be different for each layer. As such, spacer fabrics can also be compared to a 3-layer dressing system – contact layer, middle layer and outer protective layer.

Knitted spacer fabrics with elasticated yarns are stretchable and have been developed as compression bandages, as they are able to provide sufficient compression while being cushioning and allowing good air circulation (Lee et al., 2009; Rajendran & Anand, 2010). In a similar concept, spacer fabric inserts have been investigated as an alternative for thermoplastic ones used for scar treatments in pressure garments. The spacer materials were found to be promising, with better air and moisture vapour permeability, but com-parable pressure than the commercial thermoplastic material normally used (Yu, 2015; Yu et al., 2016). Several other properties of commercially avail-able spacer fabrics have been investigated in the context of them being used as a substitute for an absorbent compressive layer in advanced wound care (Tong et al., 2015). The research showed that the warp-knitted spacer fabrics can provide a good ventilated environment for wound healing, good com-pressional resistance and resilience, and adequate absorbency for wounds without heavy exudate. Another example is the use of a type of spacer fabric in the PICO◊ (Smith + Nephew) NPWT dressing. The proprietary Airlock◊

TABLE 5.4

Suitability of spacer fabrics

Best suited for	Least suited as
Thermal insulation	Low-cost disposable dressings
Compression therapy	
Requirements for micro-pockets	

technology layer is illustrated as typical of spacer fabrics, and is described as being able to distribute pressure equally over the wound, maintaining an open airflow to keep a uniform pressure over the wound area while holding its structure and without collapsing (Smith + Nephew, 2020a, 2020b). Table 5.4 indicates areas where spacer fabrics would be the most and least useful. Due to the involved manufacturing route (compared, for instance, with nonwovens), the cost of spacer fabrics does not make them the most economically advantageous as disposable dressings. Where they are used as a disposable dressing, the product would have to command a premium, for example, in NPWT treatment.

Despite the complex manufacturing structure, several research studies have been reported on the development of spacer fabrics for advanced wound care. A spacer fabric with an SAP fibre spacer layer was found to have superior absorbent properties to foams, better wettability and higher air permeability (Yang & Hu, 2018). A multi-layer composite structure of spacer fabrics with an added electrospun membrane was compared with commercial PU foams and alginate dressings and found to have good water vapour and air permeability and in some cases better absorption that the comparative products (Yang & Hu, 2017). An antimicrobial spacer fabric with a silver concentration higher in the spacer layer, to minimise silver contact with the wound bed, has also been developed by Yang et al. (2017). The absorbent spacer layer was designed to be able to pull in fluids and bacteria into the centre of the dressing structure, where it performs its antibacterial action. A 100% reduction in bacterial viability was observed within an hour in *in vitro* tests.

5.2.5 Nanofibres

Nanofibres are fibres that are generally well under a micron in diameter. Interest in this topic grew after work on microfibres (fibres of a few microns in diameter) demonstrated that due to their greater surface area per ratio, enhanced absorption, wettability, filtration, active release of ingredients, and other interesting properties linked to the fibre sizes were achievable. There are various ways of forming nanofibres, including drawing, spinneret engineering, phase separation, self-assembly, template synthesis, freeze-drying synthesis, interfacial polymerisation, and even mechanical fibrillation (Alghoraibi & Alomari, 2018). The process that really expanded the development of nanofibres and its large scale production is electrospinning, where charged polymer solutions are drawn out into nanofibres using an electric force. Electrospun fibres are deposited onto a moveable collecting device, forming a mat of varying porosity. In essence, electropinning is a nonwoven process, whereby the fibre formation, drawing, deposition and sheet formation occurs in one process. However, electrospun nanofibre mats have different properties to conventional nonwoven fabrics. Standard electrospun mats tend to be two-dimensional and look more like a lightweight and thin membrane rather than a fibrous pad. With modifications to the process, three-dimensional structures have also been produced, opening up the pores and making the nanofibres more receptive for cell infiltration and growth (Leong et al., 2016; Chen et al., 2017).

Microscopically, the morphology of electrospun nanofibres is said to mimic the extracellular matrix, and partly for this reason, it has been a structural form of interest in the development of scaffolds for advanced wound care. The other main reason why the research literature is exploding with electrospun nanofibres development is that the process enables endless combinations of raw materials and actives to be used, whether it is through blending at the solution stage, or by layering afterwards. Thus, a large body of research exists on the topic of electrospinning most of the polymers outlined in Chapter 4. All the synthetic polymers mentioned and some of the natural ones (notably collagen, chitosan, hyaluronic acid and dextran) have been reported to have been successfully electrospun, mostly for the development of wound dressings and scaffolds. There are a large number of reports with *in vivo* results on the wound healing properties of nanofibres of various polymers. These properties are likely caused by a combination of both the material used and the nanofibre structure presented. The inherent structural benefits of nanofibres themselves on wound healing are mostly speculated and few research studies compare like for like polymers in nanofibre and non-nanofibre form, for a true investigation of the effect of fibre size. An indication of the benefits of the physical structure of nanofibres is at best suggested and *in vivo* (Ghanavati et al., 2015).

With the much higher surface area per volume ratio, nanofibres can make excellent bases for cell growth, and release of actives incorporated into the structure (Table 5.5). This is particularly the case for bioresorbable and

TABLE 5.5

Suitability of nanofibres

Best suited for	Least suited for
As a layer to stimulate cell growth	Fluid handling
Scaffold base	Thermal insulation
Drug delivery layer	Providing strength

biodegradable polymers. A number of bioactives and pharmaceuticals have already been successfully incorporated into electrospun materials, with positive outcomes in terms of immediate and sustained release (Chen et al., 2017). The faster release from nanofibres is expected due to the higher surface area. This has been demonstrated compared to films, for example, in the case of PVP loaded with antibiotics (Contardi et al., 2017). Polymers that can naturally biodegrade on the wound bed have been prevalent in the development of controlled release materials, e.g., PLA, PGA, PLGA, PCL and PVP. However, non-biodegradable polymers have also been used. In both types, the mechanism of release is a combination of several processes including diffusion, drug partitioning and drug dissolution (Chou et al., 2015). The speed of water penetration and diffusion through the nanofibres and the properties of the active ingredient as it moves through the polymer affect the release rate. In the case of biodegradable polymers, the degradation rate of the fibres also contributes significantly to how quickly actives are released, as it also not only exposes more actives, but also affects the geometry and surface area available.

5.3 Foams

A highly used structure in wound care, foams are characterised by having a continuous three-dimensional matrix structure containing pores, pockets or spaces for air and fluids. The pores can be completely enclosed by the polymer matrix, in which case the foam is more resistant to fluids and gases, less compressible, and described as closed-cell. Or, they can interconnect and enable fluid or gas to move through the structure through different mechanisms such as squeezing, suction, evaporation, etc., in which case they are characterised as being open-cell. The matrix polymer is normally, but not exclusively, a synthetic polymer, which can be hydrophobic or hydrophilic. It is continuous, and typically does not shed small particles or fibres in the wound when it is removed, unlike some textiles. The properties of the polymer used, the process parameters and the thickness can all be varied and together they determine the strength of the matrix and its porosity. In turn, the structural features of the porous structure determine the absorbency, the fluid retention, the compressibility, the thermal insulation and many other characteristics.

5.3.1 Open-Cell Foams for Exudate Management

Most foams used in wound care are made up of a PU open-cell soft structure. The majority are indicated for moderate to heavily exuding wounds, as they are able to absorb large amounts of fluid into their pores, and allow its evaporation through a semi-occlusive or non-occlusive backing. Foam dressings can appear to be thicker and less conformable than some other flexible structures (Figure 5.4), but they are soft and compressible, giving a sense of gentleness, protection and cushioning when used. In addition, because of the porous structure, they make good thermal insulators, which when combined with a longer wear time, results in better thermal insulation for the wound. Dressing changes can lead to a temporary drop in wound temperature, which can have an adverse effect on wound healing, so the ability to maintain the correct skin temperature for as long as possible is beneficial.

Some foams are manufactured with additional layers such as an adhesive layer to keep the dressing in place, or a semi-occlusive or closed-cell outer layer to prevent external contamination while enabling moisture to evaporate – examples are given in Box 4.9 of Chapter 4, and shown in Figure 5.4. There is a large body of *in vitro*, *in vivo* and clinical evidence demonstrating the moderate to high absorption properties, and the safety and efficacy of foam dressings on a range of wounds, including chronic wounds and partial-thickness burns. Cochrane and other reviews however concluded that there is insufficient evidence to demonstrate that they are superior in healing diabetic foot ulcers, venous leg ulcers, pressure ulcers and burns than other treatments (Dumville et al., 2013a; O'Meara & Martyn-St James, 2013; Walker et al., 2017; Chagranti et al., 2019). Interestingly, foams were noted to have the benefit of reducing pain in the early treatment phase of partial-thickness burns. A summary of the key benefits of foams is given in Table 5.6.

Open-cell foams (PU and PVA versions) are used significantly in NPWT as an interface between the device and the wound bed. More detail about this therapy is provided in Section 5.7.2 and an example of the type of foam that is used in shown in Figure 5.4(b). Open-cell foams are well suited for

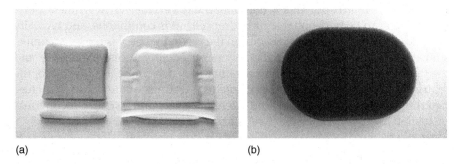

(a)   (b)

FIGURE 5.4
Examples of foam dressings (a) top views and cross-sections of foams with an outer film layer, on the left without adhesive border and on the right with a border, (b) an open-cell foam for NPWT use

TABLE 5.6

Suitability of foams

Best suited for	Least suited for
Absorbing high levels of exudate	When a thin profile is required
Cushioning and comfort	Dry wounds (unless otherwise indicated)
Thermal insulation	
Pain relief	

this device for two reasons. Firstly, they are able to re-distribute the pressure across the dressed area, and secondly, as the wound fluid is being sucked out of the wound bed, it can easily travel through the interconnected spaces and out into the fluid collecting device. Although in theory large pores can facilitate this fluid transfer, fibroblast ingrowth into the foam has been found to occur, leading to trauma upon removal of the dressing (Borgquist et al., 2009; Wiegand et al., 2013). By contrast, finer pored foams and gauze, or the use of a drainage film between the foam and the wound do not lead to the same cell-ingrowth issue.

5.3.2 Foams with Added Functionalities

As advanced wound care has expanded into providing additional functionalities in dressings, foams have also been developed with extra benefits such as incorporating various antimicrobial actives, analgesics, SAPs and other wound healing actives. The main purpose of the foam still remains as a way to manage exudate, but added benefits are becoming more mainstream. Foams are able to act as a reservoir for actives, whether they are deposited on the surface of the pores or sitting inside the pores themselves, ready to be activated or released when in contact with fluids.

In the most common form of added functionality, many commercial foam dressings are available in an antibacterial version for the prevention and management of wound infections while absorbing the fluids and enabling its evaporation. The antibacterial active of choice for these dressings has been silver, in the form of silver sulfadiazine, ionic silver, nanocrystalline silver and metallic silver. Another singular addition to a foam is that of ibuprofen, such as in Biatain® Ibu (Coloplast), which has been demonstrated to reduce or even nearly eliminate pain and discomfort on leg ulcers and split-thickness skin grafts (Cigna et al., 2009; Sibbald et al., 2007; Fogh et al., 2012).

With a more complex combination, the PolyMem® range is defined as polymeric membrane dressings with a hydrophilic PU matrix (foam), containing a mild tissue-friendly wound cleanser, a soothing moisturiser, SAP particles and a semi-permeable film backing. This combination is intended to facilitate healing, relieve pain, reduce inflammation, as well as manage exudate and cleanse the wound. From a review by Benskin (2016), the cleanser is able to loosen slough, dirt or other substances from the wound bed; the PU matrix and SAP particles absorb and trap fluids into the dressing; the moisturiser (glycerol) prevents desiccation of exposed areas and in conjunction with the other moisture-loving components of the dressing pulls nutrient-filled, enzyme-rich fluid from the body into the wound bed to enhance healing and autolytic debridement. Benskin (2016, 2018) also highlights various reports that demonstrate the ability of the polymeric membrane dressings to help in autolytic debridement, reduction of pain and inflammation, better comfort and assist in wound healing. Kim et al. (1999) reported on its efficacy on burns and donor sites.

5.4 Hydrogels

Hydrogels are high water content, soft, semi-solids or solids, which are used in the wound care setting as amorphous gels, impregnated gels onto textile structures, or gelled sheets. Their structure consists of a network of cross-linked hydrophilic polymers in water. They can be made in several ways, with the simplest process – for synthetic materials – being to polymerise monomers and crosslink them in parallel in a single step. Other multi-step procedures require to firstly synthesise the polymer (or prepare and modify the polymer molecules in the case of natural raw materials), and their subsequent crosslinking.

The starting point for hydrogels can be synthetic monomers or blends of, or natural polymers, or a mix of natural and synthetic polymers. This versatility in preparation and endless possible combinations have been well explored in research across the world. The physical and biophysical properties and characteristics of hydrogels can thus vary significantly, depending on the polymer(s) and blends used. Some are suitable for applications as diverse as agricultural aids, contact lenses, supercapacitors, sensors, drug delivery and wound dressings. In wound care, the healing benefits of hydrogels are commonly associated with the ability of the dressing or gel to maintain a moist wound healing environment, but also with other characteristics, such as those brought in by the polymers used and the active or biological ingredients incorporated within the structure. Several *in vivo* studies of hydrogels of different compositions have been found to promote specific phases of wound healing, such as epithelialisation, cell proliferation, neovascularisation and skin regeneration (Sangjun et al., 2003; Shingel et al., 2006; Sun et al., 2011; Mohamad et al., 2014; Öri et al., 2017; Kawabata et al., 2018). Biopolymers such as collagen, gelatine, fibrin and hyaluronic acid tend to encourage many cellular functions, which along with the high water content of the network, is advantageous for the viability, proliferation and development of many cell types (Tibbitt & Anseth, 2009). Other natural polymers used include chitosan, which can bring in haemostatic, antibacterial and antifungal benefits, and dextran, which can positively influence wound healing (Sun et al., 2011; Ribeiro et al., 2013; Shariatina & Jalali, 2018). Hydrogels formed from purely synthetic materials may lack the ability to actively promote cell growth in the same way some biopolymers can; however, they provide a permissive environment for the cells to be healthy and grow. Common raw materials used for hydrogels in the man-made polymer category include PVA, PAA, PEG and PVP. Their benefits and limitations have been discussed in Chapter 4, where many polymer combinations in this format have been reported. A mix of two or more components is frequently done to try to combine the properties of each component. Particularly, the mixture of a biopolymer with a synthetic one is regularly seen, as this combination tends to bring in the wound healing properties of the natural polymer, with the mechanical stability or ease of processing of a water-soluble synthetic one.

Water-soluble synthetic polymers are indeed materials of choice in the making of hydrogels. Such polymers can be crosslinked via chemical reactions, ionising radiation (which generates free radicals that can recombine as crosslinks), and physical interactions such as entanglements, electrostatics and crystallite formations (Ahmed, 2015). In the wound care sector, physical and radiation crosslinks are preferred over chemical ones to minimise the risks of cytotoxicity that the latter could lead to. Crosslinks make the structure insoluble in water, yet open to the movement of fluids. The degree of crosslinking stabilises the network and determines whether the hydrogel is a gel (amorphous) or whether it has sufficient integrity to be formed into a sheet, which is the common form of hydrogel dressings. It also determines how much more fluid the hydrogel is able to absorb until it reaches equilibrium. Typically, hydrogel sheet dressings are able to absorb only a small amount of exudate, and this moisture in some cases is able to evaporate through the backing layer. The absorption properties of the structure depend on the quantity and presence of hydrophilic functional groups in the polymer backbones. Hence, different polymer hydrogels will lead to different absorptive capacities. Hydrogels not only absorb, but the moisture movement is reversible and they are therefore also able to donate moisture to areas that lack it. This ability to absorb and donate water is in response to a physical or chemical environmental stimulus such as temperature, pH or ionic strength (Madaghiele et al., 2014; Ahmed, 2015).

The high water content (up to 95%) of hydrogels gives them certain wound care benefits (Table 5.7). Their unique selling point in the arena of wound dressings is their soothing and cooling effect, which is attributed to the level of moisture in the dressing, and their soft gel-like conformable form, even in sheet version. Hydrogels are also claimed to offer drug-free pain relief. A number of small clinical studies on the use of hydrogel sheet dressings

TABLE 5.7

Suitability of hydrogels

Best suited for	Least suited for
Soothing and cooling effect	High levels of exudate
Pain relief	Areas of high friction and movement
Atraumatic dressing removal	

on chronic and painful wounds have shown that when used, a reduction in pain has been observed (Hampton, 2004; Young & Hampton, 2005; Bradbury et al., 2008). A review of 43 clinical studies concluded that hydrogel dressings can effectively alleviate pain – particularly in second-degree burns – as well as promote wound healing on several types of wounds (Zhang et al., 2019). In terms of wound healing, the moist environment is able to enhance healing for certain types of wounds. A Cochrane review concluded that hydrogels were no better than other dressings it was compared with for pressure ulcers; however, in the case of diabetic ulcers, there was some evidence to suggest that they are more effective than some basic wound contact dressings (Dumville et al., 2013b, 2015).

Removal of the dressings is mostly atraumatic as hydrogels do not normally adhere to the wound bed. If it has been allowed to dry out on the wound, and adhere to it, re-hydrating with saline solution returns the hydrogel to its soft, easily removable version. Hydrogels are more suitable for dry and low exuding wounds as their absorption capacity is limited, particularly if they are backed by an occlusive or semi-occlusive film. On dry and necrotic tissues, hydrogels are believed to help rehydrate scabs and tissues and provide the right environment for autolytic debridement. The speed of debridement compared to more direct methods is significantly lower and the costs greater (Waycaster & Milne, 2013). However, this is sometimes an option to be considered when other methods are unsuitable. A review of several studies on the effect of debridement interventions on healing concluded that the combined effect of the slow debridement and moist wound healing increases healing rates in diabetic ulcers compared to standard care (Edwards & Stapley, 2010; Elraiyah et al., 2016).

The moisture donating properties of hydrogel have also made it a structure of interest for the delivery of actives to the wound bed. Chitosan-containing hydrogels have been significantly used in research and development for the delivery of actives such as antimicrobials (antibiotics, silver, zinc, and other metals), growth factors, stem cells, peptides, anti-inflammatories, antioxidants, vitamins, nutrients and other substances (Liu et al., 2018). Therapeutic molecules can be incorporated into the polymer solution during the making of the hydrogel, or they can be bonded to the polymer (i.e., functionalising the polymer chain). The mechanism of release of the actives mostly relies on diffusion, but in some cases, it relies on further water penetration to modify

BOX 5.1 EXAMPLES OF COMMERCIALISED HYDROGEL DRESSINGS AND TECHNOLOGIES

	Unique Selling Points
• ActiFormCool® (Lohmann & Rauscher) – sheet with 70% water	Pain relief
• Hydrosorb® range (Hartmann) – sheet with 60% water and semi-occlusive backing sheet	Soothing and cooling
• Intrasite◊ Conformable (Smith + Nephew) – nonwoven impregnated with gel	Moisture donating
• KerraLite Cool (Crawford Healthcare)	
• Soft-Pro® technology (Scapa) – sheet with 10–70% water	

the hydrogel structure and enable the movement of the actives out of the network, and in other cases, it depends on the degradation of the polymer to be released into the wound bed (Veld et al., 2020).

In the consumer goods industry, hydrogels are commonly used as blister plasters, for the prevention and treatment of superficial blisters. The plasters may include a separate adhesive border to secure it in place. In advanced wound care, a number of amorphous gels and dressings are available for the treatment of chronic and acute wounds including burns. Amorphous gels need a secondary dressing to keep it in place, e.g., a film dressing. The various versions of sheet dressings include those with or without a backing film to act as a barrier layer and those with or without an adhesive border to keep them secure. Non-adhesive sheet dressings require a secondary dressing to hold them in place. Some examples of sheet dressings for advanced wound care are provided in Box 5.1.

5.5 Films

Films are thin flexible sheets that are occlusive or semi-occlusive (semi-permeable), and act as a barrier, protecting the wound from external contaminations such as bacteria, dust, dirt and liquids. Occlusive films do not allow liquids to permeate from either direction, nor do they allow evaporation of moisture from the wound bed. Semi-occlusive ones prevent liquids from permeating but allow water vapour and gases to pass through their structure. Generally, wound dressing films are waterproof from the external side, which enables the patient to wash without risk of disrupting the wound. Films are typically transparent or semi-transparent, coated with an adhesive on one side, and can be used directly on wounds, or as a secondary dressing to hold another dressing such as a foam or absorbent nonwoven

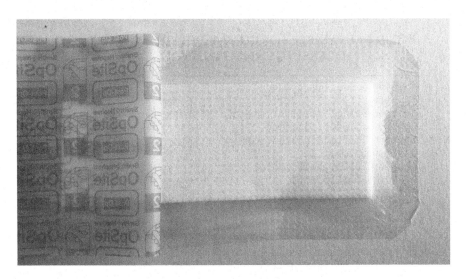

FIGURE 5.5
Clear film dressing with a central pad, with the upper release liner seen in blue

pad in place. They are also frequently used as a component of multi-layered wound dressings, typically as the outer layer, to provide an effective barrier and when coated with an adhesive, a way to keep the dressing in place. An example of a film/central pad combination is shown in Figure 5.5. When on their own and fully transparent, they enable the clinician to monitor the status of the wound without having to remove the dressing for inspection.

Because of their ability to occlude or partially occlude, films and film-containing dressing combinations can help in the autolytic debridement of necrotic wounds. This occurs very slowly over time as the minimisation of water evaporation keeps the wound moist with exudate and encourages the body's own enzymes and neutrophils to cleanse the wound. Films are thus suitable for dry wounds. They are also indicated for superficial shallow wounds with no exudate. However, with their typically lower moisture vapour transmission rate compared to open-structure dressings, they are unsuitable for wet wounds without the use of a primary absorbent dressing or central pad, as they may lead to maceration of the wound tissues. Table 5.8 sums up the suitability of film dressings as used on their own. Many dressings include a film backing as part of their design, to provide the benefits that films can bring, while at the same time delivering other benefits such as cushioning and exudate management through other structural formats such as foams and nonwovens.

Films are manufactured using polymer solutions or dispersions, spread out evenly and thinly over a base or carrier, and treated to remove the liquid fractions. In the case of polymer solutions, the film is formed by evaporation

TABLE 5.8

Suitability of film dressings

Best suited for	Least suited for
Barrier or sterile layer (or secondary layer)	Cushioning
Occlusion	Exudate management
Autolytic debridement of eschar	Patients with sensitive skin
Visibility of wound	

of the solvent; in the case of polymer dispersion, coalescence of the polymer is required first, which can only occur above the glass transition temperature (Felton, 2013). The viscosity of the solution or dispersion is an essential controllable parameter that alters the properties of the film, including its thickness, quality and strength.

Most commercial film dressings are made of hydrophilic PU, and some examples are given in Box 4.9 of Chapter 4. The films tend to be fully coated with an acrylic adhesive, which is known to adhere strongly to dry skin but can be aggressive for sensitive or fragile skin. Clear PU films are commonly used as surgical wound protection. The transparency, elasticity, waterproofness and bacteria barrier properties make it ideal for dressing such wounds, enabling patients to move and wash, and facilitating post-surgery inspection by the surgeon when used without a central absorbent pad. It has been linked to faster wound healing, decreased pain and less scaring (Rubio, 1991). Its use as a secondary dressing for surgical wounds has also been shown to be more beneficial compared to other dressings, leading to less complications such as skin blistering and signs of infection (Ravenscroft et al., 2006). In combination with gauze, the use of clear PU films has been demonstrated to be as effective in preventing surgical site infections in hip and knee arthroplasty as in other published outcomes, at a fraction of the cost of advanced bio-occlusive dressings (Chowdhry et al., 2017). One challenge however is in the handling of the film. Due to them being very thin and adhesive, without proper training and experience, it can be difficult to apply smoothly without the film sticking onto itself. This has led to the addition of backing and release layers to assist in the process. An example of an upper release layer can be seen in Figure 5.5.

5.6 Hydrocolloids

The term hydrocolloid is used to describe a crosslinked matrix that contains hydrophilic colloidal particles, typically CMC, pectin and gelatine, contained in elastomers, all in various proportions. Commercially in the wound care

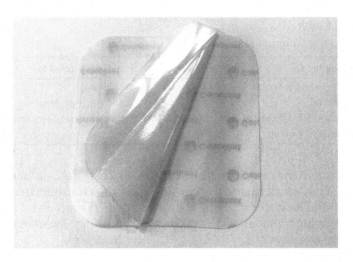

FIGURE 5.6
A hydrocolloid dressing

BOX 5.2   EXAMPLES OF COMMERCIALISED HYDRO-COLLOID DRESSINGS

	Unique Selling Points
• Duoderm® range (Convatec) • Granuflex® range (Convatec) • Comfeel® Plus range (Coloplast) • Tegaderm™ Hydrocolloid range (Acelity) • Hydrocoll® (Hartmann) • REPLICARE◊ range (Smith + Nephew)	Self-adhesive barrier Non-adherent to wound Long wear time

industry, they are available as gels or pastes, or self-adhesive thin sheet dressings (also referred to as wafers in some instances, shown in Figure 5.6) with an occlusive or semi-occlusive film backing such as a PU film. The latter acts as a barrier against contamination, making hydrocolloid sheet dressings suitable both as a stand-alone or secondary dressing. Some examples of products are provided in Box 5.2.

Despite their hydrophilic nature, hydrocolloids are typically not intended to absorb large amounts of fluids, but upon contact with wound exudate, the hydrophilic particles absorb the fluid, swell and gel, and help to maintain a moist environment for the wound bed. Thicker hydrocolloid dressings are able to absorb more fluids, but their capacity is normally much less than that of other absorbent dressings such as foams. Moisture at the wound bed and the ensuing gelation of the contact layer ensure that the dressing does not normally adhere to the wound bed itself – only to intact skin – making dressing

TABLE 5.9

Suitability of hydrocolloids

Best suited for	Least suited for
Adhesive barrier layer (or secondary dressing)	High levels of exudate
Occlusion	Odour sensitivities
Autolytic debridement	Sensitive skin
Long wear times	

removal less damaging to wound. In fact, in the presence of too much exudate, many self-adhering hydrocolloids will lose their adhesiveness and may lead to maceration of healthy surrounding tissues, if left unattended.

Hydrocolloids are indicated for a range of wounds, such as dry and necrotic wounds, partial or full-thickness, light to moderately exuding wounds (depending on the absorption capacity of the dressing), chronic and acute wounds, and for the protection of intact skin or newly healed wounds. Table 5.9 shows what they are best suitable for. In dry wounds, the moisture retention properties of the dressing are able to provide a moist wound healing environment due to the occlusive or semi-occlusive backing. These properties can further be used to help in the gradual autolytic debridement of dry, sloughy or necrotic wounds. Hydrocolloids are widely used for the treatment of pressure ulcers of different stages (Fletcher et al., 2011). They can also be used on venous leg ulcers, which require secondary compression bandages. However, they have only been found to lead to better clinical outcomes when compared with traditional dressings in the treatment of pressure ulcers and other wounds (Fletcher et al., 2011; Pott et al., 2014). Compared with other advanced dressings such as collagen or foams, hydrocolloids were found to be similar or less effective in wound healing. One of the small disadvantages of hydrocolloids is that they tend to generate an unpleasant odour, particularly when worn over several days. This may lead to discomfort, stress and worry to the patient if unexplained or unprepared. Another downside is that although they tend not to adhere to a wet wound bed, the bond to surrounding intact dry skin can be quite strong. If this periwound skin area is sensitive, it can cause an issue with difficult and painful removal from the surrounding skin area.

5.7 Therapies and Diagnostics for Advanced Wound Care

The development of wound care has moved from passive to active and from reactive to proactive, and in the same way, diagnostics in wound care will follow the same trend. Early days wound care passively protected a wound and managed the symptoms reactively, as they appeared. Then, therapies, systems and dressings were developed that could address the cause of the problem in order to help heal the wound faster. In more recent years, wound care actively encourages healing, either through physical methods and therapies or through the delivery of actives. Some of these methods include the use of dressings as part of the wound care system; in other treatments, such as light therapy, dressings do not play a critical part of the therapy itself, but may be required alongside the treatment or after, as with any wound.

5.7.1 Compression

Compression is not new as a therapy, but it is worth discussing here to illustrate how structural aspects of a flexible material and layering systems can be used to assist in wound care. There are two main ways where compression by a textile material is used. Firstly, in compression therapy for leg ulcers, it is used as a secondary dressing to manage an underlying condition in order to help a wound heal better. Secondly in keloidal scar management, compression is used in compression sleeves or garments to provide constant pressure on a raised scar, or on freshly healed wounds to prevent scar formation.

5.7.1.1 Compression Therapy for Venous Insufficiency

In the case of compression therapy for leg ulcers, the underlying condition is venous insufficiency, or ineffective venous walls and/or valves in the legs, which make it difficult for blood to return to the heart from the lower limbs. Instead, the blood has a tendency to pool at the bottom of the leg. The pressure in the leg becomes elevated as a result. Ulcers developing from this condition can be superficially managed with a primary dressing. However, without dealing with the underlying venous difficulties and the hypertension in the leg, the wound is likely to remain chronic or return. Surgery, exercise and keeping the legs elevated are some of the solutions, but compression therapy remains one of the standard treatments. Through the application of compression at the ankles and legs, the vein support is strengthened and blood flow activity can be re-stimulated. Traditionally, compression therapy is delivered with the use of special stretch bandages made with a knitted textile structure, or specially designed stockings that provide a degree of compression to the lower leg, sometimes with a graduated pressure profile. When the wound is healed, compression hosiery is recommended as a preventative measure to prevent the recurrence of another ulcer.

Depending on the materials used, the compression delivered by bandages may be constant, or may be lower during sedentary periods and higher during active periods, by increasing calf muscle activity (Sackheim et al., 2006). Inelastic bandages (also termed 'short stretch') have a lower resting compression, and high active compression due to the relatively fixed volume created when the bandage is on. When the patient walks, compression is increased, reinforcing and supporting the calf muscle pump. Because they are unable to shrink back after application, inelastic bandages lose the compression level as the oedema decreases. They therefore need to be reapplied when the volume of the leg reduces, in order to continue to provide the required level of compression. Most are made of cotton or cotton-rich knitted textiles and do not contain high stretch material such as elastane.

Elastic bandages (long stretch) provide sustained pressures which are similar at rest and during activity as they are able to accommodate changes to the geometry of the leg due to their elasticity (Marston & Vowden, 2003). They can be single or multi-layered, high compression or low compression, and can be used to maintain a higher pressure at the ankle, decreasing towards the thigh. Elastic bandages typically are made of an elastomeric material, which, in a knitted structure, is able to provide the stretch and repeated recovery necessary for the desired and sustained compression level, both at rest and during activity. They do however require more training for their application and are normally not used on their own, but with additional layers. To help judge the level of compression, a visual indicator can be incorporated in the form of a knitted or printed rectangle, which stretches to a square when the compression level is appropriate. Dual or multi-layered systems, which are more complex in application, mostly include both elastic and non-elastic bandages in order to make the most of the properties of both types. They may also involve a cohesive outer compression bandage to prevent slippage and increase compliance, and a padding inner layer for comfort. Some examples of inelastic, elastic and multicomponent compression systems are provided in Box 5.3.

Although not dressing-related, intermittent pneumatic compression (IPC) is a therapy that has been investigated as a dynamic alternative to compression bandages. The system, using a durable medical device, is electromechanical and uses an air pump to inflate and deflate a bag wrapped

BOX 5.3 EXAMPLES OF COMPRESSION BANDAGES

Inelastic bandages	Elastic bandages	Multi-layered systems
• Actico® (Lohmann & Rauscher) • Circaid® (Medi) • LoPress® (Hartmann) • Comprilan® (BSN Medical) • Elastocrepe® (BSN Medical)	• Elodur® (BSN Medical) • Setopress® (Mölnlycke)	• Proguide◊ (Smith + Nephew) • Profore◊ (Smith + Nephew) • DYNA-FLEX™ (Acelity) • JOBST® Comprifore (BSN Medical) • UrgoK2 (Urgo Medical)

around the leg. This compressing and relaxing action stimulates the venous return and lymphatic drainage and helps in reducing oedema. This system manages the venous insufficiency and a separate wound dressing is required underneath to help manage and heal any ulcers that have been formed.

A Cochrane review of compression bandages and stockings on the healing of venous leg ulcers concluded that the healing rate is better when compression is used, compared to when none was used (O'Meara et al., 2012). The authors also found that multicomponent systems (including two-components) are more effective than single layer compression and that multi-layered systems with elastic components perform better than those with only inelastic bandages. Another review found that the use of IPC is more beneficial to healing than using no compression, but could not conclude if it could be used instead of compression bandages (Nelson et al., 2011).

5.7.1.2 3D Compression Garments for Scar Management

Hypertrophic scarring is a common complication that occurs after injury, particularly after severe burns. It presents itself as raised skin tissue, which has different properties to unscarred tissue surrounding it, notably in elasticity, pigmentation, vascularity, smoothness and hardness. The impact can be both aesthetic and functional, in the latter case limiting mobility and movement in areas such as joints. There are several ways of reducing scars. Compression is one of the least invasive therapies but one that takes the longest time for noticeable outcomes. Compression garments are actually used for several conditions, including lymphoedema, vascular disease, for post-surgical support as well as for scar management. In the context of scar treatment, pressure garment therapy (PGT) is the term employed to refer to the use of elasticised garments or garment parts (such as sleeves) to apply cylindrical pressure onto a scar area. The treatment necessitates continuous application of pressure over a long period of time. Typically, patients are required to wear the garment or garment part, which provides between 15 and 30 mmHg of pressure, for 23 hours a day, and over 6–24 months (Atiyeh et al., 2013; Ai et al., 2017; DeBruler et al., 2018).

The fabric components, design and structure, and the 3D shaping of the fabric are essential in creating the right fit to provide the correct pressure at the scar location. The construction of the garment can involve direct seamless knitting, for example, of tubular sleeves and gloves. For more complex forms, it could also involve turning flat textile material into any 3D shape using accurate patterns that minimise seams and their thickness. Seamless knitting has the benefit of not having extra bulk at the seams, which can put extra pressure on the skin. Where they are present, seams are normally machine stitched, keeping the raw edges sealed and keeping them as thin as possible.

Standard sizes are available for generic garments or garment parts such as sleeves, gloves, torso cover, leggings, etc., but custom-made garments are more likely to provide the correct pressure at the right location. The garments are typically made from fabrics containing high-stretch high-recovery elastomeric fibres such as elastane, in stable warp knitted structures such as powernet and sleeknit. It is speculated that the high compression restricts blood flow to the scar area, and prevents the growth of the hypertrophic tissue by reducing collagen production (Atiyeh et al., 2013). In some cases, a plastic, or spacer fabric insert is used on top of the scar, as a means to increase or maintain localised compression.

PGT has been used for over 40 years, prophylactically after wound closure and as a treatment for mature scars, mostly due to empirical evidence. Due to the difficulties in conducting suitable trials, in ensuring patient compliance, in accurately measuring scarring, and in accurately delivering the right pressure, until recently, evidence in the effectiveness of the treatment has been deemed insufficient to recommend its widespread use for all scar types (Atiyeh et al., 2013). In a review of PGT for the prevention of scarring, meta-analysis of 4 clinical trials showed a small decrease in scar height for the pressure garment therapy group; however, the authors concluded that the beneficial effects of the therapy remain unproven (Anzarut et al., 2009). More recently though, a review concluded that burn patients managed with PGT at 15–25 mmHg showed significant improvements (Ai et al., 2017).

The difficulties in assessing efficacy are compounded by the risk of non-compliance. The intensity of wear can lead to various issues, such as discomfort, overheating, skin irritation and abnormal bone growth. This can eventually result in the patient ceasing the treatment earlier, or not conforming to the protocol of care, and therefore to a reduction in the effectiveness of the treatment. *In vivo*, it was found that if treatment is ceased early, the scars continue to evolve, resulting in more contracture, scar hardness, thickness and roughness (DeBruler et al., 2018).

5.7.2 Negative Pressure Wound Therapy (NPWT)

NPWT, also referred to as vacuum-assisted closure, or topical negative pressure therapy is a wound care technique utilising a continuous or intermittent suction or vacuum (negative pressure) on a sealed wound bed. In essence, this pressure is the opposite to the one applied by compression therapy. The system typically constitutes of several components, which can each affect its wound healing and wound care efficacy. A schematic diagram of a basic NPWT device is shown in Figure 5.7. A wound filler or dressing, for example, an open-cell foam or gauze, is used to fill the wound gap and acts as a conduit for exudate to flow through. In some cases, a separate a wound contact layer is used, which can be impregnated gauze, silicone or low-density polyethylene. An occlusive adhesive dressing or layer is used on top of the filler, sealing the wound bed to enable the vacuum to form. A pump is utilised to create the suction effect at the wound bed, draining fluids away through the

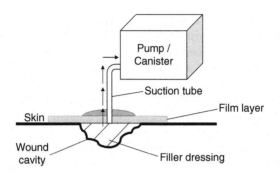

FIGURE 5.7
Schematic diagram of a basic NPWT device

filler dressing via a flexible tubing into a collecting canister. In instillation NPWT (NPWTi), a wound care liquid such as sterile water, saline, or antibiotics is streamed into the wound bed when the pump stops and the wound restores to atmospheric pressure. This liquid is then sucked out with exudate when the pump goes back on.

NPWT and NPWTi are used to treat chronic wounds such as ulcers and pressure sores, and have been recommended for a range of other lesions including abdominal wounds, open fractures, burns, post-traumatic wounds and more recently on clean surgical wounds including skin grafts (Webster et al., 2014; KCI, 2015). The treatment goals and expected outcomes could however be different for each condition. NPWT is used to manage exudate and protect wounds, to prepare a wound for surgical closure, to improve the outcome after a skin graft, to improve patient comfort, or to reduce costs (Birke-Sorensen et al., 2011). Prophylactically, it is used after surgery to prevent surgical site infections.

The mechanism of action of NPWT on the speed of healing, as for many materials and treatments, is not fully elucidated, but may be linked to several activities occurring in parallel. The negative pressure, normally between 80 and 150 mmHg, drains exudate and mechanically stimulates the wound bed, reduces oedema, contracts wound edges, diminishes bacterial count and stimulates angiogenesis, cell-induced immune response and the formation of granulation tissue (Vikatmaa et al., 2008; Borgquist et al., 2009; Birke-Sorensen et al., 2011; Webster et al., 2014; Boateng & Cantanzano, 2015). It is also widely believed that NPWT increases blood flow to the area treated. However, there are debates over the effect of the negative pressure on local perfusion, and there are reports of reduced perfusion with increased negative pressure (Kairinos et al., 2009, 2017). Kaironos and co-workers instead believe that the reduction of oedema is one of the most important contributors to NPWT's efficacy, whereby the reduction in interstitial hydrostatic pressure improves oxygen and nutrient diffusion to the cells.

It has been found that several aspects of the NPWT mechanism of action can be achieved irrespective of the type of dressing filler used. However, the structure and properties of the filler dressing are still important in distributing the pressure uniformly over the wound bed and in managing the outcome at the wound/dressing interface. In the case of foam fillers, the pore size of the foam is typically larger than that of other foam wound dressings (as illustrated in Figure 5.4), to enable fluid to flow through easily (Boateng & Cantanzano, 2015). However, with the larger pore size, cell in-growth has been observed in clinical practice on the foam at the wound-dressing interface, which can then lead to adherence, trauma and pain upon removal. Gauze by contrast is noted to result in comparatively less cell growth, as well as in denser and thinner granulation tissue. An *in vivo* study at different negative pressures compared foam and gauze, confirming the clinical observations of greater adherence by the foam material (Borgquist et al., 2009). The study also showed more leukocyte infiltration in the foam, more tissue disorganisation, disruption of contact among cells and greater differences in size among cells. For this reason, a wound contact layer that does not promote cell in-growth is sometimes used in combination with foams, when rapid granulation is expected and a high degree of wound contraction is required (Birke-Sorensen et al., 2011).

Clinically, trials indicate that NPWT is as good or better than other treatment protocols, with more positive benefits seen on chronic leg ulcers and post-traumatic ulcers (Vikatmaa et al., 2008). There is some evidence to show that it can accelerate healing in the treatment of diabetic leg ulcers, and possibly of other wounds (Xie et al., 2010). A Cochrane review concluded that patients treated prophylactically with NPWT following surgery experienced less surgical site infections than those who were not (Norman et al., 2020). However, from the review, the evidence for other outcomes such as death, dehiscence, quality of life and pain was insufficient to be conclusive. Another review of studies, on the prophylactic use of NPWT on caesarean wounds, found that results were varied but there were indications of a reduction in surgical site infections and overall wound complications (Yu et al., 2018). The WHO guidelines on the reduction of surgical site infections suggest the use of prophylactic NPWT (pNPWT) in adult patients on primary closed surgical incisions in high-risk wounds (World Health Organization, 2018).

In recent years, dressings utilised as part of NPWT have evolved and no longer simply perform the physical role of a filler, pressure leveller, or sealing layer. Antibacterial foams, gauzes and separate wound contact layers are now available to assist in the prevention and management of infections. Adhesive seals have also been improved, and have become friendlier to the skin and less painful to remove, without compromising on the seal quality. Other developments in dressing design have led to replacement of the canister for some NPWT systems – with the dressing itself acting as the reservoir for the exudate, and integrating the outer sealing and protective barrier layer. Examples of such dressings are given in Box 5.4.

BOX 5.4   EXAMPLES OF MULTIFUNCTIONAL NPWT SYSTEMS

Canister-free NPWT systems	Antimicrobial NPWT systems
• PICO◊ (Smith + Nephew)	• Granufoam® Silver (Acelity)
• Avelle™ (Convatec)	• Renasys◊ Antimicrobial gauze (Smith + Nephew)
• Nanova™ (Acelity)	• Invia® Silverlon® (Medela Healthcare)

Canister-free NPWT dressings are multi-layered – consisting typically of an absorbent core, an outer membrane, and an adhesive layer or border to provide the seal. These dressings are normally used with short-term use pumps, which are intended to be used over a period of several days or weeks and disposed of. This is in contrast with static pump systems which are durable devices used in hospital settings and re-used with different patients. PICO◊ (Smith + Nephew, 2020a, 2020b) was the first example of a canister-free NPWT dressing and consists of a silicone adhesive wound contact layer, a spacer fabric layer (air lock layer), an absorbent layer and an outer film with high moisture vapour transmission rate to help with the moisture management. The small battery-powered hand-held pump creates the negative pressure through the dressing but fluid remains trapped in the absorbent layer and evaporates through the backing layer. Nanova™ (Acelity, 2020), which uses a hand-held non-battery-powered disposable pump, has a silicone non-adherent wound contact layer, an absorbent layer and an outer film, with a silicone-acrylic adhesive border to provide the seal. Avelle™ (Convatec, 2020) is another example of a multi-layer dressing using a portable disposable battery-powered pump to create the negative pressure through a semi-occlusive backing layer, a foam layer for pressure distribution, a CMC fibrous layers for absorption and gelling wound contact layer, and a perforated silicone adhesive border. While the disposable NPWT systems ensure that there is no cross-contamination, the impact of waste and the potential for recycling must be taken into consideration.

5.7.3 Dressings Providing Electrical Stimulation

Electrical stimulation (ES) therapy is the use of an electric current through electrodes placed on the skin near or within the wound, to accelerate healing. The theory is based on the observation that when the skin's integrity is compromised, it naturally generates an electric field on the wound edge that promotes healing. An external application of an electric current is therefore believed to be able to assist in wound closure. This can be done with different modalities, such as direct current, alternating current, high-voltage pulsed current, low-intensity direct current and electrobiofeedback. It can be achieved using a wired power pack, or wirelessly whereby the current is generated within a dressing itself or within micro and nanogenerators integrated inside the dressing (bioelectric dressings).

In vitro and *in vivo* studies using ES have shown that the therapy can help to decrease inflammation by reducing oedema, lowering bacterial bioburden on the wound site, inducing pre-angiogenic cellular responses, improving blood circulation, and promoting fibroblast proliferation, cell migration and collagen deposition (Kloth, 2005; Yu et al., 2014). Several clinical studies and trials using ES have been conducted, demonstrating augmented wound angiogenesis and better tissue oxygenation; many trials demonstrating the positive outcome of using the therapy on chronic wounds including diabetic, venous leg ulcers and other hard-to-heal wounds (Kloth, 2005; Barnes et al., 2014; Ofstead et al., 2020). A Cochrane review on the effect of ES on pressure ulcers concluded that it is likely to increase the proportion of ulcers healed and rate of healing, but that the evidence was insufficient to support its widespread use for pressure ulcers (Arora et al., 2020).

Expanding the concept of ES into dressings, electroceutical dressings have been developed. However, despite some evidence on the effect of ES on wound healing, commercially, the focus of the claims of the dressings has been mostly on its antimicrobial effects. These effects are attributed to several mechanisms: changes in the pH conditions near the electrode, electrolytic generation of toxic compounds such as hydrogen peroxide, disruption of bacterial cell division, overstimulation of cell membranes and interference with adhesion and cohesion of biofilm structures (Roy et al., 2019). One example of a wireless bioelectric antimicrobial dressing is Procellera® (Vomaris, 2020), which is a single layer polyester dressing embedded with a matrix of microcell batteries that are activated by moisture. The integrated batteries are made of elemental silver and zinc, used in a pattern of alternating dots and locked by a biocompatible binder. When in contact with fluids such as wound exudate or saline, a direct current voltage of 0.5–0.8 V is generated between the silver and zinc dots. *In vitro*, the antimicrobial effects, in particular the bactericidal, bacteriostatic and anti-biofilm activities have been demonstrated by several studies (Kim et al., 2014; Kim & Izadjoo, 2015; Banerjee et al., 2015). Laboratory research has also shown that the bioelectric dressing can increase the migration of keratinocytes, generate hydrogen peroxide and improve mitochondrial function (Banerjee et al., 2014). *In vivo* studies on deep partial-thickness wounds have demonstrated the better healing rates obtained from the use of the bioelectric dressings compared to when controls were used (Harding et al., 2012). Likewise, in small clinical studies, the dressing was also found to result in faster healing, with additional benefits such as superior scar quality on split-thickness skin donor sites and increased comfort and less erythema for wounds arising from curettage and electrodessication (Sheftel & Drenten, 2009; Blount et al., 2012). Another prototype with a similar configuration of silver nanoparticle and zinc particle dot pattern onto medical cotton was also found to promote wound healing by reducing the inflammation stage and increasing growth factor expressions in an *in vivo* study (Yu et al., 2019).

In a further example of a wireless bioelectric dressing, mechanical displacement from skin movements is converted into electricity, via nanogenerators integrated into a bandage with two electrodes (Long et al., 2018). The nanogenerator is made by overlapping copper/PTFE with another copper layer on different sides of a PET substrate. The voltage generated between the two electrodes varies with the skin movement. *In vivo* studies demonstrated rapid closure of full-thickness wounds, which was attributed to enhanced fibroblast migration, proliferation and transdifferentiation.

The above non-wired versions of microcurrent dressings have the benefits of being simple and easy to use, without any accessories or wires in the way. Externally powered dressings on the other hand have the benefit of being able to actively provide a specific level of current as and when required and irrespective of the presence of exudate or saline. Although no longer available, Posifect®RD by Biofisica was one of the early developments in this field. The dressing consisted of a miniature electric circuit, two electrodes, and powered by two lithium cell batteries. One of the electrodes was incorporated into a hydrogel in the dressing, and the other was placed directly on the wound. Several small studies showed positive wound healing results, with an indication of the dressing's effect on biofilm disruption (Morris, 2006). More recently, a battery-powered clinical prototype of a patterned electroceutical dressing has been demonstrated to be safe to use on chronic wounds (Roy et al., 2019). Manufactured from silk, silver ink and medical tape backing, and with encased circuit and batteries, the prototype dressing has been demonstrated to inhibit biofilm formation *in vitro*, and could therefore be used for wounds with deeper infections.

5.7.4 Diagnostics and Theranostics

As the boundaries of advanced wound dressings are being pushed forward, the idea that dressings could to do more than care for or heal a wound is under exploration. The ability to assist in monitoring and diagnosis, which are essential parts of wound management, has been one of the areas of interest for R&D. There are a number of biochemical and physical biomarkers that can be used to monitor an area or provide an indication of the status of a wound, e.g., MMPs, uric acid, pH, bacteria, nitric oxide, oxygen, impedance, moisture, pressure and temperature (Mehmood et al., 2015; Derakhshandeh et al., 2018; Gianino et al., 2018). There are also a number of potential sensors for these markers, providing opportunities for the development of so-called smart dressings.

In the area of dressings providing diagnostics, one of the most developed field is the detection of infection *in situ*. When the bacterial bioburden increases significantly towards infection, the environmental conditions of the wound bed alter and stimuli-responsive dressings have been developed to react to some of these changes. The simplest way, which does not require any integrated electronics, is utilising colorimetric pH sensors. This is illustrated by the development of a hydrogel dressing that changes to a fluorescent colour when in contact with pathogenic wound biofilms (Thet et al., 2016). The dressing contains fluorescent self-quenching dye-bearing vesicles that undergo lysis in response to toxins and enzymes that are released by the bacteria under biofilm conditions. Another example also utilises similar dye-containing vesicles, but which are plasma-deposited on fabrics (Zhou et al., 2011). A visual cue is again used for the detection of hydrogen peroxide, believed to be a potential marker for inflammation or infections, using Europium (III) coordination polymers loaded onto polyacrylonitrile nanofibre mats (Wu et al., 2020).

Recently, theranostic (combining diagnostics and therapeutics) solutions have been developed for the detection and treatment of infection. For instance, a smart hydrogel wound dressing, where the bacterial infection is detected via pH changes using fluorescence resonance energy transfer, and an antibiotic release is triggered by exposure to near-infrared (NIR) light exposure, has been described (Qiao et al., 2020). *In vitro* studies showed obvious fluorescence transitions and the capability of the NIR light to convert to UV light to trigger the release of the drug. In another embodiment, methacrylated gelatine has been used to encapsulate both antimicrobial and fluorescent vesicles, which only activate in the presence of bacteria (Zhou et al., 2018). For their part, Singh et al. (2019) developed a PU scaffold dressing loaded with a prodrug and a chromogenic probe. A colour change and the release of the active occur in the presence of lipase, an extracellular enzyme secreted by certain bacteria. Another example is a multifunctional alginate-based dressing, developed with an array of colorimetric porous pH sensors, 3D-printed onto the substrate (Mirani et al., 2017). The changes in pH are correlated to the detection of infection. An image capture system such as a smartphone is used to quantify the colour changes over the matrix of sensors in the dressing, indicating zones of abnormal skin pH. The dressing also incorporates a 3D printed patch which gradually releases gentamicin at the wound site to manage any infection. *In vitro* and *ex vivo* tests demonstrated the ability of the sensors to react with bacterial bioburden, and the antimicrobial activity of the released antibiotic.

5.7.5 Actuated Wound Dressings for Active Drug Release

Many dressings that are loaded with actives deliver them either in bulk at the beginning (when just placed on a wound bed) followed by a slower release over time, or gradually and steadily over time. Some, which are less passive and more reactive, will only delivery their actives when there is a change in the wound environment, as in some of the theranostic solutions described above. The delivery of actives only when prompted, or to the level desired, has also been a topic of exploration in the last couple of decades. With this type of system, the clinician can decide when is the most appropriate time to release the actives, how much to deliver and when to stop.

Various mechanisms have been used for the active controlled release of drugs from wound dressings. Despite the integration of certain components within the dressing (e.g., responsive vesicles) for active control, a separate powered actuating system is normally required. Pumping requires a reservoir and pumping mechanism linked to the dressing; it is used in instillation NPWT, which uses negative pressure with intermittent release of cleansing solutions or actives such as antibiotics. Iontophoresis, which is the use of an electronic current to drive the movement of drugs, requires a controllable source of current to trigger and stop the delivery. Some mechanisms rely on modifying the immediate environment within the dressing instead (e.g., a change in temperature, pH, etc.) to create a structural or chemical change in the dressing that enables drug molecules to be delivered. Hydrogels, because of their ability to be inherently stimuli-responsive, to have good conductivity, and/or to be an easy medium into which many types of micro and nano structures can be incorporated, have been well explored to this effect.

In one example, drug-loaded chitosan nanoparticles contained within a pH-sensitive hydrogel can be made to release their actives using a DC voltage between electrodes (Kiaee et al., 2018). Applying the voltage results in a local increase in pH near the electrodes, which causes the nanoparticles to release their load due to the dehydration process. Turning off the voltage results in immediate pH recovery and puts a stop to the drug release. In another case, a hydrogel is used to contain thermo-responsive microparticles encapsulating drug molecules (Bagherifard et al., 2016). The hydrogel layer is heated electronically to trigger the release of the drugs from the microparticles. Tamayol et al. (2017) reported on the development of a nanofibrous platform with integrated flexible heaters for on-demand drug delivery. The metallic heater is patterned directly onto the substrate, which upon application of an electric voltage, generates heat which in turn releases the drugs loaded onto nanoparticles. These are early examples of developments in the field of actuating and sensing/actuating dressings, which are stepping stones into the integration of artificial intelligence in wound care, to be discussed in the concluding chapter.

References

Acelity. (2020, July). *NanovaTM Therapy System*. Retrieved from Acelity: https://www.acelity.com/healthcare-professionals/global-product-catalog/catalog/nanova-therapy

Ahmed, E. M. (2015, March). Hydrogel: Preparation, Characterization, and Applications: A Review. *Journal of Advanced Research, 6*(2), 105. doi:10.1016/j.jare.2013.07.006

Ai, J.-W., Liu, J.-T., Pei, S.-D., Liu, Y., Li, D.-S., Lin, H.-M., & Pei, B. (2017, January). The Effectiveness of Pressure Therapy (15–25 mmHg) for Hypertrophic Burn Scars: A Systematic Review and Meta-Analysis. *Scientific Reports, 7*, 40185. doi:10.1038/srep40185

Alghoraibi, I., & Alomari, S. (2018). Different Methods for Nanofiber Design and Fabrication. In A. Barhoum, M. Bechelany, & A. Makhlouf (Eds.), *Handbook of Nanofibers* (p. 1). Cham: Springer. doi:10.1007/978-3-319-42789-8_11-2

Anzarut, A., Olson, J., Singh, P., Rowe, B. H., & Tredget, E. E. (2009, January). The Effectiveness of Pressure Garment Therapy for the Prevention of Abnormal Scarring after Burn Injury: A Meta-Analysis. *Journal of Plastic, Reconstructive and Aesthetic Surgery, 62*(1), 77. doi:10.1016/j.bjps.2007.10.052.

Arora, M., Harvey, L. A., Glinsky, J. V., Nier, L., Lavrencic, L., Kifley, A., & Cameron, I. D. (2020, January 22). Electrical Stimulation for Treating Pressure Ulcers. In C. W. Group (Ed.), *Cochrane Database of Systematic Reviews*. John Wiley & Sons Ltd. doi:10.1002/14651858.CD012196.pub2

Atiyeh, B. S., El Khatib, A. M., & Dibo, S. A. (2013, December). Pressure Garment Therapy (PGT) of Burn Scars: Evidence-Based Efficacy. *Annals of Burns and Fire Disasters*, 205. Retrieved July 22, 2020, from https://www.ncbi.nlm.nih.gov/pmc/articles/PMC3978593/

Bagherifard, S., Tamayol, A., Mostafulu, P., Akbari, M., Comotto, M., Annabi, N., Ghaderi, M., Sonkusale, S., Dokmeci, M. R., & Khademhosseini, A. (2016, January). Dermal Patch with Integrated Flexible Heater for on Demand Drug Delivery. *Advanced Healthcare Materials, 5*(1), 175. doi:10.1002/adhm.201500357

Banerjee, J., Ghatak, P. D., Roy, S., Khanna, S., Hemann, C., Deng, B., Das, A., Zweier, J. L., Wozniak, D., & Sen, C. K. (2015). Silver-Zinc Redox-Coupled Electroceutical Wound Dressing Disrupts Bacterial Biofilm. *PLoS One*, e0119531. doi:10.1371/journal.pone.0119531

Banerjee, J., Ghatak, P. D., Roy, S., Khanna, S., Sequin, E. K., Bellman, K., Dickinson, B. C., Suri, P., Subramaniam, V. V., Chang, C. J., & Sen, C. K. (2014, March). Improvement of Human Keratinocyte Migration by a Redox Active Bioelectric Dressing. *PLoS One, 9*(3), e89239. doi:10.1371/journal.pone.0089239

Barnes, R., Shahin, Y., Gohil, R., & Chetter, I. (2014). Electrical Stimulation vs. Standard Care for Chronic Ulcer Healing: A Systematic Review and Meta-Analysis of Randomised Controlled Trials. *European Journal of Clinical Investigation, 44*(4), 429. doi:10.1111/eci.12244

Benskin, L. (2016). Polymeric Membrane Dressings for Topical Wound Management of Patients with Infected Wounds in a Challenging Environment: A Protocol with 3 Case Examples. *Wound Management & Prevention, 62*(6), 42.

Benskin, L. L. (2018). Evidence for Polymeric Membrane Dressings as a Unique Dressing Subcategory, Using Pressure Ulcers as an Example. *Advances in Wound Care, 7*(12), 419. doi:10.1089/wound.2018.0822

Birke-Sorensen, H., Malmsjo, M., Rome, P., Hudson, D., Krug, E., Berg, L., Bruhin, A., Caravaggi, C., Chariker, M., Depoorter, M., Dowsett, C., Dunn, R., Duteille, F., Ferreira, F., Martinez, J. M. F., Grudzien, G., Ichioka, S., Ingemansson, R., Jeffery, S., Lee, C., Vig, S., Runkel, N., Martin, R., & Smith, J. (2011). Evidence-Based

Recommendations for Negative Pressure Wound Therapy: Treatment Variables (Pressure Levels, Wound Filler and Contact Layer) – Steps Towards an International Consensus. *Journal of Plastic, Reconstructive & Aesthetic Surgery, 64,* S1. doi:10.1016/j.bjps.2011.06.001

Blount, A. L., Foster, S., Rapp, D. A., & Wilcox, R. (2012, May-June). The Use of Bioelectric Dressings in Skin Graft Harvest Sites: A Prospective Case Series. *Journal of Burn Care & Research, 33*(3), 354. doi:10.1097/BCR.0b013e31823356e4

Boateng, J., & Cantanzano, O. (2015). Advanced Therapeutic Dressings for Effective Wound Healing. *Journal of Phamaceutical Sciences, 104*(11), 3653.

Borgquist, O., Gustafsson, L., Ingemansson, R., & Malmsjö, M. (2009, November). Tissue Ingrowth into Foam But Not into Gauze during Negative Pressure Wound Therapy. *Wounds: A Compendium of Clinical Research and Practice, 21*(11), 302. Retrieved July 24, 2020, from https://www.woundsresearch.com/content/tissue-ingrowth-into-foam-not-into-gauze-during-negative-pressure-wound-therapy

Bradbury, S., Ivins, N., Harding, K., & Turner, A. (2008, September). Measuring Outcomes with Complex Patients: An Audit of the Effect of Actiform Cool on Painful Wounds. *Wounds UK, 4*(3), 22.

Chagranti, P., Gordon, I., Chao, J. H., & Zehtabchi, S. (2019, June). A Systematic Review of Foam Dressings for Partial Thickness Burns. *The American Journal of Emergency Medicine, 37*(6), 1184. doi:10.1016/j.ajem.2019.04.014

Chen, S., Liu, B., Carlson, M. A., Gombart, A. F., Reilly, D. A., & Xie, J. (2017, June). Recent Advances in Electrospun Nanofibers for Wound Healing. *Nanomedicine (London), 12*(11), 1335. doi: 10.2217/nnm-2017-0017

Chou, S.-F., Carson, D., & Woodrow, K. A. (2015, December 28). Current Strategies for Sustaining Drug Release from Electrospun Nanofibers. *Journal of Control Release, 220*(Part B), 584. doi:10.1016/j.jconrel.2015.09.008

Chowdhry, M., Dipane, M., & McPherson, E. J. (2017, December). Bio-Occlusive Gauze with Tegaderm: A Dressing for Surgical Wounds in Primary THA and TKA. *Reconstructive Review, 7*(4), 19. doi:10.15438/rr.7.4.197

Cigna, E., Tarallo, M., Bistoni, G., Anniboletti, T., Trignano, E., Tortorelli, G., & Scuderi, N. (2009, December). Evaluation of Polyurethane Dressing with Ibuprofen in the Management of Split-Thickness Skin Graft Donor Sites. *In Vivo, 23*(6), 983.

Contardi, M., Heredia-Guerrero, J. A., Perotto, G., Valentini, P., Pompa, P. P., Spanò, R., Goldoni, L., Bertorelli, R., Athanassiou, A., & Bayer, I. S. (2017, June 15). Transparent Ciprofloxacin-Povidone Antibiotic Films and Nanofiber Mats as Potential Skin and Wound Care Dressings. *European Journal of Pharmaceutical Sciences, 104,* 133. doi:10.1016/j.ejps.2017.03.044

Convatec. (2020, July). *Avelle NPWT System.* Retrieved from Convatec: https://www.convatec.co.uk/wound-skin/avelle-negative-pressure-wound-therapy/

DeBruler, D. M., Zbinden, J. C., Baumann, M. E., Blackstone, B. N., Malara, M. M., Bailey, J. K., Supp, D. M., & Powell, H. M. (2018, June 13). Early Cessation of Pressure Garment Therapy Results in Scar Contraction and Thickening. *PLoS One,* e0197558. doi:10.1371/journal.pone.0197558

Derakhshandeh, H., Kashaf, S. S., Aghabaglou, F., Ghanavati, I., & Tamayol, A. (2018, December). Smart Bandages: The Future of Wound Care. *Trends in Biotechnology, 36*(12), 1259. doi:10.1016/j.tibtech.2018.07.007

Dumville, J. C., Deshpande, S., O'Meara, S., & Speak, K. (2013a, June 6). Foam Dressings for Healing Diabetic Foot Ulcers. In C. W. Group (Ed.), *Cochrane Database of Systematic Reviews*. John Wileys & Sons Ltd. doi:10.1002/14651858. CD009111.pub3

Dumville, J. C., O'Meara, S., Deshpande, S., & Speak, K. (2013b, July 13). Hydrogel Dressings for Healing Diabetic Foot Ulcers. In C. W. Group (Ed.), *Cochrane Database of Systematic Reviews*. John Wiley & Sons Ltd. doi:10.1002/14651858. CD009101.pub3

Dumville, J. C., Stubbs, N., Keogh, S. J., Walker, R. M., & Liu, Z. (2015, February 15). Hydrogel Dressings for Treating Pressure Ulcers. In C. W. Group (Ed.), *Cochrane Database of Systematic Reviews*. John Wiley & Sons Ltd. doi:10.1002/14651858. CD011226.pub2

Edwards, J., & Stapley, S. (2010, January 20). Debridement of Diabetic Foot Ulcers. In C. W. Group (Ed.), *Cochrane Database of Systematic Reviews*. John Wiley & Sons Ltd. doi:10.1002/14651858.CD003556.pub2

Elraiyah, T., Domecq, J. P., Prutsky, G., Tsapas, A., Nabhan, M., Frykberg, R. G., Hasan, R., Firwana, B., Prokop, L. J., & Murad, M. H. (2016, February). A Systematic Review and Meta-Analysis of Débridement Methods for Chronic Diabetic Foot Ulcers. *Journal of Vascular Surgery, 63*(2), 37S. doi:10.1016/j.jvs.2015.10.002

Felton, L. A. (2013, December 5). Mechanisms of Polymeric Film Formation. *International Journal of Pharmaceutics, 457*(2), 423. doi:10.1016/j.ijpharm.2012.12.027.

Fletcher, J., Moore, Z., Anderson, I., & Matsuzaki, K. (2011, November). Pressure Ulcers and Hydrocolloids Made Easy. *Wounds International, 2*(4), 1.

Fogh, K., Andersen, M. B., Bischoff-Mikkelsen, M., Bause, R., Zutt, M., Schilling, S., Schmutz, J.-L., Borbujo, J., Jimenez, J. A., Cartier, H., & Jørgensen, B. (2012, November–December). Clinically Relevant Pain Relief with an Ibuprofen-Releasing Foam Dressing: Results from a Randomized, Controlled, Double-Blind Clinical Trial in Exuding, Painful Venous Leg Ulcers. *Wound Repair and Regeneration, 20*(6), 815. doi:10.1111/j.1524-475X.2012.00844.x

Ghanavati, Z., Neisi, N., Bayahi, V., & Makvandi, M. (2015, December). The Influence of Substrate Topography and Biomaterial Substance on Skin Wound Healing. *Anatomy & Cell Biology, 48*(4), 251. doi:10.5115/acb.2015.48.4.251

Gianino, E., Miller, C., & Gilmore, J. (2018, September). Smart Wound Dressings for Diabetic Chronic Wounds. *Bioengineering (Basel), 5*(3), 51. doi:10.3390/bioengineering5030051

Grand View Research. (2019). *Medical Textiles Market Size, Share & Trends Analysis Report by Fabric (Non-Woven, Knitted, Woven), by Application and Segment Forecasts, 2019–2025*. San Francisco: Grand View Research.

Hampton, S. (2004, July). A Small Study in Healing Rates and Symptom Control Using a New Sheet Hydrogel Dressing. *Journal of Wound Care, 13*(4), 297. doi:10.12968/jowc.2004.13.7.26639

Harding, A. C., Gil, J., Valdes, J., Solis, M., & Davis, S. C. (2012, September). Efficacy of a Bio-Electric Dressing in Healing Deep, Partial-Thickness Wounds Using a Porcine Model. *Ostomy Wound Management*, 50. Retrieved July 2020, 2020, from https://pdfs.semanticscholar.org/818f/bda1c13d709d65752094362d859689be9e29.pdf

Kairinos, N., Solomons, M., & Hudson, D. A. (2017). Negative-Pressure Wound Therapy I: The Paradox of Negative Pressure Wound Therapy. *Wound Healing South Africa, 10*(2), 6.

Kairinos, N., Voogd, A. M., Botha, P. H., Kotze, T., Kahn, D., Hudson, D. A., & Solomons, M. (2009, February). Negative-Pressure Wound Therapy II: Negative-Pressure Wound Therapy and Increased Perfusion. Just an Illusion? *Plastic and Reconstructive Surgery*, 123(2), 601. doi: 10.1097/PRS.0b013e318196b97b

Kawabata, S., Kanda, N., Hirasawa, Y., Noda, K., Matsuura, Y., Suzuki, S., & Kawai, K. (2018, May). The Utility of Silk-Elastin Hydrogel as a New Material for Wound Healing. *Plastic and Reconstructive Surgery – Global Open*, 6(5), e1778. doi:10.1097/GOX.0000000000001778

KCI. (2015). *V.A.C.® Therapy: Clinical Guidelines, A Reference Source for Clinicians*. KCI. Retrieved June 13, 2020, from https://www.acelity.com/-/media/Project/Acelity/Acelity-Base-Sites/shared/PDF/2-b-128h-vac-clinical-guidelines-web.pdf/#EN

Kiaee, G., Mostafalu, P., Samandari, M., & Sonkusale, S. (2018, September). A pH-Mediated Electronic Wound Dressing for Controlled Drug Delivery. *Advanced Healthcare Materials*, 7(18), e1800396. doi:10.1002/adhm.201800396

Kim, H., & Izadjoo, M. J. (2015, February). Antibiofilm Efficacy Evaluation of a Bioelectric Dressing in Mono- and Multi-Species Biofilms. *Journal of Wound Care*, 24(Suppl. 2), S10. doi:10.12968/jowc.2015.24.Sup2.S10

Kim, H., Makin, I., Skiba, J., Ho, A., Housler, G., Stojadinovic, A., & Izadjoo, M. (2014). Antibacterial Efficacy Testing of a Bioelectric Wound Dressing against Clinical Wound Pathogens. *The Open Microbiological Journal*, 8, 15. doi:10.2174/1874285801408010015

Kim, Y. J., Lee, S. W., Hong, S. H., Lee, H. K., & Kim, E. K. (1999). The Effects of PolyMem(R) on the Wound Healing. *Journal of the Korean Society of Plastic and Reconstructive Surgeons*, 26(6), 1165.

Kloth, L. C. (2005). Electrical Stimulation for Wound Healing: A Review of Evidence from In Vitro Studies, Animal Experiments and Clinical Trials. *Lower Extremity Wounds*, 4(1), 23. Retrieved July 28, 2020, from https://www.researchgate.net/profile/Luther_Kloth/publication/7878545_Electrical_Stimulation_for_Wound_Healing_A_Review_of_Evidence_From_In_Vitro_Studies_Animal_Experiments_and_Clinical_Trials/links/0deec528b6a9c7d107000000.pdf&hl=en&sa=X&scisig=AAGBfm1Ui

Lee, G. A., Rajendran, S., & Anand, S. (2009). New Single-Layer Compression Bandage System for Chronic Venous Leg Ulcers. *British Journal of Nursing*, 18(5), S4. doi:10.12968/bjon.2009.18.Sup5.43568

Leong, W. S., Wu, S. C., Ng, K. W., & Tan, L. P. (2016). Electrospun 3D Multi-Scale Fibrous Scaffold for Enhanced Human Dermal Fibroblasts Infiltration. *International Journal of Bioprinting*, 2(1), 81.

Liu, H., Wang, C., Li, C., Qin, Y., Wang, Z., Yang, F., Li, Z., & Wang, J. (2018). A Functional Chitosan-Based Hydrogel as a Wound Dressing and Drug Delivery System in the Treatment of Wound Healing. *RSC Advances*, 8, 7533. doi:10.1039/C7RA13510F

Long, Y., Wei, H., Li, J., Yao, G., Yu, B., Ni, D., Gibson, A. L. F., Lan, X., Jiang, Y., Cai, W., & Wang, X. (2018, November). Effective Wound Healing Enabled by Discrete Alternative Electric Fields from Wearable Nanogenerators. *ACS Nano*, 12(12), 12533. doi:10.1021/acsnano.8b07038

Madaghiele, M., Demitri, C., Sannino, A., & Ambrosio, L. (2014). Polymeric Hydrogels for Burn Wound Care: Advanced Skin Wound Dressings and Regenerative Templates. *Burns & Trauma, 2*, 153. Retrieved July 9, 2020, from https://burnstrauma.biomedcentral.com/articles/10.4103/2321-3868.143616

Marston, W., & Vowden, K. (2003). Compression Therapy: A Guide to Safe Practice. In *Understanding Compression Therapy: EWMA Position Document* (p. 11). Medical Education Partnership Ltd.

Mehmood, N., Hariz, A., Templeton, S., & Voelcker, N. H. (2015). A Flexible and Low Power Telemetric Sensing and Monitoring System for Chronic Wound Diagnostics. *BioMedical Engineering Online, 14*, 17. doi:10.1186/s12938-015-0011-y

Mirani, B., Pagan, E., Currie, B., Siddiqui, M. A., Hosseinzadeh, R., Mostafalu, P., Zhang, Y. S., Ghahary, A., & Akbari, M. (2017, October). An Advanced Multifunctional Hydrogel-Based Dressing for Wound Monitoring and Drug Delivery. *Advances in Healthcare Materials, 6*(19). doi:10.1002/adhm.201700718

Mohamad, N., Amin, M. C., Pandey, M., Ahmad, N., & Rajab, N. F. (2014, December 19). Bacterial Cellulose/Acrylic Acid Hydrogel Synthesized via Electron Beam Irradiation: Accelerated Burn Wound Healing in an Animal Model. *Carbohydrate Polymers, 114*, 312. doi:10.1016/j.carbpol.2014.08.025

Morris, C. (2006). Bio-Electrical Stimulation Therapy Using POSiFECT® RD. *Wounds UK, 2*(4), 112. Retrieved July 30, 2020, from https://www.woundsinternational.com/uploads/resources/content_9099.pdf

Nelson, E. A., Mani, R., Vowden, K., & Thomas, K. (2011, February 16). Intermittent Pneumatic Compression for Treating Venous Leg Ulcers. In C. W. Group (Ed.), *Cochrane Database of Systematic Reviews*. John Wiley & Sons Ltd. doi:10.1002/14651858.CD001899.pub3.

Norman, G., Goh, E. L., Dumville, J. C., Shi, C., Liu, Z., Chiverton, L., Stankiewicz, M., & Reid, A. (2020, June 15). Negative Pressure Wound Therapy for Surgical Wounds Healing by Primary Closure. In C. W. Group (Ed.), *Cochrane Database of Systematic Reviews*. John Wiley & Sons Ltd. doi:10.1002/14651858.CD009261.pub6

O'Meara, S., Cullum, N., Nelson, E. A., & Dumville, J. C. (2012, November 14). Compression for Venous Leg Ulcers. In C. W. Group (Ed.), *Cochrane Database of Systematic Reviews*. John Wiley & Sons Ltd. doi:10.1002/14651858.CD000265.pub3

O'Meara, S., & Martyn-St James, M. (2013, May 13). Foam Dressings for Venous Leg Ulcers. In C. W. Group (Ed.), *Cochrane Database of Systematic Reviews*. John Wiley & Sons Ltd. doi:10.1002/14651858.CD009907.pub2

Ofstead, C. L., Buro, B. L., Hopkins, K. M., & Eiland, J. E. (2020, July). The Ompact of Continuous Electrical Microcurrent on Acute and Hard-To-Heal Wounds: A Systematic Review. *Journal of Wound Care, 29*(Suppl. 7), S6. doi:10.12968/jowc.2020.29.Sup7.S6

Öri, F., Dietrich, R., Ganz, C., Dau, M., Wolter, D., Kasten, A., Gerber, T., Frerich, B. (2017, January). Silicon-Dioxide–Polyvinylpyrrolidone as a Wound Dressing for Skin Defects in a Murine Model. *Journal of Cranio-Maxillofacial Surgery, 45*(1), 99. doi:10.1016/j.jcms.2016.10.002

Pott, F. S., Meier, M. J., Stocco, J. G., Crozeta, K., & Ribas, J. D. (2014, May–June). The Effectiveness of Hydrocolloid Dressings versus Other Dressings in the Healing of Pressure Ulcers in Adults and Older Adults: A Systematic Review and Meta-Analysis. *Revista Latino-Americana Enfermagem, 22*(3), 511. doi:10.1590/0104-1169.3480.2445

Qiao, B., Pang, Q., Yuan, P., Luo, Y., & Ma, L. (2020). Smart Wound Dressing for Infection Monitoring and NIR-Triggered Antibacterial Treatment. *Biomaterials Science, 8,* 1649. doi:10.1039/C9BM02060H

Rajendran, S., & Anand, S. C. (2010). Development of Three-Dimensional Structures for Single-Layer Compression Therapy. In S. C. Anand, J. F. Kennedy, M. Miraftab, & S. Rajendran (Eds.), *Medical and Healthcare Textiles* (p. 279). Woodhead Publishing. doi:10.1533/9780857090348.279

Ramazan, E. (2019). Advances in Fabric Structures for Wound Care. In S. Rajendran (Ed.), *Advanced Textiles for Wound Care* (p. 509). Woodhead Publishing. doi:10.1016/B978-0-08-102192-7.00018-7

Ravenscroft, M. J., Harker, J., & Buch, K. A. (2006). A Prospective, Randomised, Controlled Trial Comparing Wound Dressings Used in Hip and Knee Surgery: Aquacel and Tegaderm versus Cutiplast. *Annals of the Royal College of Surgeons of England, 88,* 18. doi:10.1308/003588406X82989

Ribeiro, M. P., Morgado, P. I., Miguel, S. P., Coutinho, P., & Correia, I. J. (2013, July 1). Dextran-Based Hydrogel Containing Chitosan Microparticles Loaded with Growth Factors to Be Used in Wound Healing. *Materials Science and Engineering: C, 33*(5), 2958. doi:10.1016/j.msec.2013.03.025

Roy, S., Prakash, S., Mathew-Steiner, S. S., Ghatak, P. D., Lochab, V., Jones, T. H., Sundaram, P. M., Gordillo, G. M., Subramanian, V. V., & Sen, C. K. (2019). Disposable Patterned Electroceutical Dressing (PED-10) Is Safe for Treatment of Open Clinical Chronic Wounds. *Advances in Wound Care, 8*(4), 149. doi:10.1089/wound.2018.0915

Rubio, P. A. (1991, October). Use of Semiocclusive, Transparent Film Dressings for Surgical Wound Protection: Experience in 3637 Cases. *International Surgery, 76*(4), 253.

Sackheim, K., de Araujo, T. S., & Kirsner, R. S. (2006). Compression Modalities and Dressings: Their Use in Venous Ulcers. *Dermatologic Therapy, 19,* 338.

Sangjun, N., Phulsuksombati, D., Pilakasiri, K., Parichatikanond, P., Muensoongnoen, J., Koedpuech, K., Janvikul, W., & Tanodekaew, S. (2003). Animal Study of the Effect of Chitin-PAA and Carboxymethylchitosan Hydrogels on Healing of Deep Thickness Wounds. *Armed Forces Research Institute of Medical Sciences: Annual Progress Report,* 128. Retrieved June 16, 2020, from https://www.afrims. go.th/uploads/report/AR11.pdf

Shariatina, Z., & Jalali, A. M. (2018, August). Chitosan-Based Hydrogels: Preparation, Properties and Applications. *International Journal of Biological Macromolecules, 115,* 194. doi:10.1016/j.ijbiomac.2018.04.034

Sheftel, S. N., & Drenten, C. E. (2009). *Bioelectric vs Standard Wound Care: A Comparative Study. Symposium on Advanced Wound Care* (p. S20). Texas. Retrieved July 29, 2020, from http://www.warriorwoundcare.com/pdf/Bioelectric_vs_ Standard_Wound_Care_A_Randomized_Comparative_Study_Presented_ at_2009_SAWC.pdf

Shingel, K. I., Di Stabile, L., Marty, J.-P., & Faure, M.-P. (2006, December). Inflammatory Inert Poly(Ethylene Glycol)–Protein Wound Dressing Improves Healing

Responses in Partial- and Full-Thickness Wounds. *International Wound Journal*, 3(4), 332. doi:10.1111/j.1742-481X.2006.00262.x

Sibbald, R. G., Coutts, P., Fierheller, M., & Woo, K. (2007, March). A Pilot (Real-Life) Randomised Clinical Evaluation of a Pain-Relieving Foam Dressing: (Ibuprofen-Foam versus Local Best Practice). *International Wound Journal*, 4(S1), 16. doi:10.1111/j.1742-481X.2007.00308.x

Singh, H., Li, W., Kazemian, M. R., Yang, R., Yang, C., Logsetty, S., & Liu, S. (2019). Lipase-Responsive Electrospun Theranostic Wound Dressing for Simultaneous Recognition and Treatment of Wound Infection. *ACS Applied Bio Materials*, 2(5), 2028. doi:10.1021/acsabm.9b00076

Smith + Nephew. (2020a, November). *PICO Single Use Negative Pressure Wound Therapy*. Retrieved from Smith + Nephew: https://www.smith-nephew.com/key-products/advanced-wound-management/pico/

Smith + Nephew. (2020b, July). *PICO◊ Single Use Negative Pressure Wound Therapy*. Retrieved from Smith + Nephew: https://www.smith-nephew.com/new-zealand/healthcare/products/product-types/negative-pressure-wound-therapy/pico/

Sun, G., Zhang, X., Shen, Y.-I., Sebastian, R., Dickinson, L. E., Fox-Talbot, K., Reinblatt, M., Steenbergen, C., Harmon, J. W., & Gerecht, S. (2011, December 27). Dextran Hydrogel Scaffolds Enhance Angiogenic Responses and Promote Complete Skin Regeneration during Burn Wound Healing (R. Langer, Ed.). *Proceedings of the National Academy of Sciences of the U.S.A.*, 108(52), 20977. doi:10.1073/pnas.1115973108

Tamayol, A., Najafabadi, A. H., Mostafalu, P., Yetisen, A. K., Commotto, M., Aldhahri, M., Abdel-Wahab, M. S., Najafabadi, Z. I., Latifi, S., Akbari, M., Annabi, N., Yun, S. H., Memic, A., Dokmeci, M. R., & Khademhosseini, A. (2017). Biodegradable Elastic Nanofibrous Platforms with Integrated Flexible Heaters for On-Demand Drug Delivery. *Scientific Reports*, 7, 9220. doi:10.1038/s41598-017-04749-8

Thet, N. T., Alves, D. R., Bean, J. E., Booth, S., Nzakizwanayo, J., Young, A. E., Jones, B. V., & Jenkins, A. T. (2016, June 22). Prototype Development of the Intelligent Hydrogel Wound Dressing and Its Efficacy in the Detection of Model Pathogenic Wound Biofilms. *ACS Applied Materials Interfaces*, 8(24), 14909. doi:10.1021/acsami.5b07372

Tibbitt, M. W., & Anseth, K. S. (2009, July 1). Hydrogels as Extracellular Matrix Mimics for 3D Cell Culture. *Biotechnology and Bioengineering*, 103(4), 655. doi:10.1002/bit.22361

Tong, S.-F., Yip, J., Yick, K.-L., & Yuen, C.-W. M. (2015, July 1). Exploring Use of Warp-Knitted Spacer Fabric as a Substitute for the Absorbent Layer for Advanced Wound Dressing. *Textile Research Journal*, 85(12), 1258. doi:10.1177/0040517514561922

Veld, R. C., Walboomers, X. F., Jansen, J. A., & Wagener, A. D. (2020, June). Design Considerations for Hydrogel Wound Dressings: Strategic and Molecular Advances. *Tissue Engineering Part B: Reviews*, 26(3), 230. doi:10.1089/ten.teb.2019.0281

Vikatmaa, P., Juutilainen, V., Kuukasjärvi, P., & Malmivaara, A. (2008, October). Negative Pressure Wound Therapy: A Systematic Review on Effectiveness and Safety. *European Journal of Vascular and Endovascular Surgery*, 36(4), 438. doi:10.1016/j.ejvs.2008.06.010

Vomaris. (2020, July 29). *Procellera® by Vomaris Wound Care, Inc.* Retrieved from Vomaris: https://vomaris.com/products/procellera/

Walker, R. M., Gillespie, B. M., Thalib, L., Higgins, N. S., & Whitty, J. A. (2017, October 12). Foam Dressings for Treating Pressure Ulcers. In C. W. Group (Ed.), *Cochrane Database of Systematic Reviews.* John Wiley & Sons Ltd. . doi:10.1002/14651858. CD011332.pub2

Waycaster, C., & Milne, C. T. (2013). Clinical and Economic Benefit of Enzymatic Debridement of Pressure Ulcers Compared to Autolytic Debridement with a Hydrogel Dressing. *Journal of Medical Economics, 16*(7), 976. doi:10.3111/13696 998.2013.807268

Webster, J., Scuffham, P., Stankiewicz, M., & Chaboyer, W. P. (2014, October 7). Negative Pressure Wound Therapy for Skin Grafts and Surgical Wounds Healing by Primary Intention. In C. W. Group (Ed.), *Cochrane Database of Systematic Reviews.* John Wiley & Sons Ltd. doi:10.1002/14651858.CD009261.pub3

Wiegand, C., Springer, S., Abel, M., Wesarg, F., Ruth, P., & Hipler, U.-C. (2013, September–October). Application of a Drainage Film Reduces Fibroblast Ingrowth into Large-Pored Polyurethane Foam during Negative-Pressure Wound Therapy in an in Vitro Model. *Wound Repair and Regeneration, 21*(5), 697. doi:10.1111/wrr.12073

World Health Organization. (2018). *Global Guidelines for the Prevention of Surgical Site Infection.* Geneva: World Health Organization. Retrieved April 2, 2020, from https://apps.who.int/iris/bitstream/handle/10665/277399/9789241550475-eng.pdf?ua=1

Wu, K., Wu, X., Chen, M., Wu, H., Jiao, Y., & Zhou, C. (2020, May 1). H_2O_2-Responsive Smart Dressing for Visible H_2O_2 MonitoringMand Accelerating Wound Healing. *Chemical Engineering Journal, 387*, 124127. doi:10.1016/j.cej.2020.124127

Xie, X., McGregor, M., & Dendukuri, N. (2010, November). The Clinical Effectiveness of Negative Pressure Wound Therapy: A Systematic Review. *Journal of Wound Care, 19*(11), 490. doi:10.12968/jowc.2010.19.11.79697

Yang, Y., Bechtold, T., Redl, B., Caven, B., & Hu, H. (2017). A Novel Silver-Containing Absorbent Wound Dressing Based on Spacer Fabric. *Journal of Materials Chemistry B, 33*(5), 6786. doi:10.1039/c7tb01286a

Yang, Y., & Hu, H. (2017, July 1). Spacer Fabric-Based Exuding Wound Dressing – Part II: Comparison with Commercial Wound Dressings. *Textile Research Journal, 87*(12), 1481. doi:10.1177/0040517516654110

Yang, Y., & Hu, H. (2018, February). Application of Superabsorbent Spacer Fabrics as Exuding Wound Dressing. *Polymers (Basel), 10*(2), 210. doi:10.3390/polym10020210

Young, S. R., & Hampton, S. (2005). Pain Management in Leg Ulcers Using ActiFormCoolTM. *Wounds UK, 1*(3), 94.

Yu, A. (2015). *Development of Pressure Therapy Gloves for Hypertrophic Scar Treatment.* Hong Kong: The Hong Kong Polytechnic University. Retrieved from http://hdl.handle.net/10397/35460

Yu, A., Yick, K. L., Ng, S. P., & Yip, J. (2016, September 1). Orthopaedic Textile Inserts for Pressure Treatment of Hypertrophic Scars. *Textile Research Journal, 86*(14), 1549. doi:10.1177/0040517515573409

Yu, C., Hu, Z.-Q., & Peng, R.-Y. (2014). Effects and Mechanisms of a Microcurrent Dressing on Skin Wound Healing: A Review. *Military Medical Research*, *1*, 24. doi:10.1186/2054-9369-1-24

Yu, C., Xu, Z.-X., Hao, Y.-H., Gao, Y.-B., Yao, B.-W., Zhang, J., Wang, B., Hu, Z.-Q., & Peng, R.-Y. (2019). A Novel Microcurrent Dressing for Wound Healing in a Rat Skin Defect Model. *Military Medical Research*, *6*, 22. doi:10.1186/s40779-019-0213-x

Yu, L., Kronen, R. J., Simon, L. E., Stoll, C. R., Colditz, G. A., & Tuuli, M. G. (2018, February). Prophylactic Negative Pressure Wound Therapy after Cesarean Is Associated with Reduced Risk of Surgical Site Infection: A Systematic Review and Meta-Analysis. *American Journal of Obstetrics & Gynecology*, *218*(2), 200. doi:10.1016/j.ajog.2017.09.017

Zhang, L., Yin, H., Lei, X., Lau, J. N., Yuan, M., Wang, X., Wang, B., Hu, Z.-Q., & Wu, J. (2019). A Systematic Review and Meta-Analysis of Clinical Effectiveness and Safety of Hydrogel Dressings in the Management of Skin Wounds. *Frontiers in Bioengineering and Biotechnology*, *7*, 342. doi:10.3389/fbioe.2019.00342

Zhou, J., Tun, T. N., Hong, S.-H., Mercer-Chalmers, J. D., Laabei, M., Young, A. E., & Jenkins, A. T. (2011, December 15). Development of a Prototype Wound Dressing Technology Which Can Detect and Report Colonization by Pathogenic Bacteria. *Biosensors and Bioelectronics*, *30*(1), 67. doi:10.1016/j.bios.2011.08.028

Zhou, J., Yao, D., Qian, Z., Hou, S., Li, L., Jenkins, A. T., & Fan, Y. (2018, April). Bacteria-Responsive Intelligent Wound Dressing: Simultaneous In Situ Detection and Inhibition of Bacterial Infection for Accelerated Wound Healing. *Biomaterials*, *161*, 11. doi:10.1016/j.biomaterials.2018.01.024

6

Additives for Enhanced Functionality

6.1 Enhancing Dressing Functionality

The base materials and structural forms of wound dressings – foams, films, textiles, sponges, etc. – provide their core properties, particularly most of the mechanical and physical characteristics. Some materials, by virtue of their composition, also offer other biological or chemical properties beneficial for the wound healing process, e.g., collagen and other proteins can act as sacrificial materials to mop up excess MMPs in chronic wounds; calcium ions in calcium alginate fibres assist in the coagulation cascade to promote blood clotting. As wound dressings evolved and improved over the last few decades, more emphasis is currently being laid on making them an active rather than a passive part of a treatment or care. Extra processing is performed on base materials to develop additional features that add new functionality to the dressing. One of the largest categories of additional functionality is the antimicrobial feature, which serves the aims of speeding up wound healing as well as managing odour and patient comfort. Other added functionalities to speed up wound healing include haemostatic properties, anti-inflammatory effects, proteinase management and growth factors. Functionalities that relate to patient comfort include odour control and pain relief.

In the majority of cases, additional functionalities are imparted by using additives. These can be incorporated into fibres, films, and other forms during the polymer manufacturing process, or as an after-treatment onto already formed substrates. Common techniques that are used as after-treatments consist of coating, spraying and impregnating.

6.2 Antimicrobials

In the last couple of decades, demand for antimicrobial dressings has increased significantly in certain markets, primarily North America. The latter has been the largest consumer of anti-infective products, partly due to the high number of surgical procedures and the high adoption rate of advanced wound dressings. It was recently expected that the global antimicrobial wound dressing market will grow at a CAGR of 5.56% to reach USD 4.6 billion in 2026 (Verified Market Research, 2020). This growth is somewhat driven by the need to ensure that patients heal in a timely manner and with as little complication as possible over the wound healing period. Where in some countries, antimicrobials are used prophylactically and liberally, in other countries, their use is more moderated, cautioned by the perceived risk of increasing bacterial resistance.

6.2.1 Silver, Including Nano Silver

Silver is commonly used in ointments and creams, particularly for burns, where silver sulfadiazine is one of the well-known gold standards of care. The use of silver naturally progressed from topical applications to it being attached or contained within a dressing, thus eliminating one step in the treatment, and improving the ease of care for the clinician and comfort for the patient. While it has been demonstrated that silver-containing creams have superior bactericidal effects *in vitro* (Castellano et al., 2007), the overall benefits of silver dressings need to be taken into consideration in the choice of treatment. For example, a small study showed that reported pain levels and the number of treatments required were less when a silver textile dressing was used, as compared with silver sulfadiazine on burn patients (Yarboro, 2013). In another small study, a silver foam dressing was found to result in less pain, faster wound healing and patient discharge, and less hospital and dressing costs compared with the use of silver sulfadiazine with a regular dressing (Gupta et al., 2017). Despite insufficient strong evidence in favour of silver dressings due to the small size of studies (Lo et al., 2008), the overall positive clinical experience of silver in wound dressings has made it the current leading antimicrobial agent used commercially. It is used in multiple formats – inorganic silver compounds (e.g., silver oxide, silver phosphate, silver chloride, silver sulphate, silver-calcium-sodium phosphate, silver zirconium), elemental silver (e.g., metallic silver, nanocystalline silver) and organic complexes (e.g., silver-zinc allantoinate, silver alginate, silver carboxymethylcellulose) (Wounds International, 2012). It has been successfully applied on different substrates, including nonwoven textiles, foams, meshes, sponges, hydrogels, etc., by coating, impregnating, spraying, and other techniques. Some examples of commercially available dressings with different forms of silver and different substrates are given in Box 6.1.

It is understood that whatever the format of the silver on the dressing, it is ultimately the availability of silver ions (Ag+) that has the bactericidal effect (Wilkinson et al., 2011; Mondal et al., 2020). In some dressings, these silver cations are attached to the substrate, and act when the bacteria-containing exudate gets absorbed into its structure. In others, the silver ions are released

---

BOX 6.1   EXAMPLES OF COMMERCIALLY AVAILABLE SILVER-CONTAINING DRESSINGS

- AQUACEL® Ag range (Convatec) – silver chloride on CMC textile substrate
- Mepilex® Ag range (Mölnlycke) – silver sulphate particles in PU foam substrate
- Silverlon® range (Argentum Medical) – metallic silver coated onto nylon textile substrate
- Tegaderm™ Ag range (3M) – silver sulphate coated onto cotton mesh substrate
- ACTICOAT◊ range (Smith + Nephew) – nanocrystalline silver onto multicomponent textile substrate
- ALLEVYN◊ Ag range (Smith + Nephew) – hydrocellular PU foam with silver sulfadiazine
- TRITEC® Silver (Milliken) – ceramic (complexed) silver zirconium phosphate, onto micro-knit textile substrate
- V.A.C.® GRANUFOAM SILVER™ (Acelity) – micro-bonded metallic silver impregnated in foam sponge
- PolyMem® Silver (Ferris Mfg. Corp.) – nanocrystalline silver particles in foam layer

---

onto the wound bed, with the exudate or other fluids (such as added saline) acting as the carrying medium. The presence of fluids is essential for the release of the silver ions. When a wound is dry, the application of a saline solution is advocated to assist in the release of the ions, and to help with moist wound healing in parallel. The silver cations can be released during an ion exchange process in the wound fluid or saline; or can be released through oxidation of elemental silver particles, which is made faster in an aqueous environment (Kostenko et al., 2010; Wounds International, 2012).

6.2.1.1 Mechanisms of Action

The presence of silver ions $Ag+$ is believed to have several effects on bacteria (Lo et al., 2008; Wilkinson et al., 2011; Wounds International, 2012; Mölnlycke, 2020). Firstly, when the cation binds to the surface of the bacteria, it can cause disruption and rupture of the cell walls, cell leakage and subsequent damages to the cell. Secondly, the ion can also bind to the bacteria's proteins and enzymes, preventing it from performing essential functions efficiently. Thirdly, $Ag+$ could also bind with cell DNA and RNA and interfere with cell multiplication. Finally, it can also interfere with thiol groups and provoke the generation of ROS, a major contributor to antibacterial efficacy.

Because of the generic way its positive ions interfere with the proteins and enzymatic systems of microorganisms, silver has a broad-spectrum activity, which makes it a popular choice as antimicrobial treatment. Although it can be argued that not all silver dressings have the same antimicrobial efficacy, several *in vitro* studies have demonstrated the effectiveness of silver ions and nanoparticles at inhibiting the growth of a large number of aerobic and anaerobic bacteria, yeast and fungi, and antibiotic-resistant bacteria (Bowler et al., 2004; 3M, 2006; Rai et al., 2014). The variations in bactericidal properties of different dressings are attributed mainly to differences in silver content, silver release profiles, types of silver, shape and size of particles and the bacteria itself. It is noted for example that gram-negative bacteria seem to be more prone to the effects of Ag+ on cell wall disruption than gram-positive bacteria due to the difference in their cell wall structure (Liao et al., 2019). In addition, in the case of nano silver wound dressings, the bactericidal effects would seem to depend on the nanoparticle characteristics – size, shape, surface charge, dose and particle dispersion state. In their 2019 review, Liao and colleagues summed up that silver nanoparticles that were well dispersed performed better than agglomerated ones, that smaller sized particles exhibited the highest antibacterial activity, that truncated triangular silver nanoplates were more efficacious than spherical and rod-shaped nano particles, and that positively charged particles had better bactericidal activity than negatively charged or neutral ones.

The potentially rapid availability of the ions to the wound bed (particularly in the case of nano silver and soluble silver compounds), combined with the fact that natural equilibrium of silver ion content is maintained at the wound bed means that rapid and long-term sustained release are also possible for the right combination of silver/substrate format (Bowler et al., 2004; 3M, 2006; Bradford et al., 2009).

6.2.1.1.1 Silver and Biofilms

In the case of efficacy against non-planktonic bacteria in biofilms, silver dressings have been found to be bactericidal to some extent, but the long-term efficacy varies as does the potency of the effect on different bacteria strains. Silver cations can bind to electron donor groups of bacterial cells and extracellular polymeric substances (EPS), and thereon interfere with the intermolecular forces in the biofilm, and facilitate the biofilm dispersion. It has been found that a small concentration of silver ions (50 ppb) is sufficient to destabilise the biofilm matrix in this way by reducing the number of binding sites available (Chaw et al., 2005). The combined result of this destabilisation and the bactericidal action of silver ions can be seen *in vitro* in the first day or two of dressing application (Percival et al., 2008; Thorn et al., 2009; Kostenko et al., 2010). However, depending on the *in vitro* model used, biofilms have been found to recover after 7 days, consistent with some clinical findings (Kostenko et al., 2010).

6.2.1.2 Silver Safety and Risks

In general, the amount of silver from wound dressings that a patient is likely to be in contact with for the duration of a treatment is considered to be low enough not to be a serious health hazard, compared to the potential benefits.

Silver is not listed as a carcinogen (National Toxicology Program (NTP), 2016) and it has been commonly and historically used in the medical care and in consumer goods. However, there have always been concerns about various potential risks of the use of silver, and about the unknown effects of nanosized silver.

6.2.1.2.1 Known Reactions to Silver

There is no evidence in the literature to suggest that silver has a toxic effect on the immune, cardiovascular, nervous or reproductive system in humans (Wilkinson et al., 2011). There is a low potential for skin irritation: rare occurrences of skin reactions (irritation or allergy) have been reported, although this seems to be correlated with higher occupational exposure to silver (Group & Lea, 2010). The irritation presents itself as a contact dermatitis, which is an inflammatory skin reaction that can manifest in different ways such as erythema, oedema, vesiculation and pruritus. However, only one case of reaction with a silver product (silver sulfadiazine cream) has been reported so far (Group & Lea, 2010), and none yet with a silver dressing.

A rare reported side effect of the use of silver dressings is argyria-like symptoms. Argyria itself is an infrequent, permanent, but non-life-threatening discolouration of the skin caused by silver deposition and often linked with the ingestion of colloidal silver. The effect may be exacerbated when the skin is exposed to the sun. Related symptoms with the use of silver wound dressings have tended to be temporary or semi-permanent, therefore not considered argyria itself (Trop et al., 2006; Zweiker et al., 2014). The total body content of silver necessary to cause argyria has been suggested to be in the range of 3.8–6.4 g, which is unlikely to be achieved with systemic absorption of silver via wound dressings (Wounds International, 2012).

6.2.1.2.2 Silver Levels in the Body

Linked with temporary argyria-like symptoms, Trop et al. (2006) also reported concurrent but temporary elevated levels of silver in plasma, urine and liver enzymes. In an *in vivo* study, Wang et al. (2009) also found silver depositions in porcine internal organs, and found from their paediatric burns clinical study that overall serum silver levels were correlated with burn size, with a few exceptions. A study of 30 patients by Vlachou et al. (2007) supported the evidence of elevated serum silver levels during the use of a nanocrystalline silver dressing on burns. The silver levels subsequently dropped down at the 6 months follow up. The authors concluded from their study that there were no haematological or biochemical indicators of toxicity associated with the absorption of silver. Another small study on patients with chronic wounds also found elevated silver levels in half of the patients after a month of treatment but no toxicity was detected (Brouillard et al., 2018). A propensity for higher systemic silver absorption was linked to wound size, anaemia, malnutrition and possibly on wound vascularisation. The study also emphasised the slow elimination of silver from the body.

Silver is not normally absorbed in the central or peripheral nervous systems, but it can be absorbed systemically through biological membranes. The two main factors that affect how easily silver can penetrate the membranes are the particle size and the degree of ionisation (Wilkinson et al., 2011). Soluble silver compounds would therefore diffuse more easily than metallic or insoluble particles. Silver ions are believed to traverse membranes by binding onto intracellular proteins, particularly serum albumins and macroglobulins, and they are normally excreted via the biliary route in faeces and urine (Langsdown, 2010).

6.2.1.2.3 Nanosized Silver

Much of the above-mentioned work on the silver levels in the body has been done with nanocrystalline silver dressings, which is also where a lot of the current concerns have been. The ionisation of metallic silver is in proportion to the size of the particle – the smaller the particle, the greater the surface area, and the greater the release of Ag+ (Langsdown, 2010). This suggests that while the initial bactericidal properties of nano silver particles would be high, the total amount of silver released and absorbed by the body may also follow. It was also observed that the uptake of nano silver by the body is influenced by the size of the nanoparticles. Wu et al. (2019) showed that *in vitro*, the size of nano silver particles affects the efficiency of cellular uptake and the type of endocytosis. 5 nm particles were found in both cytoplasm and nucleus half an hour after incubation; 100 nm particles migrated with more difficulty, but were found in the nucleus 12 hours after incubation. Once free inside the cytoplasm, silver nanoparticles have the potential to initiate oxidative damage. While this effect raises some concerns regarding the cytotoxicity of nano silver particles, it also provides an additional mechanism of action for faster and enhanced bactericidal effects. The rapid penetration of nano particles inside the bacterial cells results in faster interaction with proteins and DNA and eventually bacterial cell death (Liao et al., 2019). This would be in addition to a faster release of Ag+ ions to the bacterial environment.

6.2.1.2.4 Cytotoxicity and Wound Healing

The bactericidal and tissue cytotoxity of silver nano particles (and indeed of silver compounds) seem to go hand in hand, as they follow a similar mode of action. An *in vitro* study by Singh and Ramarao (2012) showed that silver nanoparticles can cause mitochondrial damage, induce cell apoptosis and lead to cell death by releasing silver ions inside the cytoplasm. AshaRani et al. (2009) also demonstrated that silver nanoparticles reduced the ATP[1] content of cells, which in turn caused mitochondrial damage and an increased production of ROS, in a dose-dependent manner. The net effect of excessive ROS can result in oxidative damage to DNA. It can be argued however that as the body already has its own cellular antioxidant mechanism to protect the cells from oxidative damage, the net effect of tissue cell death via excess ROS is moderated by the body's natural defence mechanism and only adversely affected when these defences are overwhelmed (Wilkinson et al., 2011).

A number of cell culture *in vitro* studies have therefore unsurprisingly reported the varying cytotoxic effects of silver dressings (Lam et al., 2004; Paddle-Ledinek et al., 2006; Burd et al., 2007; Wiegand et al., 2009; Zou et al., 2013; Boonkaew et al. 2014; Hajská et al., 2017). The results often depend on the test model used, and silver dressings show a range of variations in *in vitro* cytotoxic effects. Cell viability, morphology and proliferation and protein synthesis were reported to be affected by a range of silver dressings, compared to non-silver controls. In some *in vivo* models, an inhibition of reepithelialisation has also been observed with some dressings (Burd et al., 2007). However, in other models, wound healing has been found to be accelerated with silver dressings (Wright et al., 2002; Hiro et al., 2012). The mechanisms of this effect could be linked to a moderation of the inflammatory stage, through the generation of ROS from silver ions, which can also stimulate cell proliferation, the inhibition of certain proteinases by the silver ions, and to the induced apoptosis of inflammatory cells (Wilkinson et al., 2011). Evidence from *in vitro* cytotoxicity tests should therefore not be used in isolation in assessing the risks, and especially the risks/benefits balance associated with silver. The use of silver prophylactically is not generally recommended where the risk of infection can be managed otherwise, e.g., with surgical wounds (World Health Organization, 2018).

6.2.1.2.5 Bacterial Resistance

There are two common concerns linked to bacterial resistance: that bacteria will develop resistance to silver by genetically modifying itself, and that excessive use of silver dressing will increase the prevalence of bacteria resistant to antibiotics. According to the consensus group from Wounds International (2012), although theoretically possible, there has been no evidence so far to prove the latter and bacterial resistance to silver appears to be very rare. This is due to the way silver ions generically interact with microbial cells, and the fact that silver does not target any specific bacteria but instead is indiscriminate in its action. Resistance of a wound to a silver treatment however does exist – but this could be linked to other issues, including the presence of recalcitrant biofilms, or inappropriately managed underlying comorbidities.

6.2.1.2.6 Environment

There are concerns about the effect of the excessive use of silver, particularly as it is also used in consumer goods such as washable antimicrobial fabrics, paint, plastics, cosmetics and domestic appliances. Principally, the concerns revolve around the release of silver into the environment from the manufacturing process or disposal, and the potential impact of silver ions on the aquatic environment and in the food chain (Wilkinson et al., 2011).

A greater concern is felt regarding the increasing use of nano-sized silver particles, as these can be toxic even at low concentrations and tend to be difficult to detect and characterise in environmental waters (Walters et al., 2014; McGillicuddy et al., 2017). The impact of silver nanoparticles depends on the volume released in the environment, the particle size, the particle coating and aggregation effects, if any. Aggregation is thought to reduce the toxicity of nanoparticles, and the environment in which the particles are released affects the aggregation or disaggregation (Walters et al., 2014). For example, aggregation is enhanced in marine waters compared with fresh water. In the context of silver dressings, the highest risk to the aquatic environment is during the manufacturing process. As a finished product, the majority of silver-containing dressings ends up in landfills, either as decontaminated soiled dressings, unused cut or whole dressings, or manufacturing waste.

A study of the impact of silver nanoparticles and silver ions on the operations of a landfill bioreactor concluded that silver ions had minimal impact on methane production at a concentration of 10 mg/Kg (Yang et al., 2013). Currently, the majority of silver-containing dressings and the largest volumes are those that utilise silver compounds. The study however showed that nano silver is more toxic and inhibits methanogenesis due to a slow and long-term Ag+ release. It can be argued that the wound dressing sector accounts for only a small amount of the total global silver and nano silver consumption (Wounds International, 2012) and that therefore contributes proportionately to only a small amount released in the aquatic and landfill environment. However, it does play a part alongside other users and therefore further monitoring of the usage and disposal trends and the effects on the environment are required. The variability in the characteristics of silver and its nanoparticles currently results in a degree of uncertainty in the ecological assessments of silver wound dressings, adding to the lack of solid and long-standing evidence on this topic. It is nevertheless essential that environmental risks related to the manufacture of silver dressings are mitigated. The impact of silver on landfill as decontaminated or unused dressings should also be regularly reviewed.

6.2.2 Iodine

Iodine has been used in household first aid, pre-surgery skin preparations and wound care for decades due to its antiseptic abilities. Initially used as aqueous or alcoholic solutions, they were then associated with staining, irritation, and instability of solution. Subsequently, iodophors – iodine-releasing agents – were developed. They are typically complexes of iodine and a solubilising agent, which act as a reservoir of active iodine. In the same token, bonding the iodine with another molecule reduces its toxicity and makes it more gradually released into the wound environment (Sibbald et al., 2011). The antimicrobial mode of action is not exactly known, but it is believed that it is molecular iodine (I_2) which imparts the antimicrobial effects. In their review of published literature, McDonnell and Russell (1999) sum up the iodine-caused bacterial cell death to be linked to the penetration of molecular iodine into microorganisms and its interaction with key groups of proteins, particularly free-sulphur amino acids, nucleotides and fatty acids. Like silver, iodine impairs the metabolic activities of key enzymes, denaturing DNA and disrupting the cell membrane (Smith + Nephew, 2020). Also, like silver, because of the way the iodine molecules interact with cells, they have a broad-spectrum activity, against bacteria, viruses, fungi, spores, protozoa, and amoebic cysts (Bigliardi et al., 2017; Acelity, 2020; Gillam et al., 2021; Smith + Nephew, 2020).

Povidone-iodine (also known as iodopovidone), poloxamer iodine and cadexomer iodine are the commonly used iodophors for the disinfection of skin and minor wounds. They are available as ointments and gels and are also used impregnated in dressings for the treatment of various types of wounds. Examples of iodine-containing wound dressings are provided in Box 6.2. Iodine dressings make up the second largest category of antimicrobial dressings after silver, in terms of market size, but concerns over the cytotoxicity of iodine, based on early experiences with tinctures and animal studies, have limited its market size and growth. The evidence on *in vitro* and *in vivo* cytotoxicity is conflicting (Sibbald et al., 2011; Bigliardi et al., 2017; Sood et al., 2014). *In vitro* tests of a range of antimicrobial dressings, including povidone-iodine impregnated gauze showed that the sensitivity of cells differed according to test cell types (Hajská et al., 2017). The model using murine fibroblasts showed the iodine product to be more cytotoxic after 24 hours, but by contrast, the human dermal fibroblasts model showed better cell adherence.

A systematic review of the use of iodine products for the treatment of different contaminated wounds concluded that iodine was an effective antiseptic agent, not inferior to other antiseptic products, and not associated with adverse side effects or delays in healing, particularly for chronic and burn wounds (Vermeulen et al., 2010). Leaper and Durani (2008), and Sibbald et al.

BOX 6.2 EXAMPLES OF COMMERCIALLY AVAILABLE IODINE-CONTAINING DRESSINGS

- IODOFLEX◊ pads (Smith + Nephew) – cadexomer iodine in microbeads, on textile pads
- Iodosorb* sheet dressings (Smith + Nephew) – cadexomer iodine with PEG on textile base
- INADINE™ (Acelity) – 10% povidone-iodine with PEG on knitted textile base
- Povitulle® (CD Medical) – povidone-iodine on textile tulle base

(2011) reviewed the *in vitro*, *in vivo* and clinical evidence on iodophors and concluded that they are safe, can improve healing rates and are effective antimicrobials. Bacterial resistance was noted to be very rare and debatable, and evidence on cytotoxicity on animal studies seems to be counteracted by effective healing rates in human studies. With regard to safety in use, Sibbald et al. (2011) advised medical supervision in patients with thyroid diseases and iodine sensitivity, pregnant and breastfeeding women, newborns, infants and children with large burn areas. Proven allergies to povidone iodine are rare, but some reactions to iodinated contrast media can occur (Bigliardi et al., 2017).

6.2.2.1 Iodine and Biofilms

An interesting aspect of the antimicrobial efficacy of iodine is its reported good performance on biofilms, particularly in comparison with silver dressings (Fitzgerald et al., 2017; Roche et al., 2019). A systematic literature review of the effect of topical agents on biofilms found that from an *in vitro* perspective, iodine had the highest log reduction observed compared to other antimicrobials, including silver (Schwarzer et al., 2020). A comparison of an iodine hydrogel dressing with a silver dressing found that with the *in vitro* model used, the iodine dressing demonstrated superior anti-biofilm efficacy in 24 hours of test (Thorn et al., 2009). Over this same test timeframe, povidone-iodine formulations of different concentrations were also found to exhibit superior anti-biofilm activity *in vitro* than other tested antimicrobial agents (Hoekstra et al., 2017). Using a slightly more mature biofilm (3 days), another study on the efficacy of different antimicrobials on porcine explant biofilms concluded that cadexomer iodine was the most effective, and even outperformed its povidone-iodine counterpart (Phillips et al., 2009). Iodine was also observed *in vitro* to be able to disrupt 7-day mature biofilms, an effect which could not be achieved with the comparable silver dressings or antibiotic treatments in the study (Hill et al., 2010). This long-term efficacy was noted for the iodine-containing dressings only, not for the equivalent solution treatment. Presumably, this was because of a sustained release of the antimicrobial over the test period; but it could also be linked to the effect of the gel-based carrier of the iodine complex on the dressings.

6.2.3 Honey

Honey has been used both as a wound healing and antimicrobial agent, applied directly onto wounds or impregnated onto dressings (some examples are given in Box 6.3). As a natural product, there are significant differences between different honey types, depending on the sources and the associated environmental conditions, including the flora type, bee species, their nutritional behaviour and geographical location, the harvesting process, storage

---

BOX 6.3   EXAMPLES OF COMMERCIALLY AVAILABLE HONEY DRESSINGS AND OINTMENTS

Dressings
- Actilite (Advancis Medical) – Manuka honey and oil onto a viscose textile net
- L-Mesitran® Net (H&R Healthcare) – unspecified medical-grade honey with antioxidants on textile net base

Ointments
- Medihoney® (Comvita) – Manuka honey
- Activon® (Advancis Medical) – Manuka honey
- L-Mesitran® (H&R Healthcare) – unspecified medical-grade honey

---

conditions and so on (Cooper, 2014). This makes it difficult to generalise on the efficacy of honey and could be a reason for the lack of sufficient data to support its more widespread use. The type of honey with the most reported therapeutic benefits is Manuka honey (*Leptospermum scoparium*), which is available as food-grade, or as medical-grade ointments or impregnated on dressings (examples of which are provided in Box 6.3). Medical-grade honey is processed with full traceability and stricter controls on the local environmental and processing factors, thus resulting in reduced variability of batches within the same source.

As an antimicrobial, the activity of honey is generally broad spectrum and the mechanism of action on bacterial and fungal cells is linked to several factors. The osmolarity of this supersaturated solution of sugars make it bacteriostatic to start with – few water molecules are freely available for bacteria to grow in. However, even when diluted, some honey varieties still inhibit bacterial growth. It is believed that this effect is caused by a combination of the acidic environment with the production of hydrogen peroxide by the enzyme glucose oxidase, and additionally by phytochemical factors and likely the synergistic effects of all (Cooper et al., 1999; French et al., 2005; Olaitan et al., 2007; Kwakman et al., 2010; Oryan et al., 2016; Alnaimat et al., 2018). Indirect antimicrobial effects have also been suggested, through immunomodulation via the stimulation of lymphocytes and antibody production, and through the presence of nitric oxide metabolites (Lee et al., 2011; Oryan et al., 2016).

Honey has also been reported to have some anti-biofilm properties, interfering with the biofilm formation process, as well as disrupting and penetrating the network of existing structures to directly affect bacterial cells (Cooper, 2014; Lu et al., 2014; Phillips et al., 2015). These latter studies reported that bacterial resistance has not been identified from microorganisms isolated directly from patients nor from *in vitro* experiments of prolonged exposure to planktonic bacteria, but Cooper (2014) noted that a reduced susceptibility to antibiotics and honey has been observed in persister cells of treated biofilms.

One active ingredient in honey that has been identified as being a key player, particularly in Manuka honey is methylglyoxal (MGO). This compound was demonstrated to be strongly linked to the pronounced antibacterial activity of the honey, even in a diluted state (Mavric et al., 2008). It is typically found in larger amounts in Manuka honey, which has been used as an explanation for its more potent antimicrobial properties. An *in vitro* study of the antibacterial effects of MGO-containing textile wound dressings demonstrated the ability of the compound to inhibit the growth of bacteria (Bulman et al., 2017). MGO has also been identified as one of the components that contributes to the anti-biofilm properties of honey (Cooper, 2014). Interestingly, Lu et al. (2014) reported that on its own, MGO is ineffective as an anti-biofilm agent, which indicates that a synergistic effect with other components of the honey is required. From a wound healing perspective, Majtan (2011) highlighted that high levels of MGO may pose a potential risk for the healing of wounds of diabetic patients due to its role as a protein-glycating agent and being a precursor of advanced glycation end products.

With regard to other risks, compared to iodine and silver, the mechanism of antimicrobial action is less likely to demonstrate honey to be cytotoxic in *in vitro* tests. A comparison of untreated control, honey dressing and nano-crystalline silver dressing conducted *in vitro* using human keratinocyte and fibroblast cultures showed that the honey-based product had excellent cyto-compatibility compared with the silver counterpart (Du Toit & Page, 2009). The *in vitro* cytotoxic effect of honey may however be variable, depending on the test method used and, on the formulation used in the dressing. For example, Hajská et al. (2017) found that two honey dressings from the same manufacturer performed significantly differently in their model; viable cell counts of one after 24 hours was under 10% and the other above 70%.

6.2.3.1 Honey and Wound Healing

Honey has been reported to be beneficial for wound healing, aside from its antimicrobial effect. It can be used for gentle debridement and to reduce oedema. It has been shown to have some anti-inflammatory effect through the reduction of ROS production, stimulation of cytokine production and enhanced TNF-alpha release (Tonks et al., 2001, 2003, 2007). The low pH of honey may also assist in the wound healing process by increasing the amount of oxygen off-loaded from haemoglobin and suppressing excessive protease activity (Simon et al., 2009). *In vivo* testing of topical honey has shown the potential of faster healing compared to a control (Bergman et al., 1983; Iftikhar et al., 2010).

Clinically, the wound healing properties of honey have been investigated in several small trials and honey was found to be a safe treatment, with varying efficacy (Oryan et al., 2016). Reviews of topical honey used in superficial burns and wounds found that despite positive outcomes being observed, the evidence was not strong enough due to the size and quality of studies (Moore et al., 2001; Bull et al., 2015; Aziz & Hassan, 2017). In their Cochrane review, Bull et al. (2015) do however point out that honey appears to heal partial-thickness burns and post-operative wounds faster than conventional treatments.

6.2.4 Other Antibacterial Agents

6.2.4.1 Polyhexamethylene Biguanide (PHMB)

PHMB, also known as polyhexanide and polyaminopropyl biguanide, is an antiseptic and preservative commonly used in the cosmetic and personal care industry, including in contact lens solutions. It is also used as an antibacterial in wound care solutions and wound dressings (examples in Box 6.4). A number of *in vitro* and case studies have shown that PHMB is able to reduce bacteria load compared to an untreated control (Cazzaniga et al., 2002; Moore & Gray, 2007; Mulder et al., 2007; Gray et al., 2010). Comparing with silver dressings, a small clinical study found that both types of dressings reduced bioburden and pain, but the bacterial critical load was reduced faster and better in the PHMB group (Eberlein et al., 2011). The mechanism of action of PHMB is linked to its similarity to naturally occurring antimicrobial peptides and is understood to be at its best over a pH of 5–6 (Mulder et al., 2007; Gray et al., 2010). The positively charged polymer works against negatively charged microorganisms: it is believed to be able to adhere and disrupt cell membranes, causing them to leak, and to eventually penetrate cells and affect bacterial DNA. This interference with cells is reported to be stronger with the acidic lipids within bacterial membranes, and only weak with the neutral lipids of human cell membranes (Ikeda et al., 1984), helping to prevent damage to surrounding healthy tissues. In *in vitro* studies, Müller and Kramer (2008) calculated the ratio of cytotoxicity on cultured murine fibroblasts and antibacterial activity against two test organisms and concluded that PHMB was one of the better performing agents, with more antimicrobial than cytotoxic effects. Its performance in the test was better than povidone-iodine, silver nitrate and silver sulfadiazine.

BOX 6.4   EXAMPLES OF COMMERCIALLY AVAILABLE PHMB-CONTAINING DRESSINGS

- Suprasorb® X+PHMB (Lohmann & Rauscher) – biocellulose dressing with PHMB
- AMD range with PHMB (Cardinal Health) – dressings and foams with 0.2 and 0.5% PHMB
- ACTIVHEAL® PHMB Foam (Advanced Medical Solutions) – PU foam dressing with PHMB

The performance of PHMB on biofilms varies depending on the assessment method. An *ex vivo* study with porcine implants and *in vitro* biofilm model showed PHMB to be ineffective towards biofilms (Woods et al., 2012; Phillips et al., 2015), but a small study using a PHMB dressing concluded from healing data that the dressing was able to reduce biofilms in chronic wounds (Lensenlink & Andriessen, 2011). The use of PHMB in an irrigation solution was also found to be effective at reducing bacterial count on 24 hour *in vivo* biofilms, compared with other solutions (Davis et al., 2017).

6.2.4.2 Other Metal Nanoparticles (NPs)

While silver nanoparticles have been at the forefront of the nanoparticle route of dealing with the management of infections due to the prior commercial success of silver in wound care, other heavy metal nanoparticles have also been investigated in recent years as alternatives. Examples of metal and metal oxide NPs with demonstrated antimicrobial properties include zinc oxide (ZnO), copper, copper oxide, gold, iron oxide, aluminium oxide, titanium dioxide and silicon dioxide (Ren et al., 2009; Seil & Webster, 2012; Jamnongkan et al., 2015; Fernando et al., 2018; Mohandas et al., 2018; Negut et al., 2018). Antibiofilm properties have been reported for silver NPs, rhamnolipid-coated silver and iron oxide NPs and zinc oxide NPs (Markowska et al., 2013; Velázquez-Velázquez et al., 2015; Khalid et al., 2019; Kaur et al., 2020). The antimicrobial properties of metal NPs are believed to be caused by a combination of factors, some linked to the morphology of the particles and others to the metal component itself. For example, like silver, zinc and copper also exhibit antibacterial properties in their bulk form, but other materials such as iron oxide are not normally antimicrobial, but may exhibit some antimicrobial properties in their nanoparticulate form (Seil & Webster, 2012). Several mechanisms of action have been reported, with most NPs able to interfere, disrupt and penetrate cell membranes and generate ROS. Other mechanisms that are also believed to take place in combination with the previous are: (a) having a physical form that is abrasive to bacterial cell membranes, (b) protein inactivation and (c) bacterial flocculation/agglomeration leading to reduced cell viability. Several research groups have also combined metal NPs with other materials that have mild antibacterial properties, such as chitosan, thus creating antimicrobial materials with synergistic mechanisms of action.

With regard to the physical properties of the NPs, the smaller the particles, the greater their penetration into the bacteria's cells. The higher surface area per volume of smaller NPs leads to a larger and faster release of metal ions, which are the key instruments to affect the cell membrane and cell processes as well as accumulate ROS. A positive zeta potential creates an electrostatic interaction that promotes cell membrane penetration. On the other hand, as discussed with silver NPs in Section 6.2.1.2, the enhanced ability of the

NPs to penetrate biological membranes and generate ROS could also lead to increased potential toxicity to tissue cells. Several cell culture studies have demonstrated that similar to the antimicrobial effect, the higher the dose of NPs released, the less the cell viability (Seil & Webster, 2012). A degree of caution must therefore be exercised in the use of any NPs in wound care.

6.2.4.3 Essential Oils and Plant Extracts

Another recent area of research activity is the incorporation of natural antimicrobials or healing agents (oils and other extracts) into dressings as an alternative way of combatting or preventing infection. Essential oils are extracted from plants and their antimicrobial action is linked to the quality of the source, extraction and distillation process. It is also associated to the sufficient presence of certain components such as phenolic compounds thymol and carvacrol in oregano oil, linalool and linalyl in lavender oil, terpinene-4-ol and 1,8-cineole in tea tree oil and hyperforin in St John's wort (Negut et al., 2018). The mechanism of action has been associated with a disruption in the cell wall integrity and of certain cellular processes. A large number of natural essential oils have attracted interest in the development of new wound dressings recently and no single compound has been the focus of more intense scrutiny or commercial exploration. Examples investigated include cinnamon, lavender, tea tree, lemongrass, peppermint, eucalyptus, pepper, thyme, clove, chamomile blue, lemon, St John's Wort, rosemary, oregano, Zataria multiflora, Elicriso italico, orange and combinations thereof (Muthaiyan et al., 2012; Liakos et al., 2014, 2015; Rosa et al., 2018; Negut et al., 2018; Ardekani et al., 2019; Unalan et al., 2019; Liu et al., 2020; Qin et al., 2020). Many of these exploratory studies were able to demonstrate an effective zone of inhibition or reduction in bacterial count, and low *in vitro* cytotoxicity. However, some studies report a cytotoxic effect from certain oils, such as thyme and clove ones (Junka et al., 2019).

Taking inspiration from traditional medicine, a large number of natural plant extracts have been experimentally incorporated onto base substrates, and reported to result in antimicrobial dressings. Some examples include Moringa leaf extracts, curcumin (from turmeric), neem extracts, papaya leaf extracts, Tecomella undulate bark extracts, chamomile, henna, *Centella asiatica*, propolis and hinokitiol (Hussain et al., 2017; Fayemi et al., 2018; Pilehvar-Soltanahmadi et al., 2018; Rebia et al., 2019). The extracts contain or are phytochemicals such as phenolics, zeatin, kaempferom, quercetin and amino acids, and in some cases are reported to not only have an antibacterial effect, but to also contribute to improved wound healing. For example, the incorporation of curcumin into PCL/PEG nanofibre mats generated an antibacterial activity *in vitro*, and demonstrated faster wound closure on a murine wound model compared to the control without the natural active agent (Bui et al., 2014).

For many of the above natural ingredients, the base substrates of choice have been films, hydrogels, and electrospun nanofibres, for the relative ease with which the actives can be incorporated. The appeal of using natural actives often means that they are incorporated into other biodegradable or natural base materials, such as chitosan, PCL, alginates, zein, gelatine, PVA and their combinations. However, combinations and blends with other non-biodegradable materials or actives have also been developed, with the aim of obtaining multi-functional, synergistic benefits for wound care.

6.2.4.4 Antibiotics

As the prescription of antibiotics is a common treatment for infections, it is unsurprising to observe that there has also been some activity in the incorporation of various antibiotics into wound dressings, particularly nanofibrous structures. Compounds such as amoxicillin, ciprofloxacin, gentamicin, among many others have been impregnated onto standard textiles or foam dressings, or incorporated into films and nanofibrous mats, with some degree of success (Simões et al., 2018; Negut et al., 2018). However, while antibiotics can be effective, they do have specific antimicrobial targets, and suffer from the issues of increasing antibiotic resistance. These disadvantages and concerns make it difficult for them to become serious commercial competitors to the existing broad-spectrum antiseptic agents discussed above and their commercially available dressings.

6.2.5 Anti-Biofilms

Today, it is well accepted that biofilms play an important role in infected wounds, particularly chronic ones. The efficacy of silver, iodine, honey and PHMB, in preventing the formation of biofilms, and/or disrupting them has been briefly discussed above. Mostly, the effect of such antimicrobials is in affecting the microorganisms themselves. Other anti-biofilms actives, which may or may not have a direct effect on bacteria itself, can also be added to increase or supplement the anti-biofilm efficacy of a dressing. The mode of action of these actives is instead to interfere with the bacterial cellular communication, disrupt the film's intercellular matrix or alter cell metabolism, with some of them doing so without impairing the growth, integrity or reproduction of the microbial cells (Rhoads et al., 2008). Several strategies can be employed for fighting biofilms and some examples of ingredients that can help with each strategy are provided in a review by Roy et al. (2018), summed up in Table 6.1.

In terms of incorporation of the above for wound dressing applications, there are some challenges regarding the cytotoxicity of some of the components (at levels required for significant efficacy) or regarding successfully

TABLE 6.1

Active ingredients for anti-biofilm strategies

Strategy	Examples of ingredients
Interfering with quorum sensing (cell-to-cell communication)	Furanones, quercetin, curcumin
Inhibition of bacterial stringent response, inhibiting their survival under stress conditions	Certain peptides such as peptide 1018 and its derivatives, peptide 1037 and 1038
Enzymatic dispersion of EPS, releasing bacteria	DNases, Dispersin B
Cleavage of peptidoglycan, disrupting cell wall functions	Tannic acid, endolysins, epigallocatechin gallate (EGCG)
Biofilm disassembly through matrix degrading enzymes	Berberine, usnic acid
Neutralisation or disassembly of liposaccharides, disrupting the integrity of the cellular membrane	Antimicrobial peptides, polymyxins
Alteration of membrane potential or permeabilisation, disrupting the cytoplasmic membrane	Chlorhexidine, PHMB, lantibiotics such as nisin
Inhibition of cell division and survival	Chitosan, sodium citrate, tetrasodium ethylenediaminetetraacetic acid (EDTA)
Inhibition of adhesion	Cadexomer iodine, lactoferrin, xylitol
Inhibition and dispersion of biofilm by exo-polysaccharides	EPS273, Psl and Pel polysaccharides, PAM galactan

Source: Roy et al. (2018) and Loimaranta et al. (2020).

incorporating the compound. A number of them have been effectively incorporated into commercial solutions, and some on an experimental basis as dressings or used in combination with dressings. Some examples are chlorhexidine (Ambrogi et al., 2017), lactoferrin and xylitol gel with an antimicrobial dressing (Ammons et al., 2011), antimicrobial peptide ε-poly-l-lysine (Tavakolian et al., 2020), and Dispersin B spray used with an antimicrobial dressing (Gawande et al., 2014).

Commercially and clinically, not many wound dressings claim to have been designed to include actives specifically to combat biofilms. One example is Aquacel® Ag+, which as well as being able to release silver ions, also contains EDTA and a surfactant to work on disrupting the biofilm structure (Convatec, 2020). It is of note that *in vitro* testing on its efficacy on biofilms demonstrated that the dressing with the EDTA and surfactant was effective, but not the EDTA or surfactant alone, suggesting a combined synergistic effect for the anti-biofilm agent to work (Said et al., 2014). Other commercially available antimicrobial dressings have been demonstrated to have anti-biofilm efficacy, with sometimes conflicting results depending on the test method used. For example, Smith + Nephew demonstrated the efficacy of their Iodoflex◊ cadexomer iodine dressing on a porcine skin explant biofilm model study, and showed only a planktonic efficacy for Coloplast's Biatain® Ag dressing (Phillips et al., 2015). However, in their own study, Coloplast demonstrated anti-biofilm efficacy for both their Biatain® Ag and Biatain® Silicone Ag products (Christiansen & Allesen-Holm, 2020). Bourdillon (2016) explains that the model and assay conditions for *in vitro* biofilm studies can significantly affect results, particularly when some of the models aim at replicating very specific clinical conditions. In particular, she concludes that *in vitro* models with low exudate/media conditions tend to favour iodine as being more efficacious, whereas those models with higher exudate/media conditions show more positive results for silver-containing wound dressings.

6.3 Wound Healing Additives

Advanced wound care aims at speeding up or preventing a slowdown in the healing process while minimising discomfort for the patient. The four stages of wound healing (haemostasis, inflammation, proliferation, and remodelling/maturation) can each be assisted, with the right choice of dressing type and components. Additives used for the management of infection also have wound healing properties by default – they help progress the wound out of the inflammation stage by dealing with the infection. Some of them have been reported to have wound healing properties even on non-infected wounds, e.g., honey and other natural ingredients such as curcumin. Likewise, many base materials used may have some wound healing benefits, through the management of moisture and exudate, or by providing the right environment for the healing stage the wound is in. In this section, additional ingredients that are added to a dressing to help enhance the wound healing stages are discussed.

6.3.1 Haemostatic Additives

The ability to quickly help reduce blood outpour at an incident site, prior to hospitalisation can make a difference in the outcome for a patient, particularly if there are no nearby hospitals. In Chapter 4, several fibrous, particulate or film-forming base materials with haemostatic properties were introduced (chitosan, oxidised cellulose and alginates). Some of these, in particular oxidised cellulose and chitosan, can be impregnated as granules into standard gauze or other substrates as an additive to provide significant haemostatic effects, e.g., with ChitoGauze® XR Pro (by Prometheus Medical), HemCon® (by Tricol Biomedical) and Celox™ (Medtrade Products Ltd). Here, other additives that can be incorporated into such base materials or others to rapidly assist in the blood clotting cascade, are discussed. Along with systemic interventions, they form part of the toolkit available for immediate trauma assistance.

Kaolin is a natural inorganic mineral (aluminium silicate) used as an active ingredient in dressings for rapidly initiating and enhancing the clotting process. As it contacts blood, it immediately activates factor XII of the clotting cascade, which leads to the transformation of factor XII, XI and prekallikrein to their activated forms, and which in turn activate the rest of the coagulation cascade (Z-Medica, 2020). In its commercially available wound dressing format (QuikClot™, by Z-Medica), kaolin is impregnated onto a polyester/ rayon nonwoven gauze, and can be used at first point of care. It has also been used post-surgery as a way to control bleeding. Studies have demonstrated that kaolin-based dressings can help achieve a reduced haemostasis time following surgical procedures compared with manual or mechanical compression (Trabattoni et al., 2011; Roberts et al., 2017). Other studies at first point of care (prehospital care) have also highlighted the dressings as an effective tool to control haemorrhage prior to hospitalisation (Shina et al., 2015; Zietlow et al., 2015; Travers et al., 2016). Kaolin has now replaced zeolites, which were the first minerals used as haemostats in the QuickClot™ range, but resulted in an exothermic reaction and risk of thermal injury (Smith et al., 2013).

While some haemostats, including kaolin, work by enhancing the coagulation cascade, they can be ineffective if the body's own natural clotting mechanism is compromised, e.g., with coagulopathic bleeding. There are other haemostats however, such as chitosan granules, which will promote adherence to tissues and are able to physically block bleeding independent of the body's clotting mechanism (Khoshmohabat et al., 2016). Likewise, procoagulant supplementers also act irrespective of how well the body's own clotting mechanism is performing, by directly kick-starting the coagulation process. These natural coagulating additives (primarily the combination of fibrinogen and thrombin) have been integrated onto base materials such as collagen to create a number of solid bioresorbable fibrin sealant dressings and patches (Teng, 2020). Thrombin is a naturally occurring enzyme that converts fibrinogen into fibrin, which then starts a blood clot. The biological nature of the mechanism of action (as opposed to a mechanical or chemical one) leads to such technologies to be sometimes referred to as 'biologics'. Early use of fibrin sealants was in liquid form, but when used in the form of a bioresorbable dressing or patch, larger cavities can be filled without the need to be removed and manual pressure can also be applied to help in controlling the bleeding (Spotnitz, 2014). Fibrin sealant patches have been used with success in internal surgical procedures, including pulmonary, cardiovascular

BOX 6.5   EXAMPLES OF COMMERCIALLY AVAILABLE FIBRIN SEALANT PATCHES

- Tachosil® (Baxter) – human fibrinogen and thrombin on equine collagen sponge
- Evarrest® (Ethicon) – human fibrinogen and thrombin with a flexible composite textile patch of oxidised cellulose and polyglactin 910

and hepatic surgery (Koea et al., 2013; Spotnitz, 2014; Romero-Velez et al., 2020). Two commercial examples are given in Box 6.5.

6.3.2 Anti-Inflammatory and Pain Relief Ingredients

The inflammation stage of the wound healing process can be prolonged or delayed for many reasons, including infection or an imbalance of the wound fluid components, particularly when there is an excess of MMPs and oxidative stress. Wound dressing components or additives intended for other functions (e.g., for absorption or as antimicrobials) can help in progressing the inflammation stage via their inherent properties and effect on the wound. For example, by dealing with an infection, antimicrobials can help in taking a wound out of the inflammation stage. Many antimicrobials, such as silver, have even been shown to have anti-inflammatory effects, and some even in the absence of infections, e.g., honey and curcumin (Hadagali & Chua, 2014; Zhao et al., 2019). EDTA, mentioned above as an active ingredient against biofilms, has also been found to have anti-inflammatory effects via its ability to bind with MMPs to deactivate them. This mechanism of action is used for dressings such as Biostep◊ (Smith + Nephew) and ColActive® Plus (Covalon).

Collagen as a base material, and additive to promote wound healing in general is also reported to be able to moderate MMPs by acting as a sacrificial protein (Metzmacher et al., 2007; Bohn et al., 2016). Likewise, several base materials intended for fluid management (e.g., Hydrofiber® and superabsorbent fibres) have been shown to have the ability to sequester and inhibit excessive MMPs, and as a result, may help to reduce inflammation too (Wiegand & Hipler, 2013; Krejner & Grzela, 2015). With regard to pain, some base materials such as hydrogels and other gelling materials are known to be soothing during wear, which helps in pain management. As complementary technologies to the above, other active ingredients have been explored as potentials to develop anti-inflammatory wound dressings or those that can help with pain management.

One way to deal with local inflammation (and by default the pain that is associated with it) via the use of additives is to incorporate anti-inflammatory pharmaceutical actives into wound dressing substrates. Non-steroidal anti-inflammatory drugs (NSAIDs) and their more powerful counterpart, steroids (also called corticosteroids) are examples that have been explored so far. NSAIDs work by inhibiting cyclooxygenase enzymes, which in turn moderate the release of prostaglandins – a biological mediator for inflammation. Ibuprofen is a well-known NSAID and analgesic and has been successfully incorporated into a soft foam dressing (Biatain® Ibu by Coloplast). However, the manufacturers make no claim regarding anti-inflammatory effects, focusing instead on its pain-relieving benefits (Coloplast, 2020). Pain is of course one of the symptoms of inflammation. Ibuprofen, as well as ketoprofen, naxopren and diclofenac, other NSAID analgesics, have also been incorporated into a range of substrates, including electrospun PVA, PVA/PVP hydrogels, PVA/chitosan hydrogel membranes, chitosan hydrogels, collagen/chitosan scaffold, carboxymethylcellulose film and fibres, sodium alginate/gelatine/hyaluronic acid/reduced graphene oxide composite films, hyaluronic acid/cyclodextrin nanofibres, PCL/gelatine nanofibre mats and PLA/PGA scaffolds (Kenawy et al., 2007; Cantón et al., 2010; Vinklárková et al., 2015; Morgado et al., 2017; Basar et al., 2017; Aycan et al., 2019; Séon-Lutz et al., 2019; Rubina et al., 2019; Maver et al., 2019; Oustadi et al., 2020). While the anti-inflammatory or pain-relieving effects of the above combinations have not all been proven, some studies have demonstrated *in vitro* or *in vivo* a reduced response of fibroblasts to pro-inflammatory stimulators, a reduction in excessive inflammation and faster wound healing (Cantón et al., 2010; Morgado et al., 2017).

The second group of anti-inflammatory pharmaceutical actives incorporated in wound dressings are steroids, which are synthetic hormones developed to reduce inflammation and the activity of the immune system. Steroids work by suppressing multiple inflammatory genes that are activated when there is an inflammation. The negative side effects of the systemic use of steroids have encouraged its use as a topical agent for localised treatment. Experimental work has been conducted on the incorporation of a hydrocortisone and an antibiotic into chitosan-PEO nanofibre mats as potential material for wound dressings (Fazli et al., 2016). Nishiguchi and Taguchi (2020) reported an anti-inflammatory tissue adhesive wound dressing containing corticosteroid-modified gelatine particles. They found that the steroid-loaded microparticles were taken up by macrophages and effectively suppressed morphological changes of activated macrophages and the expression level of inflammatory cytokine. The use of topical steroids in combination with a dressing has been shown to be effective in speeding up healing or improving healing outcomes for certain wounds. For example, absorbable nasal packing impregnated with the steroid triamcinolone was found to be associated with improved healing following endoscopic sinus surgery (Côté & Wright, 2010). Case studies using hydrocortisone also demonstrated that it can be an effective, inexpensive and noninvasive option for treating hypergranulation tissue arising from burns (Jaeger et al., 2016).

6.3.3 Biologics for Enhancing Cell Proliferation

Several strategies have been explored for enhancing cell proliferation in chronic wounds. In Chapter 4, it was highlighted that various base materials such as collagen, hyaluronic acid and some other proteinaceous materials can have a positive effect on the proliferation of fibroblasts and keratinocytes. A route to further enhance this effect, or to provide an alternative way of promoting cell growth, is to incorporate cell-promoting biological components within a dressing.

The use of live cell cultures – keratinocytes and fibroblasts – on wounds is not new and they can now be reliably harvested and reproduced *in vitro*, even to form multi-layered epithelium. This approach has been explored since the early 1980s, particularly for the treatment of large burns. The treatment is delivered through cultured skin substitutes or cultured cells application using sprays. Live cells integrated into wound dressings are in principle able to boost the epithelialisation stage and/or kick-start the process. Human fibroblasts for example have been successfully added onto a resorbable sheet for use on diabetic foot ulcers (Dermagraft® by Organogenesis). A randomised controlled multicentre study on diabetic foot ulcers comparing the fibroblast-containing dressing with conventional therapy showed that the former resulted in more wound closure over the study period, with fewer ulcer-related adverse events (Marston et al., 2003). Human keratinocytes and fibroblasts have been added to bacterial cellulose/acrylic acid hydrogels, demonstrating an increased in healing rate and greater deposition of collagen *in vivo* (Mohamad et al., 2019).

The other biologic route is using growth factors, which are naturally occurring polypeptides that form a complex signalling network able to affect cell migration, infiltration, proliferation and differentiation (Barrientos et al., 2008). With the ability to promote collagen synthesis, growth factors, alongside other biological actives such as cytokines and matrikines, have been used in advanced cosmetics and skincare products, with claims around skin rejuvenation and reduction of signs of ageing. In the context of wound healing, growth factors are essential players in the four stages of wound healing, kicking off the inflammation stage, forming new tissue and closing the wound. There is a broad range of growth factors involved in the wound healing process; key ones have been identified as EGF, transforming growth factors beta (TGF-β), fibroblast growth factors (FGF), vascular endothelial growth factor (VEGF), granulocyte macrophage colony-stimulating factor (GM-CSF), platelet-derived growth factor (PDGF), connective tissue growth factor (CTGF), interleukins (IL), and tumour necrosis factors alpha (TNF-α) (Barrientos et al., 2008). In chronic wounds in particular, an extended inflammation stage results in an excessive proteolytic environment which degrades the body's own growth factors and cytokines, leaving cells unable to proliferate sufficiently. Growth factors, particularly in a state that can resist rapid degradation from the wound's excess proteases, have therefore been explored as potential topical actives to speed up the healing of chronic wounds and some have been experimentally integrated into advanced wound dressings.

From the literature, the most popular growth factor to be incorporated into a base substrate appears to be EGF and bFGF (basic fibroblast growth factors). Despite challenges such as easy decomposition and deactivation and difficulties in achieving consistent delivery, they have been incorporated into biological substrates such as hyaluronic acid, collagen and gelatine. These base materials are also known to have inherent properties that facilitate cell proliferation, creating therefore the perfect substrate for a combined wound healing effect. Several *in vitro* and *in vivo* studies have demonstrated that when EGFs and bFGFs are added to a base material, cell growth was improved and wound healing and closure were faster (Ulubayram et al., 2001; Mizuno et al., 2003; Tanaka et al., 2005; Schneider et al., 2009; Matsumoto & Kuroyanagi, 2010; Yu et al., 2013; Choi et al., 2018; Cheng et al., 2020). There is also a small amount of clinical evidence on the safety and efficacy of EGF-containing wound dressings. A collagen-gel matrix with EGF was evaluated on hard-to-heal venous leg ulcers and was found to be well tolerated, with significant wound surface reduction (Doerler et al., 2014). A hyaluronic acid/collagen sponge with EGF was used on a range of wound types in a preliminary clinical study, also demonstrated positive healing outcomes, with rapid epithelialisation (Yu et al., 2015).

6.4 Additives for Patient Comfort

Many wound dressings benefits associated with patient comfort are delivered by the base materials and its structural forms, discussed in Chapters 4 and 5. For example, the prevention of pain upon dressing changes can be achieved by using a wound dressing with a non-adherent wound contact layer. A soothing and cooling effect can be obtained with the use of high water content hydrogels, or gelling fibres. Patient mobility and the appearance of the dressed wound can be influenced by the choice of inobtrusive and flexible dressings, if appropriate.

Some comfort-related wound dressing benefits can be enhanced with additives. For example, the provision of analgesics in the wound dressing, addressed in Section 6.3.2, helps with pain management. In the same line of thought, the control of undesirable odours arising from a wound can also be done by incorporating certain actives into the wound dressing structure.

6.4.1 Odour Management

Malodour in an acute or chronic wound is normally linked to infection, and the general consensus is that dealing with the infection is preferred over masking the odour. Hence, the antimicrobial additives discussed in Section 6.2 can indirectly assist in reducing the discomfort rising from unpleasant odours by reducing the bacterial bioburden. Many dressings with antimicrobial additives such as silver and honey are thus indicated for malodorous wounds. Malodour, like pain, particularly when it occurs over a long period of time or is chronic, can have serious impacts on the quality of life and the mental health of patients, discouraging some to have social interactions due to embarrassment. As a result, over time, there have been a number of dressings developed specifically to address the issue of odour more directly by trapping or absorbing volatile organic compounds (VOCs).

The most common material used in odour management products in wound care is activated charcoal. A survey of clinicians on the topic indicated that charcoal was the most often used strategy for reducing wound odours, but only 48% of the respondent deemed it to be effective (Gethin et al., 2014). In the same survey, silver-containing dressings were ranked second best in frequency of use, but antimicrobial agents were generally cited as most effective. The use of aromatherapy to mask odours was only used by 8% of the 1444 participants.

Activated charcoal is characterised by its highly porous surface area, which enables it to absorb and trap malodorous gases, as well as bacteria and liquids (Akhmetova et al., 2016). Typically, the activated charcoal is produced by carbonising a carbonaceous base material, which can be as varied as coconut and palm shells, wood, husks and waste fibres. This process can be used to manufacture activated carbon granules or powder, which can be integrated into a wound dressing. Alternatively, activated carbon textiles that can be sandwiched in between other layers in a wound dressing can also be produced. Example products are given in Box 6.6.

An *in vitro* study of several odour-controlling dressings was conducted using diethylamine as test material to simulate odour-producing chemicals from the wound (Thomas et al., 1998). The results indicated that different dressings have different diethylamine-absorbing capabilities, and that products with both an absorbent layer and a charcoal component performed better in trapping the molecule. Clinically, the efficacy of activated charcoal has not been fully proven. It is thought that some of the deodorising activity may be hindered by the presence of proteins in the wound fluid. However, some case studies have reported the ability of such dressings to reduce malodour, alongside other wound management properties (Williams, 2000; Haycocks & Chadwick, 2014).

Cyclodextrins are another group of materials commonly used for odour management, e.g., in air and fabric fresheners and cosmetics, and also

> **BOX 6.6 EXAMPLES OF COMMERCIALLY AVAILABLE CHAR-**
> **COAL WOUND DRESSINGS**
>
> - CarboFlex® (Convatec) – five-layer textile dressing with a central activated charcoal pad, absorbent wound contact layer and water-resistant outer layer
> - CARBONET◊ (Smith + Nephew) – multilayer textile dressing with activated charcoal layer, non-adherent wound contact layer and absorbent padding layer
> - ACTISORB™ range (Acelity) – activated charcoal with silver in a non-adherent nylon sleeve
> - CliniSorb® (Clinimed) – activated charcoal cloth sandwiched between textile layers of viscose rayon and coated with polyamide to prevent adherence
> - Askina® Carbosorb (B Braun) – activated charcoal cloth layer with absorbent nonwoven layer of viscose rayon

explored in the wound dressing sector. By nature of their molecular form, these cyclic oligosaccharides are able to trap odour molecules within their ring-shaped structure. One example of a commercialised product is Medline's Exuderm® Odorshield™, a cyclodextrin-containing sheet hydropolymer (Medline Industries Inc., 2007). Lipman and Van Bavel (2007) demonstrated the *in vitro* odour-absorbing performance of this combination and reported two case studies. Another more recent report is that of β-cyclodextrin functionalised poly (ε-caprolactone) nanofibers, also shown to have efficient *in vitro* wound odour removal (Narayanan et al., 2015).

6.5 Other Additives

In this last section, it is worth highlighting the vast possibilities for additives in wound dressings, particularly with many recent technological advances enabling actives to be encased and protected until they need to be released. Within each functional category discussed in this chapter (anti-infectives, wound healing and comfort), new active ingredients will continue to emerge and be explored, some more than others, as is currently the case with silver. There are already a large number of other additives not discussed in this chapter, but which may need to be reviewed in the future. One example is the use of natural ingredients for healing, e.g., *aloe vera* and many other herbal extracts. Other skincare agents may also be of interest, to impart dressings with a greater ability to participate in the wound healing process. PolyMem® (Ferris) is already an example of a wound dressing containing a moisturiser (glycerine), which is intended to prevent the dressing sticking to the wound bed, drawing fluid from deeper tissue into the bed to stimulate healing

(Cutting et al., 2015). The dressing also contains a cleanser that can help in autolytic debridement. As demonstrated by the PolyMem® example, combinations of additives can be made, with the intent of creating multifunctional dressings that can address several issues in parallel. As with any areas of research, evidence and technological advances in other industries may contribute to the future of additives in advanced wound dressing. The advanced cosmetic and skincare sectors in particular are of interest, especially in the context of skin repair and regeneration technologies.

Note

1 ATP: Adenosine Triphosphate, a central metabolite that plays a fundamental role as an energy transfer molecule, a phosphate donor and a signalling molecule inside the cells (Tantama & Yellen, 2014).

References

3M. (2006). *The Power of Silver: A Product Monograph*. St Paul: 3M Healthcare Division. Retrieved September 22, 2020, from https://multimedia.3m.com/mws/media/3577530/tegaderm-ag-mesh-dressin-power-of-silver-product-monograph.pdf&fn=70-2009-7137-5_R2.pdf

Acelity. (2020). *InadineTM Dressing*. Retrieved October 2, 2020, from 3M KCI: https://www.acelity.com/healthcare-professionals/global-product-catalog/catalog/inadine-dressing

Akhmetova, A., Saliev, T., Allan, I. U., Illsley, M. J., Nurgozhin, T., & Mikhalovsky, S. (2016, November/December). A Comprehensive Review of Topical Odor-Controlling Treatment Options for Chronic Wounds. *Journal of Wound, Ostomy and Continence Nursing, 43*(6), 598. doi:10.1097/WON.0000000000000273

Alnaimat, S., Wainwright, M., & Al'Abri, K. (2018). Antibacterial Potential of Honey from Different Origins: A Comparison with Manuka Honey. *Journal of Microbiology, Biotechnology and Food Sciences, 1*(5), 1328. Retrieved from https://papers.ssrn.com/sol3/Delivery.cfm/SSRN_ID3256673_code3148362.pdf?abstractid=3256673&mirid=1&type=2

Ambrogi, V., Pietrella, D., Nocchetti, M., Casagrande, S., Moretti, V., De Marco, S., & Ricci, M. (2017, April 1). Montmorillonite–Chitosan–Chlorhexidine Composite Films with Antibiofilm Activity and Improved Cytotoxicity for Wound Dressing. *Journal of Colloid and Interface Science, 265*. doi:10.1016/j.jcis.2016.12.058

Ammons, M. C., Ward, L. S., & James, G. A. (2011, June). Anti-Biofilm Efficacy of a Lactoferrin/Xylitol Wound Hydrogel Used in Combination with Silver Wound Dressings. *International Wound Journal, 8*(3), 268. doi:10.1111/j.1742-481X.2011.00781.x

Ardekani, N. T., Khorram, M., Zomorodian, K., Yazdanpanah, S., Veisi, H., & Veisi, H. (2019, March 15). Evaluation of Electrospun Poly(Vinyl Alcohol)-Based Nanofiber Mats Incorporated with Zataria Multiflora Essential Oil as Potential Wound *Dressing. International Journal of Biological Macromolecules,* 743. doi:10.1016/j.ijbiomac.2018.12.085

AshaRani, P. V., Mun, G. L., Hande, M. P., & Valiyaveettil, S. (2009). Cytotoxicity and Genotoxicity of Silver Nanoparticles in Human Cells. *ACS Nano, 3*(2), 279. doi:10.1021/nn800596w

Aycan, D., Selmi, B., Kelel, E., Yildirim, T., & Alemdar, N. (2019, December). Conductive Polymeric Film Loaded with Ibuprofen as a Wound Dressing Material. *European Polymer Journal, 121,* 109308. doi:10.1016/j.eurpolymj.2019.109308

Aziz, Z., & Hassan, B. A. (2017, February). The Effects of Honey Compared to Silver Sulfadiazine for the Treatment of Burns: A Systematic Review of Randomized Controlled Trials. *Burns, 43*(1), 50. doi:10.1016/j.burns.2016.07.004

Barrientos, S., Stojadinovic, O., Golinko, M. S., Brem, H., & Tomic-Canic, M. (2008). Growth Factors and Cytokines in Wound Healing. *Wound Repair and Regeneration, 16,* 585. doi:10.1111/j.1524-475X.2008.00410.x

Basar, A. O., Castro, S., Torres-Giner, S., Lagaron, J. M., & Sasmazel, H. T. (2017, December 1). Novel Poly(ε-Caprolactone)/Gelatine Wound Dressings Prepared by Emulsion Electrospinning with Controlled Release Capacity of Ketoprofen Anti-Inflammatory Drug. *Materials Science and Engineering: C, 81,* 459. doi:10.1016/j.msec.2017.08.025

Bergman, A., Yanai, J., Weiss, J., Bell, D., & David, M. P. (1983, March). Acceleration of Wound Healing by Topical Application of Honey: An Animal Model. *The American Journal of Surgery, 145*(3), 374. doi:10.1016/0002-9610(83)90204-0

Bigliardi, P. L., Alsagoff, S. A., El-Kafrawi, H. Y., Pyon, J.-K., Wa, C. T., & Villa, M. A. (2017, August). Povidone Iodine in Wound Healing: A Review of Current Concepts and Practices. *Surgery, 44,* 260. doi:10.1016/j.ijsu.2017.06.073

Bohn, G., Liden, B., Schultz, G., Yang, Q., & Gibson, D. J. (2016, January 1). Ovine-Based Collagen Matrix Dressing: Next-Generation Collagen Dressing for Wound Care. *Advances in Wound Care (New Rochelle), 5*(1), 1. doi:10.1089/wound.2015.0660

Boonkaew, B., Kempf, M., Kimble, R., & Cuttle, L. (2014, December). Cytotoxicity Testing of Silver-Containing Burn Treatments Using Primary and Immortal Skin Cells. *Burns, 40*(8), 1562. doi:10.1016/j.burns.2014.02.009

Bourdillon, K. (2016). Dressings and Biofilms: Interpreting Evidence from In Vitro Biofilm Models. *Wounds International, 7*(1), 9. Retrieved from https://www.researchgate.net/profile/Katie_Bourdillon/publication/317259725_Dressings_and_biofilms_interpreting_evidence_from_in_vitro_biofilm_models/links/5e9edfb64585150839eff5e4/Dressings-and-biofilms-interpreting-evidence-from-in-vitro-biofilm-models

Bowler, P. G., Jones, S. A., Walker, M., & Parsons, D. (2004, March–April). Microbicidal Properties of a Silver-Containing Hydrofiber Dressing against a Variety of Burn Wound Pathogens. *Journal of Burn Care and Rehabilitation, 25*(2), 192. doi:10.1097/01.bcr.0000112331.72232.1b

Bradford, C., Freeman, R., & Percival, S. L. (2009, December). In Vitro Study of Sustained Antimicrobial Activity of a New Silver Alginate Dressing. *The Journal of the American College of Certified Wound Specialists, 1*(4), 117. doi:10.1016/j.jcws.2009.09.001

Brouillard, C., Bursztejn, A.-C., Latarche, C., Cuny, J.-F., Truchetet, F., Goullé, J.-P., & Schmutz, J.-L. (2018, December). Silver Absorption and Toxicity Evaluation of Silver Wound Dressings in 40 Patients with Chronic Wounds. *Journal of the European Academy of Dermatology and Venereology, 32*(12), 2295. doi:10.1111/jdv.15055

Bui, H. T., Chung, O. H., Dela Cruz, J., & Park, J. S. (2014, December). Fabrication and Characterization of Electrospun Curcumin-Loaded Polycaprolactone-Polyethylene Glycol Nanofibers for Enhanced Wound Healing. *Macromolecular Research, 22*, 1288. doi:10.1007/s13233-014-2179-6

Bull, A. B., Cullum, N., Dumville, J. C., Westby, M. J., Deshpande, S., & Walker, N. (2015, March 6). Honey as a Topical Treatment for Wounds. In C. W. Group (Ed.), *Cochrane Database of Systematic Reviews*. John Wiley & Sons Ltd. doi:10.1002/14651858.CD005083.pub4

Bulman, S. E., Tronci, G., Goswami, P., Carr, C., & Russell, S. J. (2017, August 16). Antibacterial Properties of Nonwoven Wound Dressings Coated with Manuka Honey or Methylglyoxal. *Materials (Basel), 10*(8), 954. doi:10.3390/ma10080954

Burd, A., Kwok, C. H., Hung, S. C., Chan, H. S., Gu, H., Lam, W. K., & Huang, L. (2007, January–February). A Comparative Study of the Cytotoxicity of Silver-Based Dressings in Monolayer Cell, Tissue Explant, and Animal Models. *Wound Repair and Regeneration, 15*(1), 94. doi:10.1111/j.1524-475X.2006.00190.x

Cantón, I., McKean, R., Charnley, M., Blackwood, K. A., Fiorica, C., Ryan, A. J., & MacNeil, S. (2010, February 1). Development of an Ibuprofen-Releasing Biodegradable PLA/PGA Electrospun Scaffold for Tissue Regeneration. *Biotechnology and Bioengineering, 105*(2), 396. doi:10.1002/bit.22530

Castellano, J. J., Shafii, S. M., Ko, F., Donate, G., Wright, T. E., Mannari, R. J., Payne, W. G., Smith, D. J., & Robson, M. C. (2007). Comparative Evaluation of Silver-Containing Antimicrobial Dressings and Drugs. *International Wound Journal, 4*(2), 114. doi:10.1111/j.1742-481X.2007.00316.x

Cazzaniga, A., Serralta, V., Davis, S., Orr, R., Eaglstein, W., & Mertz, P. M. (2002, June). The Effect of an Antimicrobial Gauze Dressing Impregnated with 0.2-Percent Polyhexamethylene Biguanide as a Barrier to Prevent Pseudomonas Aeruginosa Wound Invasion. *Wounds, 14*(5), 169. Retrieved from https://www.woundsresearch.com/article/550

Chaw, K. C., Manimaran, M., & Tay, F. E. (2005, December). Role of Silver Ions in Destabilization of Intermolecular Adhesion Forces Measured by Atomic Force Microscopy in Staphylococcus Epidermidis Biofilms. *Antimicrobial Agents and Chemotherapy, 49*(12), 4853. doi:10.1128/AAC.49.12.4853-4859.2005

Cheng, Li Y., Huang, S., Yu, F., Bei, Y., Zhang, Y., Tang, J., Huang, Y., & Xiang, Q. (2020, July 15). Hybrid Freeze-Dried Dressings Composed of Epidermal Growth Factor and Recombinant Human-Like Collagen Enhance Cutaneous Wound Healing in Rats. *Frontiers in Bioengineering and Biotechnology, 8*, 742. doi:10.3389/fbioe.2020.00742

Choi, S. M., Lee, K.-M., Kim, H. J., Park, I. K., Kang, H. J., Shin, H.-C., Baek, D., Choi, Y., Park, K. H., & Lee, J. W. (2018, January 15). Effects of Structurally Stabilized EGF and bFGF on Wound Healing in Type I and Type II Diabetic Mice. *Acta Biomaterialia, 66*, 325. doi:10.1016/j.actbio.2017.11.045

Christiansen, C., & Allesen-Holm, M. (2020). *In Vitro Evaluation of Biatain® Silicone Ag and Biatain® Ag against Biofilms and a Broad Range of Microorganism*. Retrieved October 21, 2020, from Coloplast: https://www.coloplast.com/products/wound/articles/biatain-ag-against-biofilms/#section=Reference-list_464019

Coloplast. (2020). *Biatain®Ibu Non-Adhesive*. Retrieved October 27, 2020, from Coloplast: https://www.coloplast.co.uk/biatain-ibu-non-adhesive-en-gb.aspx#section=product-description_3

Convatec. (2020). *AQUACEL® Dressings: How MORE THAN SILVER™ Disrupts and Destroys Biofilm*. Retrieved October 21, 2020, from Convatec: https://www.convatec.co.uk/wound-skin/aquacel-dressings/aquacel-agplus-dressings/how-more-than-silver-works/

Cooper, R. (2014, August 6). Honey as an Effective Antimicrobial Treatment for Chronic Wounds: Is There a Place for It in Modern Medicine? *Chronic Wound Care Management and Research, 1*, 15. doi:10.2147/CWCMR.S46520

Cooper, R. A., Molan, P. C., & Harding, K. G. (1999, June). Antibacterial Activity of Honey against Strains of Staphylococcus Aureus from Infected Wounds. *Journal of the Royal Society of Medicine, 92*, 283. doi:10.1177/014107689909200604

Côté, D. W., & Wright, E. D. (2010, June). Triamcinolone-Impregnated Nasal Dressing Following Endoscopic Sinus Surgery: A Randomized, Double-Blind, Placebo-Controlled Study. *The Laryngoscope, 120*(6), 1269. doi:10.1002/lary.20905

Cutting, K. F., Vowden, P., & Wiegand, C. (2015). Wound Inflammation and the Role of a Multifunctional Polymeric Dressing. *Wounds International, 6*(2), 41. Retrieved from https://www.apodan.dk/media/1905/artikel-om-polymem-og-inflammation-wounds-international-2015.pdf

Davis, S. C., Harding, A., Gil, J., Parajon, F., Valdes, J., Solis, M., & Higa, A. (2017, December). Effectiveness of a Polyhexanide Irrigation Solution on Methicillin-Resistant Staphylococcus Aureus Biofilms in a Porcine Wound Model. *International Wound Journal, 14*(6), 937. doi:10.1111/iwj.12734

Doerler, M., Eming, S., Dissemond, J., Wolter, A., Stoffels-Weindorf, M., Reich-Schupke, S., Altmeyer, P., & Stücker, M. (2014, October). A Novel Epidermal Growth Factor-Containing Wound Dressing for the Treatment of Hard-to-Heal Venous Leg Ulcers. *Advances in Skin & Wound Care, 27*(10), 456. doi:10.1097/01.ASW.0000451942.39446.c2

Du Toit, D. F., & Page, B. J. (2009, September 1). An In Vitro Evaluation of the Cell Toxicity of Honey and Silver Dressings. *Journal of Wound Care, 18*(9), 383. doi:10.12968/jowc.2009.18.9.44307

Eberlein, T., Haemmerle, G., Signer, M., Gruber-Moesenbacher, U., Traber, J., Mittlboeck, M., Abel, M., & Strohal, R. (2011, January). Comparison of PHMB-Containing Dressing and Silver Dressings in Patients with Critically Colonised or Locally Infected Wounds. *Journal of Wound Care, 21*(1), 12. doi:10.12968/jowc.2012.21.1.12

Fayemi, O. E., Ekennia, A. C., Ketata-Seru, L., Ebokaiwe, A. P., Ijomone, O. M., Onwudiwe, D. C., & Ebenso, E. E. (2018, May 31). Antimicrobial and Wound Healing Properties of Polyacrylonitrile-Moringa Extract Nanofibers. *ACS Omega, 3*(5), 4791. doi:10.1021/acsomega.7b01981

Fazli, Y., Shariatinia, Z., Kohsari, I., Azadmehr, A., & Pourmortazavi, S. M. (2016, November 20). A Novel Chitosan-Polyethylene Oxide Nanofibrous Mat Designed for Controlled Co-Release of Hydrocortisone and Imipenem/Cilastatin Drugs. *International Journal of Pharmaceutics, 513*(1–2), 636. doi:10.1016/j.ijpharm.2016.09.078

Fernando, S. S., Gunasekara, T. D., & Holton, J. (2018). Antimicrobial Nanoparticles: Applications and Mechanisms of Action. *Sri Lankan Journal of Infectious Diseases, 8*(1), 2. doi:10.4038/sljid.v8i1.8167

Fitzgerald, D. J., Renick, P. J., Forrest, E. C., Tetens, S. P., Earnest, D. N., McMillan, J., Kiedaisch, B. M., Shi, L., & Roche, E. D. (2017, January/February). Cadexomer Iodine Provides Superior Efficacy against Bacterial Wound Biofilms In Vitro and In Vivo. *Wound Repair and Regeneration, 25*(1), 13. doi:10.1111/wrr.12497

French, V. M., Cooper, R. A., & Molan, P. C. (2005, July). The Antibacterial Activity of Honey against Coagulase-Negative Staphylococci. *Journal of Antimicrobial Chemotheray, 56*(1), 228. doi:10.1093/jac/dki193

Gawande, P. V., Clinton, A. P., LoVetri, K., Yakandawala, N., Rumbaugh, K. P., & Madhyastha, S. (2014, January 1). Antibiofilm Efficacy of DispersinB® Wound Spray Used in Combination with a Silver Wound Dressing. *Microbiology Insights, 7*, 9. doi:10.4137/MBI.S13914

Gethin, G., Grocott, P., Probst, S., & Clarke, E. (2014, June). Current Practice in the Management of Wound Odour: An International Survey. *International Journal of Nursing Studies, 51*(1), 865. doi:10.1016/j.ijnurstu.2013.10.013

Gillam, T. A., Goh, C. K., Ninan, N., Bilimoria, K., Shirazi, H. S., Saboohi, S., Al-Bataineh, S., Whittle, J., & Blencowe, A. (2021, January 30). Iodine Complexed Poly(Vinyl Pyrrolidone) Plasma Polymers as Broad-Spectrum Antiseptic Coatings. *Applied Surface Science, 537*, 147866. doi:10.1016/j.apsusc.2020.147866

Gray, D., Barrett, S., Battacharyya, M., Butcher, M., Enoch, S., Fumerola, S., Stephen-Haynes, J., Edwards-Jones, V., Leaper, D., Strohal, R., White, R., Wicks, G., & Young, T. (2010). PHMB and Its Potential Contribution to Wound Management. *Wounds UK, 6*(2), 40. Retrieved from https://www.woundsme.com/uploads/resources/content_9519.pdf

Group, A., & Lea, A. (2010, December). Contact Dermatitis with a Highlight on Silver: A Review. *Wounds, 22*(12), 311. Retrieved from https://www.woundsresearch.com/article/contact-dermatitis-highlight-silver-review

Gupta, S., Kumar, N., & Tiwari, V. K. (2017). Silver Sulfadiazine versus Sustained-Release Silver Dressings in the Treatment of Burns: A Surprising Result. *Indian Journal of Burns, 25*(1), 38. doi:10.4103/ijb.ijb_22_17

Hadagali, M. D., & Chua, L. S. (2014, December). The Anti-Inflammatory and Wound Healing Properties of Honey. *European Food Research and Technology, 239*, 1003. doi:10.1007/s00217-014-2297-6

Hajská, M., Dragúňová, J., & Koller, J. (2017). Cytotoxicity Testing of Burn Wound Dressings: First Results. *Cell Tissue Bank, 18*, 143. doi:10.1007/s10561-017-9621-x

Haycocks, S., & Chadwick, P. (2014). Using an Activated Charcoal Dressing with Silver for Malodour, Infection and Overgranulation in Diabetic Foot Ulcers. *The Diabetic Foot Journal, 17*(2), 74. Retrieved from https://www.researchgate.net/profile/Samantha_Haycocks/publication/270759015_Using_an_activated_charcoal_dressing_with_silver_for_malodour_infection_and_overgranulation_in_diabetic_foot_ulcers_Importance_of_appropriate_dressing_selection_for_diabetic_foot

Hill, K. E., Malic, S., McKee, R., Rennison, T., Harding, K. G., Williams, D. W., & Thomas, D. W. (2010, June). An In Vitro Model of Chronic Wound Biofilms to Test Wound Dressings and Assess Antimicrobial Susceptibilities. *Journal of Antimicrobial Chemotherapy, 65*(6), 1195. doi:10.1093/jac/dkq105

Hiro, M. E., Pierpont, Y. N., Ko, F., Wright, T. E., Robson, M. C., & Payne, W. G. (2012). Comparative Evaluation of Silver-Containing Antimicrobial Dressings on In

Vitro and In Vivo Processes of Wound Healing. *EPlasty*, *12*, E48. Retrieved from https://www.ncbi.nlm.nih.gov/pmc/articles/PMC3471607/

Hoekstra, M. J., Westgate, S. J., & Mueller, S. (2017, February). Povidone-Iodine Ointment Demonstrates In Vitro Efficacy against Biofilm Formation. *International Wound Journal*, *14*(1), 172. doi:10.1111/iwj.12578

Hussain, F., Khurshid, M. F., Masood, R., & Ibrahim, W. (2017, December 2). Developing Antimicrobial Calcium Alginate Fibres from Neem and Papaya Leaves Extract. *Journal of Wound Care*, *26*(12), 778. doi:10.12968/jowc.2017.26.12.778

Iftikhar, F., Arshad, M., Rasheed, F., Amraiz, D., Anwar, P., & Gulfraz, M. (2010, April). Effects of Acacia Honey on Wound Healing in Various Rat Models. *Phytotherapy Research*, *24*(4), 583. doi:10.1002/ptr.2990

Ikeda, T., Ledwith, A., Bamford, C. H., & Hann, R. A. (1984, January 11). Interaction of a Polymeric Biguanide Biocide with Phospholipid Membranes. *Biochimica et Biophysica Acta (BBA)–Biomembranes*, *769*(1), 57. doi:10.1016/0005-2736(84)90009-9

Jaeger, M., Harats, M., Kornhaber, R., Aviv, U., Zerach, A., & Haik, J. (2016). Treatment of Hypergranulation Tissue in Burn Wounds with Topical Steroid Dressings: A Case Series. *International Medical Case Reports Journal*, *9*, 241. doi:10.2147/IMCRJ.S113182

Jamnongkan, T., Sukumaran, S. K., Sugimoti, M., Hara, T., Takatsuka, Y., & Koyama, K. (2015). Towards Novel Wound Dressings: Antibacterial Properties of Zinc Oxide Nanoparticles and Electrospun Fiber Mats of Zinc Oxide Nanoparticle/Poly(Vinyl Alcohol) Hybrids. *Journal of Polymer Engineering*, *35*(6), 575. doi:10.1515/polyeng-2014-0319

Junka, A., Zywicka, A., Chodaczek, G., Dziadas, M., Czajkowska, J., Duda-Madej, A., Bartoszewicz, M., Mikolajewicz, K., Krasowski, G., Szymczyk, P., & Fijalkowski, K. (2019). Potential of Biocellulose Carrier Impregnated with Essential Oils to Fight against Biofilms Formed on Hydroxyapatite. *Scientific Reports*, *9*, 1256. doi:10.1038/s41598-018-37628-x

Kaur, T., Putatunda, C., Vyas, A., & Kumar, G. (2020, September 12). Zinc Xide Nanoparticles Inhibit Bacterial Biofilm Formation via Altering Cell Membrane Permeability. *Preparative Biochemistry & Biotechnology*. doi:10.1080/10826068.20 20.1815057

Kenawy, E.-R., Abdel-Hay, F. I., El-Newehy, M. H., & Wnek, G. E. (2007, June 25). Controlled Release of Ketoprofen from Electrospun Poly(Vinyl Alcohol) Nanofibers. *Materials Science and Engineering: A*, *459*(1–2), 390. doi:10.1016/j.msea.2007.01.039

Khalid, H. F., Tehseen, B., Sarwar, Y., Hussain, S. Z., Khan, W. S., Raza, Z. A., Bajwa, S. Z., Kanaras, A. G., Hussain, I., & Rehman, A. (2019, February 15). Biosurfactant Coated Silver and Iron Oxide Nanoparticles with Enhanced Anti-Biofilm and Anti-Adhesive Properties. *Journal of Hazardous Materials*, *364*, 441. doi:10.1016/j.jhazmat.2018.10.049

Khoshmohabat, H., Paydar, S., Kazemi, H. M., & Dalfardi, B. (2016, February). Overview of Agents Used for Emergency Hemostasis. *Trauma Monthly*, *21*(1), e26023. doi:10.5812/traumamon.26023

Koea, J. B., Batiller, J., Patel, B., Shen, J., Hammond, J., Hart, J., Fischer, C., & Garden, O. J. (2013, January). A Phase III, Randomized, Controlled, Superiority Trial Evaluating the Fibrin Pad versus Standard of Care in Controlling

Parenchymal Bleeding during Elective Hepatic Surgery. *HPB, 15*(1), 61. doi:10.1111/j.1477-2574.2012.00583.x

Kostenko, V., Lyczak, J., Turner, K., & Martinuzzi, R. J. (2010, December). Impact of Silver-Containing Wound Dressings on Bacterial Biofilm Viability and Susceptibility to Antibiotics during Prolonged Treatment. *Antimicrobial Agents and Chemotherapy, 54*(12), 5120. doi:10.1128/AAC.00825-10

Krejner, A., & Grzela, T. (2015, October 15). Modulation of Matrix Metalloproteinases MMP-2 and MMP-9 Activity by Hydrofiber-Foam Hybrid Dressing – Relevant Support in the Treatment of Chronic Wounds. *Central European Journal of Immunology, 40*(3), 391.

Kwakman, P. H., te Velde, A. A., de Boer, L., Speijer, D., Vandenbroucke-Grauls, M. C., & Zaat, S. A. (2010, July). How Honey Kills Bacteria. *The FASEB Journal, 24*(7), 2576. doi:10.1096/fj.09-150789

Lam, P. K., Chan, E. S., Ho, W. S., & Liew, C. T. (2004). In Vitro Cytotoxicity Testing of a Nanocrystalline Silver Dressing (Acticoat) on Cultured Keratinocytes. *British Journal of Biomedical Science, 61*(3), 125. doi:10.1080/09674845.2004.11732656

Langsdown, A. B. (2010, August). A Pharmacological and Toxicological Profile of Silver as an Antimicrobial Agent in Medical Devices. *Advances in Pharmacological and Pharmaceutical Sciences*, 910686. doi:10.1155/2010/910686

Leaper, D. J., & Durani, P. (2008, June). Topical Antimicrobial Therapy of Chronic Wounds Healing by Secondary Intention Using Iodine Products. *International Wound Journal, 5*(2), 361. doi:10.1111/j.1742-481X.2007.00406.x

Lee, D. S., Sinno, S., & Khachemoune, A. (2011). Honey and Wound Healing: An Overview. *American Journal of Clinical Dermatology, 12*(3), 181.

Lensenlink, E., & Andriessen, A. (2011, November 1). A Cohort Study on the Efficacy of a Polyhexanide-Containing Biocellulose Dressing in the Treatment of Biofilms in Wounds. *Journal of Wound Care, 20*(11), 534. doi:10.12968/jowc.2011.20.11.534

Liakos, I., Rizzello, L., Hajiali, H., Brunetti, V., Carzino, R., Pompa, P. P., Athanasiou, A., & Mele, E. (2015). Fibrous Wound Dressings Encapsulating Essential Oils as Natural Antimicrobial Agents. *Journal of Materials Chemistry B* (3), 1583. doi:10.1039/C4TB01974A

Liakos, I., Rizzello, L., Scurr, D. J., Pompa, P. P., Bayer, I. S., & Athanassio, A. (2014, March 25). All-Natural Composite Wound Dressing Films of Essential Oils Encapsulated in Sodium Alginate with Antimicrobial Properties. *International Journal of Pharmaceutics, 463*(2), 137. doi:10.1016/j.ijpharm.2013.10.046.

Liao, C., Li, Y., & Tjong, S. C. (2019, January 21). Bactericidal and Cytotoxic Properties of Silver Nanoparticles. *International Journal of Molecular Science, 20*(2), 449. doi:10.3390/ijms20020449

Lipman, R., & Van Bavel, D. (2007). Odor Absorbing Hydrocolloid Dressings for Direct Wound Contact. *Wounds, 19*(5), 138. Retrieved from https://www.researchgate.net/profile/Roger_Lipman2/publication/228480125_Odor_Absorbing_Hydrocolloid_Dressings_for_Direct_Wound_Contact/links/56f12c9608aedbe21877218e.pdf

Liu, J.-X., Dong, W.-H., Mou, X.-J., Liu, G.-S., Huang, X.-W., Yan, X., Zhou, C.-F., Jiang, S., & Long, Y.-Z. (2020). In Situ Electrospun Zein/Thyme Essential Oil-Based Membranes as an Effective Antibacterial Wound Dressing. *ACS Applied Bio Materials, 3*(1), 302. doi:10.1021/acsabm.9b00823

Lo, S.-F., Hayter, M., Chang, C.-J., Hu, W.-Y., & Lee, L.-L. (2008, August). A Systematic Review of Silver-Releasing Dressings in the Management of Infected Chronic Wounds. *Journal of Clinical Nursing*, 17(15), 1973. doi:10.1111/j.1365-2702.2007.02264.x

Loimaranta, V., Mazurel, D., Deng, D., & Söderling, E. (2020). Xylitol and Erythritol Inhibit Real-Time Biofilm Formation of Streptococcus Mutans. *BMC Microbiology*, 20, 184. doi:10.1186/s12866-020-01867-8

Lu, J., Turnbull, L., Burke, C. M., Liu, M., Carter, D. A., Schlothauer, R. C., Whitchurch, C. B., & Harry, E. J. (2014, March 25). Manuka-Type Honeys can Eradicate Biofilms Produced by Staphylococcus Aureus Strains with Different Biofilm-Forming Abilities. *Peer Journal*, e326. doi:10.7717/peerj.326

Majtan, J. (2011). Methylglyoxal – A Potential Risk Factor of Manuka Honey in Healing of Diabetic Ulcers. *Evidence-Based Complementary and Alternative Medicines*, 2595494. doi:10.1093/ecam/neq013

Markowska, K., Grudniak, A. M., & Wolska, K. I. (2013). Silver Nanoparticles as an Alternative Strategy against Bacterial Biofilms. *Acta Biochimica Polonica*, 60(4), 523. doi:10.18388/abp.2013_2016

Marston, W. A., Hanft, J., Norwood, P., Pollak, R., & The Dermagraft Diabetic Foot Ulcer Study Group. (2003, June). The Efficacy and Safety of Dermagraft in Improving the Healing of Chronic Diabetic Foot Ulcers. *Diabetes Care*, 26(6), 1701. doi:10.2337/diacare.26.6.1701

Matsumoto, Y., & Kuroyanagi, Y. (2010). Development of a Wound Dressing Composed of Hyaluronic Acid Sponge Containing Arginine and Epidermal Growth Factor. *Journal of Biomaterials Science, Polymer Edition*, 21(6–7), 715. doi:10.1163/156856209X435844

Maver, T., Gradišnik, L., Smrke, D. M., Kleinschek, K. S., & Maver, U. (2019, January 2). Systematic Evaluation of a Diclofenac-Loaded Carboxymethyl Cellulose-Based Wound Dressing and Its Release Performance with Changing pH and Temperature. *AAPS PharmSciTech*, 29. doi:10.1208/s12249-018-1236-4

Mavric, E., Wittmann, S., Barth, G., & Henle, T. (2008, April). Identification and Quantification of Methylglyoxal as the Dominant Antibacterial Constituent of Manuka (Leptospermum scoparium) Honeys from New Zealand. *Molecular Nutrition and Food Research*, 52(4), 483. doi:10.1002/mnfr.200700282.

McDonnell, G., & Russell, A. D. (1999, January). Antiseptics and Disinfectants: Activity, Action, and Resistance. *Clinical Microbiology Reviews*, 12(1), 147. Retrieved October 1, 2020, from https://www.ncbi.nlm.nih.gov/pmc/articles/PMC88911/

McGillicuddy, E., Murray, I., Kavanagh, S., Morrison, L., Fogarty, A., Cormican, M., Dockery, P., Prendergast, M., Rowan, N., & Morris, D. (2017, January 1). Silver Nanoparticles in the Environment: Sources, Detection and Ecotoxicology. *Science of the Total Environment*, 575, 231. doi:10.1016/j.scitotenv.2016.10.041

Medline Industries Inc. (2007). *Exuderm®OdorShield™ Wound Dressing... The First Odor Control Hydropolymer*. Retrieved from http://www.medexsupply.com/images/medlineproduct.pdf

Metzmacher, I., Ruth, P., Abel, M., & Friess, W. (2007, July/August). In Vitro Binding of Matrix Metalloproteinase-2 (MMP-2), MMP-9, and Bacterial Collagenase on Collagenous Wound Dressings. *Wound Repair and Regeneration*, 15(4), 549. doi:10.1111/j.1524-475X.2007.00263.x

Mizuno, K., Yamamura, K., Yano, K., Osada, T., Saeki, S., Takimoto, N., Sakurai, T., & Nimura, Y. (2003, January 1). Effect of Chitosan Film Containing Basic Fibroblast Growth Factor on Wound Healing in Genetically Diabetic Mice. *Journal of Biomedical Materials Research, Part A, 64A*(1), 177. doi:10.1002/jbm.a.10396

Mohamad, N., Loh, E. Y., Fauzi, M. B., Ng, M. H., & Amin, M. C. (2019). In Vivo Evaluation of Bacterial Cellulose/Acrylic Acid Wound Dressing Hydrogel Containing Keratinocytes and Fibroblasts for Burn Wounds. *Drug Delivery and Translational Research, 9*, 4444. doi:10.1007/s13346-017-0475-3

Mohandas, A., Deepthi, S., Biswas, R., & Jayakumar, R. (2018, September). Chitosan Based Metallic Nanocomposite Scaffolds as Antimicrobial Wound Dressings. *Bioactive Materials, 3*, 267. doi:10.1016/j.bioactmat.2017.11.003

Mölnlycke. (2020). *Mepilex Ag.* Retrieved September 22, 2020, from Mölnlycke: https://www.molnlycke.co.uk/products-solutions/mepilex-ag/

Mondal, R., Foote, M., Canada, A., Wiencek, M., Cowan, M. E., & Acevedo, C. (2020, January). Efficient Silver Release from Ion Exchange Silver Dressings in Biologically Relevant Media. *Wounds, 32*(1), 22. Retrieved from https://www.woundsresearch.com/article/efficient-silver-release-ion-exchange-silver-dressings-biologically-relevant-media

Moore, K., & Gray, D. (2007, June). Using PHMB Antimicrobial to Prevent Wound Infection. *Wounds UK, 3*(2), 96. Retrieved from https://lohmann-rauscher.co.uk/downloads/clinical-evidence/SXP015-Moore-and-Gray-Using-PHMB-antimicrobial-to-prevent-.pdf

Moore, O. A., Smith, L. A., Campbell, F., Seers, K., McKay, H. J., & Moore, R. A. (2001, June). Systematic Review of the Use of Honey as a Wound Dressing. *BMC Complementary and Alternative Medicine, 1*, 2. doi:10.1186/1472-6882-1-2

Morgado, P. I., Miguel, S. P., Correia, I. J., & Aguiar-Ricardo, A. (2017, March 1). Ibuprofen Loaded PVA/Chitosan Membranes: A Highly Efficient Strategy Towards an Improved Skin Wound Healing. *Carbohydrate Polymers, 159*, 136. doi:10.1016/j.carbpol.2016.12.029

Mulder, G. D., Cavorsi, J. P., & Lee, D. K. (2007, July). Polyhexamethylene Biguanide (PHMB): An Addendum to Current Topical Antimicrobials. *Wounds, 19*(7), 173. Retrieved from https://www.woundsresearch.com/article/7494

Müller, G., & Kramer, A. (2008, June). Biocompatibility Index of Antiseptic Agents by Parallel Assessment of Antimicrobial Activity and Cellular Cytotoxicity. *Journal of Antimicrobial Chemotherapy, 61*(6), 1281. doi:10.1093/jac/dkn125

Muthaiyan, A., Biswas, D., Crandall, P. G., Wilkinson, B. J., & Ricke, S. C. (2012, August). Application of Orange Essential Oil as an Antistaphylococcal Agent in a Dressing *Model. BMC Complementary and Alternative Medicine,* 125. doi:10.1186/1472-6882-12-125

Narayanan, G., Ormond, B. R., Gupta, B. S., & Tonelli, A. E. (2015, December 5). Efficient Wound Odor Removal by β-Cyclodextrin Functionalized Poly (ε-Caprolactone) Nanofibers. *Journal of Applied Polymer Science, 132*(45), 42782. doi:10.1002/app.42782

National Toxicology Program (NTP). (2016). *14th Report on Carcinogens.* US Department of Health and Human Services. Retrieved September 29, 2020, from https://ntp.niehs.nih.gov/whatwestudy/assessments/cancer/roc/index.html?utm_source=direct&utm_medium=prod&utm_campaign=ntpgolinks&utm_term=roc12#S

Negut, I., Grumezescu, V., & Grumezescu, A. M. (2018, September). Treatment Strategies for Infected Wounds. *Molecules, 23*(9), 2392. doi:10.3390/molecules23092392

Nishiguchi, A., & Taguchi, T. (2020, April). Designing an Anti-Inflammatory and Tissue-Adhesive Colloidal Dressing for Wound Treatment. *Colloids and Surfaces B: Biointerfaces, 188*, 110737. doi:10.1016/j.colsurfb.2019.110737.

Olaitan, P. B., Adeleke, O. E., & Ola, I. O. (2007). Honey: A Reservoir for Microorganisms and an Inhibitory Agent for Microbes. *African Health Sciences, 7*(3), 159. Retrieved October 5, 2020, from https://www.ajol.info/index.php/ahs/article/download/7009/58269

Oryan, A., Alemzadeh, E., & Moshiri, A. (2016, May). Biological Properties and Therapeutic Activities of Honey in Wound Healing: A Narrative Review and Meta-Analysis. *Journal of Tissue Viability, 25*(2), 98. doi:10.1016/j.jtv.2015.12.002.

Oustadi, F., Nazarpak, M. H., Mansouri, M., & Ketabat, F. (2020, August 2). Preparation, Characterization, and Drug Release Study of Ibuprofen-Loaded Poly (Vinyl Alcohol)/Poly (Vinyl Pyrrolidone) Bilayer Antibacterial Membrane. *International Journal of Polymeric Materials and Polymeric Biomaterials*. doi:10.1080/00914037.2020.1798437

Paddle-Ledinek, J. E., Nasa, Z., & Cleland, H. (2006, June). Effect of Different Wound Dressings on Cell Viability and Proliferation. *Plastic and Reconstructive Surgery, 117*(7S), 110S. doi:10.1097/01.prs.0000225439.39352.ce

Percival, S. L., Bowler, P., & Woods, E. J. (2008, January–February). Assessing the Effect of an Antimicrobial Wound Dressing on Biofilms. *Wound Repair and Regeneration, 16*(1), 52. doi:10.1111/j.1524-475X.2007.00350.x

Phillips, P. L., Yang, Q., Davis, S., Sampson, E. M., Azeke, J. I., Hamad, A., & Schultz, G. S. (2015, August). Antimicrobial Dressing Efficacy against Mature Pseudomonas Aeruginosa Biofilm on Porcine Skin Explants. *International Wound Journal, 12*(4), 469. doi:10.1111/iwj.12142

Phillips, P. L., Yang, Q. P., Sampson, E. M., & Schultz, G. S. (2009). Microbicidal Effects of Wound Dressings on Mature Bacterial Biofilm on Porcine Skin Explants. *EWMA*. Helsinki, Finland.

Pilehvar-Soltanahmadi, Y., Dadashpour, M., Mohajeri, A., Fattahi, A., Sheervalilou, R., & Zarghami, N. (2018). An Overview on Application of Natural Substances Incorporated with Electrospun Nanofibrous Scaffolds to Development of Innovative Wound Dressings. *Mini Reviews in Medicinal Chemistry, 18*(5), 414. doi:10.2174/1389557517666170308112147

Qin, M., Mou, X.-J., Dong, W.-H., Liu, J.-X., Liu, H., Dai, Z., Huang, X.-W., Wang, N., & Yan, X. (2020, March). In Situ Electrospinning Wound Healing Films Composed of Zein and Clove Essential Oil. *Macromolecular Materials and Engineering, 305*(3), 1900790. doi:10.1002/mame.201900790

Rai, M., Kon, K., Ingle, A., Duran, N., Galdiero, S., & Galdiero, M. (2014, March). Broad-Spectrum Bioactivities of Silver Nanoparticles: The Emerging Trends and Future Prospects. *Applied Microbiology and Biotechnology, 98*, 1951. doi:10.1007/s00253-013-5473-x

Rebia, R. A., Sadon, N. S., & Tanaka, T. (2019). Natural Antibacterial Reagents (Centella, Propolis, and Hinokitiol) Loaded into Poly[(R)-3-Hydroxybutyrate-Co-(R)-3-Hydroxyhexanoate] Composite Nanofibers for Biomedical Applications. *Nanomaterials, 9*(12), 1665. doi:10.3390/nano9121665

Ren, G., Hu, D., Cheng, E. W., Vargas-Reus, M. A., Reip, P., & Allaker, R. P. (2009, June). Characterisation of Copper Oxide Nanoparticles for Antimicrobial Applications. *International Journal of Antimicrobial Agents*, 33(6), 587. doi:10.1016/j.ijantimicag.2008.12.004

Rhoads, D. D., Wolcott, R., & Percival, S. (2008, November). Biofilms in Wounds: Management Strategies. *Journal of Wound Care*, 17(11), 502.

Roberts, J. S., Niu, J., & Pastor-Cervantes, J. A. (2017, October). Comparison of Hemostasis Times with a Kaolin-Based Hemostatic Pad (QuikClot Radial) vs Mechanical Compression (TR Band) Following Transradial Access: A Pilot Study. *Journal of Invasive Cardiology*, 29(10), 328. Retrieved from https://www.invasivecardiology.com/articles/comparison-hemostasis-times-kaolin-based-hemostatic-pad-quikclot-radial-vs-mechanical

Roche, E. D., Woodmansey, E. J., Yang, Q., Gibson, D. J., Zhang, H., & Schultz, G. S. (2019, June). Cadexomer Iodine Effectively Reduces Bacterial Biofilm in Porcine Wounds Ex Vivo and In Vivo. *International Wound Journal*, 16(3), 674. doi:10.1111/iwj.13080

Romero-Velez, G., Kaban, J. M., Chao, E., Lewis, E. R., Stone Jr, M. E., Teperman, S., & Reddy, S. H. (2020, August). Use of the EVARREST Patch for Penetrating Cardiac Injury. *Trauma Case Reports*, 28, 100324. doi:10.1016/j.tcr.2020.100324

Rosa, J. M., Bonato, L. B., Mancuso, C. B., Martinelli, L., Okura, M. H., Malpass, G. R., & Granato, A. C. (2018, March 22). Antimicrobial Wound Dressing Films Containing Essential Oils and Oleoresins of Pepper Encapsulated in Sodium Alginate Films. *Ciência Rural*, 48(3), EPub. doi:10.1590/0103-8478cr20170740

Roy, R., Tiwari, M., Donelli, G., & Tiwari, V. (2018). Strategies for Combating Bacterial Biofilms: A Focus on Anti-Biofilm Agents and Their Mechanisms of Action. *Virulence*, 9(1), 522. doi:10.1080/21505594.2017.1313372

Rubina, M. S., Said-Galiev, E. E., Naumkin, A. V., Shulenin, A. V., Belyakova, O. A., & Vasil'kov, A. Y. (2019, December). Preparation and Characterization of Biomedical Collagen–Chitosan Scaffolds with Entrapped Ibuprofen and Silver Nanoparticles. *Polymer Engineering and Science*, 59(12), 2479. doi:10.1002/pen.25122

Said, J., Walker, M., Parsons, D., Stapleton, P., Beezer, A. E., & Gaisford, S. (2014, October 20). An In Vitro Test of the Efficacy of an Anti-Biofilm Wound Dressing. *International Journal of Pharmaceutics*, 474(1–2), 177. doi:10.1016/j.ijpharm.2014.08.034

Schneider, A., Wang, X. Y., Kaplan, D. L., Garlick, J. A., & Egles, C. (2009, September). Biofunctionalized Electrospun Silk Mats as a Topical Bioactive Dressing for Accelerated Wound Healing. *Acta Biomaterialica*, 5(7), 2570. doi:10.1016/j.actbio.2008.12.013

Schwarzer, S., James, G. A., Goeres, D., Bjarnsholt, T., Vickery, K., Percival, S. L., Stoodley, P., Schultz, G., Jensen, S. O., & Malone, M. (2020, March). The Efficacy of Topical agents Used in Wounds for Managing Chronic Biofilm Infections: A Systematic Review. *Journal of Infection*, 80(3), 261. doi:10.1016/j.jinf.2019.12.017

Seil, J. T., & Webster, T. J. (2012). Antimicrobial Applications of Nanotechnology: Methods and Literature. *International Journal of Nanomedicine*, 7, 2767. doi:10.2147/IJN.S24805

Séon-Lutz, M., Couffin, A.-C., Vignoud, S., Schlatter, G., & Hébraud, A. (2019, March 1). Electrospinning in Water and In Situ Crosslinking of Hyaluronic Acid/Cyclodextrin Nanofibers: Towards Wound Dressing with Controlled Drug Release. *Carbohydrate Polymers, 207*, 276. doi:10.1016/j.carbpol.2018.11.085

Shina, A., Lipsky, A. M., Nadler, R., Levi, M., Benov, A., Ran, Y., Yitzhak, A., & Glassberg, E. (2015, October). Prehospital Use of Hemostatic Dressings by the Israel Defense Forces Medical Corps: A Case Series of 122 Patients. *Journal of Acute Care Surgery, 79*(4 Suppl. 2), S204. doi:10.1097/TA.0000000000000720.

Sibbald, R. G., Leaper, D. J., & Queen, D. (2011). Iodine Made Easy. *Wounds International, 2*(2), S1. Retrieved from http://www.woundsinternational.com/uploads/reso urces/03983a959705d34a896ec163f7fc34d9.pdf

Simões, D., Miguel, S. P., Ribeiro, M. P., Coutinho, P., Mendonça, A. G., & Correia, I. J. (2018, June). Recent Advances on Antimicrobial Wound Dressing: A Review. *European Journal of Pharmaceutics and Biopharmaceutics, 127*, 130. doi:10.1016/j.ejpb.2018.02.022

Simon, A., Traynor, K., Santos, K., Blaser, G., Bode, U., & Molan, P. (2009, June). Medical Honey for Wound Care – Still the 'Latest Resort'? *Evidence-Based Complementary Alternative Medicine, 6*(2), 165. doi:10.1093/ecam/nem175

Singh, R. P., & Ramarao, P. (2012, September 3). Cellular Uptake, Intracellular Trafficking and Cytotoxicity of Silver Nanoparticles. *Toxicology Letter, 213*(2), 249. doi:10.1016/j.toxlet.2012.07.009

Smith + Nephew. (2020). *How IODOSORB Works: IODOSORB a Unique Dual Action.* Retrieved October 1, 2020, from Smith + Nephew: https://www.smith-nephew.com/key-products/advanced-wound-management/iodosorb/

Smith, A. H., Laird, C., Porter, K., & Bloch, M. (2013, September 7). Haemostatic Dressings in *Prehospital Care. Emergency Medicine Journal, 784*. doi:10.1136/emermed-2012-201581

Sood, A., Granick, M. S., & Tomaselli, N. L. (2014, August 1). Wound Dressings and Comparative Effectiveness Data. *Advances in Wound Care (New Rochelle), 3*(8), 511. doi:10.1089/wound.2012.0401

Spotnitz, W. D. (2014). Fibrin Sealant Patches: Powerful and Easy-to-Use Hemostats. *Open Access Surgery, 7*, 71. doi:10.2147/OAS.S41516

Tanaka, A., Nagate, T., & Matsuda, H. (2005). Acceleration of Wound Healing by Gelatine Film Dressings with Epidermal Growth Factor. *Journal of Veterinary Medical, 67*(9), 909. doi:10.1292/jvms.67.909

Tantama, M., & Yellen, G. (2014). Imaging Changes in the Cytosolic ATP-to-ADP Ratio. In A. N. Murphy & D. C. Chan (Eds.), *Methods in Enzymology: Mitochondrial Function* (Vol. 547, p. 355). Elsevier.

Tavakolian, M., Munguia-Lopez, J. G., Valiei, A., Islam, S., Kinsella, J. M., Tufenkji, N., & van de Ven, T. G. (2020, August 14). Highly Absorbent Antibacterial and Biofilm-Disrupting Hydrogels from Cellulose for Wound Dressing Applications. *ACS Applied Materials Interfaces, 12*(36), 39991. doi:10.1021/acsami.0c08784

Teng, H. T. (2020, March 25). Hemostatic Agents for Prehospital Hemorrhage Control: A Narrative Review. *Military Medical Research, 7*, 13. doi:10.1186/s40779-020-00241-z

Thomas, S., Fisher, B., Fram, P. J., & Waring, M. J. (1998, May 2). Odour-Absorbing Dressings. *Journal of Wound Care, 7*(5), 246. doi:10.12968/jowc.1998.7.5.246

Dressings for Advanced Wound Care

Thorn, R. M., Austin, A. J., Greenman, J., Wilkins, J. P., & Davis, P. J. (2009, August). In Vitro Comparison of Antimicrobial Activity of Iodine and Silver Dressings against Biofilms. *Journal of Wound Care, 18*(8), 343. Retrieved from http://www. biologiq.nl/UserFiles/In%20vitro%20comparison%20of%20antimicrobial%20 activity%20of%20iodine%20and%20silver%20dressings%20against%20bio-films%20JWC%20Aug%2009%20-%20Thorn%20Greenman%20Austin.pdf

Tonks, A., Cooper, R. A., Price, A. J., Molan, P. C., & Jones, K. P. (2001, May 21). Stimulation of TNF-Alpha Release in Monocytes by Honey. *Cytokine, 14*(4), 240. doi:10.1006/cyto.2001.0868.

Tonks, A. J., Cooper, R. A., Jones, K. P., Blair, S., Parton, J., & Tonks, A. (2003, March 7). Honey Stimulates Inflammatory Cytokine Production from Monocytes. *Cytokine, 21*(5), 242. doi:10.1016/s1043-4666(03)00092-9

Tonks, A. J., Dudley, E., Porter, N. G., Parton, J., Brazier, J., Smith, E. L., & Tonks, A. (2007, November). A 5.8-KDa Component of Manuka Honey Stimulates Immune Cells via TLR4. *Journal of Leukocyte Biology, 82*(5), 1147. doi:10.1189/jlb.1106683

Trabattoni, D., Montorsi, P., Fabbiocchi, F., Lualdi, A., Gatto, P., & Bartorelli, A. L. (2011, August). A New Kaolin-Based Haemostatic Bandage Compared with Manual Compression for Bleeding Control after Percutaneous Coronary Procedures. *European Radiology, 21*(8), 1687. doi:10.1007/s00330-011-2117-3

Travers, S., Lefort, H., Ramdani, E., Lemoine, S., Jost, D., Bignand, M., & Tourtier, J.-P. (2016, October). Hemostatic Dressings in Civil Prehospital Practice: 30 Uses of QuikClot Combat Gauze. *European Journal of Emergency Medicine, 23*(5), 391. doi:10.1097/MEJ.0000000000000318

Trop, M., Novak, M., Rodl, S., Hellbom, B., Kroell, W., & Goessler, W. (2006, March). Silver-Coated Dressing Acticoat Caused Raised Liver Enzymes and Argyria-Like Symptoms in Burn Patient. *The Journal of Trauma: Injury, Infection, and Critical Care, 60*(3), 648. doi:10.1097/01.ta.0000208126.22089.b6

Ulubayram, K., Cakar, A. N., Korkusuz, P., Ertan, C., & Hasirci, N. (2001, June 1). EGF Containing Gelatine-Based Wound Dressings. *Biomaterials, 22*(11), 1345. doi:10.1016/S0142-9612(00)00287-8

Unalan, I., Endlein, S. J., Slavik, B., Buettner, A., Goldmann, W. H., Detsch, R., & Boccaccini, A. R. (2019). Evaluation of Electrospun Poly(ε-Caprolactone)/Gelatine Nanofiber Mats Containing Clove Essential Oil for Antibacterial Wound Dressing. *Pharmaceutics, 11*(11), 570. doi:10.3390/pharmaceutics11110570

Velázquez-Velázquez, J. L., Santos-Flores, A., Araujo-Meléndez, J., Sánchez-Sánchez, R., Velasquillo, C., González, C., Martínez-Castañon, G., & Martinez-Gutierrez, F. (2015, April 1). Anti-Biofilm and Cytotoxicity Activity of Impregnated Dressings with Silver Nanoparticles. *Materials Science and Engineering: C, 49*, 604. doi:10.1016/j.msec.2014.12.084

Verified Market Research. (2020). *Global Antimicrobial Dressings Market by Product, by Application, by Geographic Scope and Forecast.* Verified Market Research.

Vermeulen, H., Westerbos, S. J., & Ubbink, D. T. (2010). Benefit and Harm of Iodine in Wound Care: A Systematic Review. In *Database of Abstracts of Reviews of Effects (DARE): Quality Assessed Reviews.* York: The University of York Centre for Reviews and Dissemination. Retrieved October 1, 2020, from https://www.ncbi.nlm.nih.gov/books/NBK80212/

Vinklárková, L., Masteiková, R., Vetchý, D., Doležel, P., & Bernatonienė, J. (2015). Formulation of Novel Layered Sodium Carboxymethylcellulose Film Wound Dressings with Ibuprofen for Alleviating Wound Pain. *Biomedical Research International*, 892671. doi:10.1155/2015/892671

Vlachou, E., Chipp, E., Shale, E., Wilson, Y. T., Papini, R., & Moeimen, N. S. (2007, December). The Safety of Nanocrystalline Silver Dressings on Burns: A Study of Systemic Silver Absorption. *Burns*, *33*(8), 979. doi:10.1016/j.burns.2007.07.014

Walters, C. R., Pool, E. J., & Somerset, V. S. (2014). Ecotoxicity of Silver Nanomaterials in the Aquatic Environment: A Review of Literature and Gaps in Nano-Toxicological Research. *Journal of Environmental Science and Health, Part A*, *49*(13), 1588. doi:10.1080/10934529.2014.938536

Wang, X.-Q., Kempf, M., Mott, J., Chang, H.-E., Francis, R., Liu, P.-Y., Cuttle, L., Olszowy, H., Kravchuk, O., Mill, J., & Kimble, R. M. (2009, March–April). Silver Absorption on Burns after the Application of ActicoatTM: Data from Pediatric Patients and a Porcine Burn Model. *Journal of Burn Care & Research*, *30*(2), 341. doi:10.1097/BCR.0b013e318198a64c

Wiegand, C., Heinze, T., & Hipler, U.-C. (2009, July/August). Comparative In Vitro Study on Cytotoxicity, Antimicrobial Activity, and Binding Capacity for Pathophysiological Factors in Chronic Wounds of Alginate and Silver-Containing Alginate. *Wound Repair and Regeneration*, *17*(4), 511. doi:10.1111/j.1524-475X.2009.00503.x

Wiegand, C., & Hipler, U.-C. (2013). A Superabsorbent Polymer-Containing Wound Dressing Efficiently Sequesters MMPs and Inhibits Collagenase Activity in Vitro. *Journal of Materials Science: Materials for Medicine*, *24*, 2473. doi:10.1007/s10856-013-4990-6

Wilkinson, L. J., White, R. J., & Chipman, J. K. (2011). Silver and Nanoparticles of Silver in Wound Dressings: A Review of Efficacy and Safety. *Journal of Wound Care*, *20*(11), 543. doi:10.12968/jowc.2011.20.11.543

Williams, C. (2000, August/September). CliniSorb Activated Charcoal Dressing for Odour Control. *British Journal of Nursing*, *9*(15), 1016. doi:10.12968/bjon.2000.9.15.5485

Woods, J., Boegli, L., Kirker, K. R., Agostinho, A. M., Durch, A. M., deLancey Pulcini, E., Stewart, P. S., & James, G. A. (2012, May). Development and Application of a Polymicrobial, In Vitro, Wound Biofilm Model. *Journal of Applied Microbiology*, *112*(5), 998. doi:10.1111/j.1365-2672.2012.05264.x

World Health Organization. (2018). *Global Guidelines for the Prevention of Surgical Site Infection*. Geneva: World Health Organization. Retrieved April 2, 2020, from https://apps.who.int/iris/bitstream/handle/10665/277399/9789241550475-eng.pdf?ua=1

Wounds International. (2012). *International Consensus: Appropriate Use of Silver Dressings in Wounds*. London: Wounds International. Retrieved September 24, 2020, from https://www.woundsinternational.com/download/resource/6010

Wright, J. B., Lam, K., Buret, A. G., Olson, M. E., & Burrell, R. E. (2002, May). Early Healing Events in a Porcine Model of Contaminated Wounds: Effects of Nanocrystalline Silver on Matrix Metalloproteinases, Cell Apoptosis, and Healing. *Wound Repair and Regeneration*, *10*(3), 141. doi:10.1046/j.1524-475X.2002.10308.x

Wu, M., Guo, H., Liu, Y., & Xie, L. (2019, June). Size-Dependent Cellular Uptake and Localization Profiles of Silver Nanoparticles. *International Journal of Nanomedicine, 14*, 4247. doi:10.2147/IJN.S201107

Yang, Y., Gajaraj, S., Wall, J. D., & Hu, Z. (2013, June 15). A Comparison of Nanosilver and Silver Ion Effects on Bioreactor Landfill Operations and Methanogenic Population Dynamics. *Water Research, 47*(10), 3422. doi:10.1016/j.watres.2013.03.040

Yarboro, D. D. (2013, June). A Comparative Study of the Dressings Silver Sulfadiazine and Aquacel Ag in the Management of Superficial Partial-Thickness Burns. *Advances in Skin & Wound Care, 26*(6), 259. doi:10.1097/01.ASW.0000431084.85141.d1

Yu, A., Niiyama, H., Kondo, S., Yamamoto, A., Suzuki, R., & Kuroyanagi, Y. (2013). Wound Dressing Composed of Hyaluronic Acid and Collagen Containing EGF or bFGF: Comparative Culture Study. *Journal of Biomaterials Science, Polymer Edition, 24*(8), 1015. doi:10.1080/09205063.2012.731375

Yu, A., Takeda, A., Kumazawa, K., Miyoshi, H., Kuroyanagi, M., Yoshitake, T., Uchinuma, E., Suzuki, R., & Kuroyanagi, Y. (2015). Preliminary Clinical Study Using a Novel Wound Dressing Composed of Hyaluronic Acid and Collagen Containing EGF. *Open Journal of Regenerative Medicine, 4*(1), 54985. doi:10.4236/ojrm.2015.41002

Zhao, Y., Dai, C., Wang, Z., Chen, W., Liu, J., Zhuo, R., Yu, A., & Huang, S. (2019). A Novel Curcumin-Loaded Composite Dressing Facilitates Wound Healing due to Its Natural Antioxidant Effect. *Drugs Design, Development and Therapy, 13*, 3269. doi:10.2147/DDDT.S219224

Zietlow, J. M., Zietlow, S. P., Morris, D. S., Berns, K. S., & Jenkins, D. H. (2015, Summer). Prehospital Use of Hemostatic Bandages and Tourniquets: Translation from Military Experience to Implementation in Civilian Trauma Care. *Journal of Special Operations Medicine, 15*(2), 48.

Z-Medica. (2020). *Frequently Asked Questions*. Retrieved October 22, 2020, from QuikClot Power to Stop Bleeding: https://quikclot.com/QuikClot/FAQ

Zou, S.-B., Yoon, W.-Y., Han, S.-K., Jeong, S.-H., Cui, Z.-J., & Kim, W.-K. (2013, June). Cytotoxicity of Silver Dressings on Diabetic Fibroblasts. *International Wound Journal, 10*(3), 306. doi:10.1111/j.1742-481X.2012.00977.x

Zweiker, D., Hoell, A., Seitz, S., Walter, D., & Trop, M. (2014, December 31). Semi-Permanent Skin Staining Associated with Silver-Coated Wound Dressing Acticoat. *Annals of Burns and Fire Disasters, 27*(4), 197. Retrieved from https://www.ncbi.nlm.nih.gov/pmc/articles/PMC4544430/

7

Development Aspects to Consider for New Wound Dressings

7.1 Wound Dressings from Idea to Market

The process of developing a wound dressing varies from business to business and from country to country. Overall, however, there are certain common elements that need to be addressed before any new product can be released in the global market. Generally, the five main organisational phases of product development are (a) concept, (b) feasibility, (c) development, (d) pre-launch/launch and (e) post market. It is common to have a stage-gated approach to control and monitor progress, where at the end of each stage, certain criteria need to have been fulfilled in order to progress further. Variations between organisations and their approaches to new product development make this process fluid, with the stages sometimes overlapping, the criteria variable between companies, and the lines between stages sometimes blurry.

A more systematic route and record of the process are normally followed by businesses supplying healthcare products globally: the design control process. This is a prescribed, established methodology to ensure that the product development and manufacture are controlled, traceable, and meet specific safety and efficacy requirements. Documentation produced out of the design control process builds up the Design History Files.

The organisational product development stages can be considered in parallel with the more regulated design control process (Figure 7.1). The concept stage could include background research, market research, idea generation, idea development, concept development and concept testing, leading to a better understanding of the user and design needs. The essential claims or benefits of the product need to be identified early on, as they are important drivers of the design requirements. During the subsequent feasibility stage, the design inputs are established based on the user and design needs, and on the knowledge obtained over that development period. Activities could include the construction of prototypes, development of test methods, preliminary testing and the identification of candidate materials, manufacturing

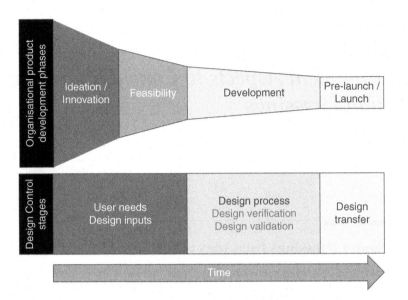

FIGURE 7.1
Organisational product development stages and design control process

processes, suppliers and collaborators. In these two early stages, consideration should be given to intellectual property regarding the new ideas and related new manufacturing processes. In the traditional product development model, a funnelling pathway is followed (as shown in Figure 7.1), whereby at the start of the process during the concept and feasibility stages, several ideas or options may be evaluated in parallel, but the output for further development and launch may only be one product.

In the development stage, a selected prototype is progressed further, the raw materials are narrowed down, chosen and validated, the process is fully developed, optimised and validated, risk assessments are conducted for the product and manufacturing, quality control measures are put in place, numerous testing is performed, including characterisation, efficacy and stability, and clinical investigations may be conducted. The development stage should ensure that any claims that were identified in the early stages can be substantiated, through various testing and if required, through user and patient trials. It is also at this stage that the bulk of the regulatory documentation is compiled, and that the design verification and validation could be conducted.

In the pre-launch stage, final design transfer to manufacturing is completed, with all manufacturing validations conducted and first launch batches produced. This stage is also likely to include the completion of all documentation for regulatory approval. The launch of a product is often accompanied or preceded by significant marketing activities, for example, presentation of the new product and the related clinical evidence at major international conferences, trade and professional shows. Finally, once a product is launched, many countries require a post-market surveillance system in place where any feedback, complaints and adverse events can be logged and investigated. The identification of issues in market may lead to product recalls, or future changes in the product or process specifications.

Whatever the regulatory classification of the wound dressing (more on this in Section 7.2.3.1), other than the Design History Files, a series of additional documentation and measures must generally be in place to satisfy the regulatory requirements. Altogether, these are needed to ensure that the process of designing and developing the dressing has been rigorous, that the clinical safety has been evaluated, that the efficacy has been demonstrated, that all risks have been assessed and mitigated, that quality controls are in place for the manufacturing process to be accurate, reliable and reproducible, and that there is full traceability of each product made. One of the many aspects to consider in the development of new advanced wound care dressings is that the above process of collating all the necessary documentation can take time, depending on how much testing and trials are required and depending on how complex the manufacturing process is. The use of documentation for a predicate dressing, i.e., a dressing which can be demonstrated to be equivalent, can speed up the process to some extent. This naturally is not applicable in the case of a completely new product, using new materials. The speed to market is also influenced by the time it takes for the regulatory body to review the documentation (where required), to provide feedback and to give the final approval. Finally, the internal organisational structure and systems in place can also play a vital part in the time to market. The launch of a new product always requires the close collaboration of several units within a business – e.g., R&D, packaging, marketing, quality, clinical, regulatory and manufacturing teams.

7.2 Challenges for Introducing New Materials and Structures

Research in the fields of new materials and new structures is quite rich and diverse in academia and technology-driven companies, but as per the funnel model of Figure 7.1, only a few will make it to a launched product. The drivers for the development of new materials are generally linked to three main aspects of improvements: costs, performance and environmental impact. Superiority in one aspect compared to existing products may justify further efforts and investments to launch, provided that the overall sum of benefits is on balance believed to be higher than the sum of investments.

Net cost reduction is always attractive, whether the savings occur at the raw material stage, processing stages or at the point of final use. If this can translate in reduced costs to the caregiver, patient, or to better profit margins, there is development and investment potential for some businesses, as long as there is a degree of equivalence in performance to other comparable materials. In recent years, there has been significant interest in better utilising our resources, in sustainability, and in the reduction of waste material from processing, manufacturing and use. New materials that make a claim towards any of these have the attention of a growing market of users who are more environmentally conscious, sometimes even willing to compromise on performance. Performance however is one major driver in healthcare, and while a small compromise may be accepted by some, a certain degree of equivalence is generally expected for commercial success. If better clinical outcomes can be demonstrated with a new material, investment interest is likely to be more forthcoming, even if initial costs are high.

In the current era, drivers for the development of new structures and hybrids are more often related to the quest for better performance and/or differentiation. Some innovation outcomes are linked to new processes being explored: for example, the development of the electrospinning process has brought to attention the nano porous membranes that they can form. Where such new structures also result in cost savings or a positive environmental impact, this is generally considered a bonus. The development of new structures and combinations using established raw materials has a faster route to market compared to developing completely new materials, provided that the materials used are already commercially available in the wound dressing arena. In the latter case, there should already be sufficient evidence on the safety of the raw material, to be used in the regulatory documentation. It is therefore not uncommon to see rapid innovation in wound dressings to revolve around manipulating materials that are already well understood and accepted to be safe for patient use. The claims of the new structure developed are often seen to piggy-back on the claims or evidence of the base materials used.

7.2.1 Evidence of Performance

One of the big challenges of new materials and structures is demonstrating sufficient evidence of an overall positive benefit in performance. For new advanced wound dressings, this means providing evidence of good clinical outcomes such as those exemplified in Table 7.1. Evidence on performance is necessary to support claims to be used by the new product. This is challenging, particularly for new materials previously unused in the medical field, because there may have been no prior work to inform its safety profile, its efficacy and its performance on a wound compared to other treatments. Any investigation to support both the regulatory documentation and the

TABLE 7.1

Examples of measurable clinical outcomes

Wound clinical outcomes	Patient clinical outcomes
Rate of healing	Pain and anxiety scores
Number of wounds closed in time frame	Time spent in hospital
Percentage reduction in wound size	Recovery time
Incidence of infection	Percentage of compliance
Scar score	
Incidence of recurrence	
Incidence of complications	
Number and type of adverse events	
Frequency of dressing changes	

marketing claims requires careful planning, consideration of the protocols, of the outcomes to be measured, of the duration of the study, the numbers required, and so on. If done incorrectly, the data from tests and investigations may be considered to be too small to be conclusive, to be biased, or not representative of real-life situations, or not providing the right information to support the desired claims.

In vitro and *in vivo* studies are commonly the starting points to gather information on the safety and performance of a new product in a relatively short time. However, such data, while informative and while even possibly comparative against other competitive products, are generally insufficient for commercial success. In some cases, for new products, they may not demonstrate the efficacy, i.e., that the product is achieving the intended results during use. Large, multi-centred randomised clinical trials provide better evidence of efficacy and performance, but they are expensive and time-consuming. For many small companies, the cost of such trials may be prohibitive or can only be achieved with significant financial strains and high risks. Nowadays, clinicians are encouraged to take an evidence-based approach in order to include a new product in their protocols of care, and if the evidence is insufficient, they may be more reluctant to try something new with an unproven track record.

7.2.2 Global Market Penetration and Differentiation

New products, particularly those with new materials, need substantial regulatory and marketing efforts in order to be able to penetrate successfully in multiple markets. From a regulatory perspective, documentation is required for each separate market (or block of markets, such as the European Union) before the product can be made available for sale. Markets around the world also have different healthcare objectives and priorities. Competition within each country may also be quite different, with each needing a different strategic approach for penetration. From a marketing perspective, the classic strategies for market penetration (e.g., starting with a lower price point and increasing as market share increases) may not always work for advanced wound care products where potentially high costs have already been incurred in the design and development and securing the appropriate intellectual property. Product performance and differentiation then become essential to support the launch.

The global market for advanced wound dressings is dominated by a handful of large corporations, which are highly competitive. There are over 400 vendors globally supplying this market, with the large and diversified companies accounting for nearly half of the share (Report Linker, 2019). A new product may be as good as other existing products, but without any specific differentiation, successful penetration into a market becomes a huge challenge. There are several strategies that can be taken upon launch in order to differentiate a new product to existing ones. One of them is emphasising the unique selling points of the new product (which could be as simple as a lower cost, or as complex as better clinical outcomes); another is demonstrating its superiority over leading competitors. With the vast number of new advanced wound care products on the markets, it becomes more and more difficult to identify a truly unique benefit. Unique features are very easy to create; however, the challenge is demonstrating the true positive effect and value of such features. A deep understanding of all aspects of wound care is essential in order to be able to truly identify genuine benefits that resonate with the practitioners.

Comparison with competitor products is a common route taken by many manufacturers, as evidenced by the number of randomised controlled trials comparing a new product with standard protocol of care or best practice. This strategy seems to be popular, particularly since clinicians mostly take an evidence-based approach in their decision-making. Proving clinical equivalence to a leading competitor or gold standard treatment can be positive as well, particularly if there are additional benefits or unique selling points such as a net financial benefit. As discussed above, providing clinical equivalence and superiority over competitor products from large trials is a lengthy and costly process. Case studies and smaller-sized patient studies can give early indications of the benefits, but without the required numbers to be statistically sound, the evidence may be considered insufficient.

7.2.3 Regulatory Challenges Around New Wound Dressings

In all major markets, wound dressings are subjected to regulatory controls, and the right documentation and evidence must be in place before the product can be released in the market. The requirements for different countries may be slightly or significantly different, even down to how the product is classified. A regulatory roadmap developed at the beginning of a project can inform the overall launch plans, the timeframe for launch and the regulatory side of development costs. The roadmap could include for example the order of countries where the product will be launched and the requirements that need to be in place prior to the submissions of documents. The claims that the business wants to associate with the new product are closely interlinked to the classification of the product, and therefore to its regulatory pathway.

7.2.3.1 Classifications of Wound Dressings

The majority of wound dressings are classified as medical devices in the key commercial regions of the world. The definitions of a medical device by the EU Medical Device Regulation (MDR) and by the Food and Drug Administration (FDA) in the US are provided in Table 7.2. Some wound dressings may be borderline with pharmaceutical products or classified as such, if they contain ingredients or have intended mechanisms of actions that are pharmacological, immunological or metabolic in nature. Within the overarching medical device category, the products can be further classified according to the level of risks associated with them, and this is also linked to the intended use and the indication for use. This classification varies

TABLE 7.2

EU and US definitions of medical devices

EU MDR definition	US FDA definition
An article intended by the manufacturer to be used for: - diagnosis, prevention, monitoring, prediction, prognosis, treatment or alleviation of a disease - for diagnosis, monitoring, treatment, alleviation of or compensation for, an injury or disability - for investigation, replacement or modification of the anatomy, or of a physiological or pathological process or state - for providing information by means of in vitro examination of specimens derived from the human body and which does not achieve its principle intended action by pharmacological, immunological or metabolic means, but which may be assisted in its functions by such means.	An article recognised in the official National Formulary or the US Pharmacopoeia or any supplement to them, which is intended: - for diagnosis of disease of other conditions, or in the cure, mitigation, treatment, or prevention of disease - to affect the structure or any function of the body and which does not achieve its primary intended purposes through chemical action within or on the body, and which is not dependent upon being metabolised for the achievement of any of its primary intended purposes.

Source: Medical Device Regulation (2017b) and FDA (2018).

slightly from region to region, but follows the same principle. For example, for both the EU and the US, devices are classified from Class I to Class III, with III having the highest risks. As the risk category increases, the controls that need to be in place to ensure the safety and effectiveness of the dressing need to be more detailed and rigorous and the regulatory requirements become more complex. Hence the classification of the product has an impact on the development of a new product and on the regulatory preparations and submissions.

In the EU, the MDR (Medical Device Regulation, 2017a) classifies all non-invasive wound dressings in contact with injured skin or mucous membrane as Class I, if they are intended to be used as a mechanical barrier, for compression or for absorption of exudates. Examples are non-sterile dressings, absorbent pads, island dressings, gauze dressings, adhesive bandages and compression hosiery. However, they are categorised as Class IIa if they are principally intended to manage the micro-environment of injured skin or mucous membrane, such as with polymer film dressings, hydrogel dressings and non-medicated impregnated gauze dressings. Wound dressings are classified as Class IIb if they are intended to be used principally for injuries to skin which have breached the dermis, or mucous membrane and can only heal by secondary intent (i.e., where the edges are not closed and the wound heals from bottom up). Examples in this category are dressings for extensive chronic ulcerated wounds, for severe burns, severe decubitis wounds, and dressings that can augment tissue and provide a temporary skin substitute. Class III devices in the MDR are typically surgically invasive devices that are in contact with the heart, the central circulatory system or central nervous system or which have a biological effect or are mainly absorbed. Other features that push devices into the Class III category, and which have more relevance to advanced wound dressings are: if they contain nanomaterials that present a high to medium potential for internal exposure, if they utilise tissues or cells of human or animal origins or their derivatives, or if they incorporate an integral medicinal substance that is liable to act in an ancillary way on the body. For example, dressings that contain an antimicrobial agent which provides an ancillary action on the wounds are classed as Class III medical devices. Xenografts and dressings which contain collagen and hyaluronic acid of animal origins are also Class III devices in the EU.

In the US (FDA, 2019), the classification is also based on risks, but takes a different approach. Class I devices are those that do not present an unreasonable risk of illness or injury, and are not life-supporting or life-sustaining. Except for some exemptions, only general controls are deemed necessary in the manufacturing process of US Class I devices to provide assurance that the device is safe and effective. For this category, the documentary evidence for regulatory controls is faster to compile. Simple bandages, non-resorbable gauzes and sponges, compression bandages, and a number of basic wound dressings (e.g., occlusive, hydrogel and hydrophilic dressings) fall into this group. Class II devices are those where general manufacturing controls are deemed insufficient to provide assurance of safety and effectiveness, and additional special controls are required. An example is an antimicrobial dressing with pDADMAC,[1] where the additive is permanently attached to the textile substrate. Class III devices are those for which insufficient information exists to determine that general controls and special controls provide assurance of safety and effectiveness, and if the device is in addition life-supporting, life-sustaining and presents a potential unreasonable risk of illness or injury. Wound dressings that are 'unclassified' by the FDA are also automatically considered Class III (FDA, 2016b). Examples are wound dressings that are intended to accelerate the normal rate of wound healing, serve as a replacement for full-thickness skin grafting, or treat full-thickness burns, such as artificial skin substitutes and collagen dressings.

7.2.3.2 Regulations Around the World

Regulations on wound dressings can vary significantly from country to country, which can make it challenging for businesses that sell globally. However, there are some global standards that are followed worldwide, and some initiatives working towards harmonisation. Typically, there are three main elements in a country's regulatory space:

1) a set of regulations, setting out the directives and rules that manufacturers anywhere in the world need to comply with in order to be able to sell the product in the country;
2) a regulatory body or competent authority, which is normally governmental and responsible for transposing regulations into law, i.e., imposing the necessary requirements and standards and enforcing compliance and
3) a series of standards, which the manufacturers can follow in order to meet the regulations.

In some cases, as in the EU, there are also a number of notified bodies that carry out the assessments and verification operations, as per the required regulations. The grouping of economic areas, for example, the EU and the Eurasian region, where several countries within the zone follow a single directive, massively helps in making a new product more widely accessible within that economic zone. However, in the development and launch of a new product globally, the differences in regulation must be taken into consideration for the planning.

Where they are followed, regulations are generally in three stages (Lamph, 2012). Firstly, pre-market regulations ensure that a new product being developed will meet minimum safety and effectiveness standards. In the majority of cases, this takes the form of a conformity assessment or declaration, which the manufacturer prepares to demonstrate that the product meets the requirements, and which a regulatory body may need to assess. On-market regulations ensure that products currently being sold are correctly labelled and advertised. Post-market regulations ensure that the safety and effectiveness is continued over time. Some countries have multiple governmental bodies that look after these three different stages. For others, a single regulatory body is responsible. A number of regulatory bodies and their regulations are given as examples in Table 7.3. Launching and selling a new product in a global market can therefore be a challenge if the right internal structures and expertise are not in place to support the business.

7.3 Considerations for the Practitioner

Aside from the technical, clinical and regulatory challenges, it is worth mentioning the interaction of the product with its user in the development of new dressing. Several trends are driving the need for products to be easy to use, intuitive, require minimal training, and be disposed of easily. Some of these trends are: expectations for simpler instructions and faster plug-and-play driven by the consumer electronics sector, less time available for training or for changing of dressings, and wound care increasingly happening in a home setting. The latter also implies that dressing changes and disposal in a home environment need to be simple and safe, with low risk of contaminating others. These considerations must be applied to all the components of the wound care product. Typically, this consists at a minimum, of the wound dressing itself, the primary packaging, the instructions for use and the secondary packaging. Some practitioners will also have to deal with tertiary packaging. In addition, the user considerations have to be met at all the different stages of using the product: e.g., opening a secondary packaging, opening a primary packaging, taking a dressing out, applying onto a patient's wound and disposing of all packaging materials. A more detailed breakdown of a simple adhesive dressing change journey is provided in Figure 7.2. The process is longer where more than one dressing is applied (e.g., a primary and a secondary dressing) and where NPWT or other devices are used.

7.3.1 Human Factors

Human factors (HF) is a discipline taking into consideration all aspects of human interaction with the product, the environment and each other (in the context of a task at hand) in order to ensure that the task is conducted with the best chance of success. It is one way of ensuring the safety of patients,

TABLE 7.3

Regulatory bodies and regulations across the world

Country	Regulatory body/competent authority	Regulations followed
UK	MHRA (Medicines and Healthcare Products Regulatory Agency)	Medical Device Regulation (MDR), leading to submission and approval for CE Marking
EU	Each country has its own competent authority, e.g., Bundesinstitut für Arzneimittel und Medizinprodukte (BfArM) for Germany, Agence Nationale de Sécurité du Médicament et des Produits de Santé (ANSM) for France, Agencia Española de Medicamentos y Productos Sanitarios (AEMPS) for Spain, the Norwegian Medicines Agency (NoMA) for Norway, and the Medical Products Agency (MPA) in Sweden	MDR, as above
US	Food and Drugs Administration (FDA), Center for Devices and Radiological Health (CDRH)	Code of Federal Regulations (CFR) Title 21, subchapter H, leading to a 510 K, Premarket Approval (PMA) or de Novo submission and approval
Canada	Health Canada, Medical Device Directorate (MDD)	Canadian Medical Device Regulations (CMDR) SOR/98-282, leading to a Medical Device Establishment Licence (MDEL)
Australia	The Therapeutic Goods Administration (TGA)	Australian Regulatory Guidelines for Medical Devices (ARGMD), Therapeutic Goods (Medical Devices) Regulation
Brazil	Agência Nacional de Vigilância Sanitária (ANVISA, Brazilian Health Regulatory Agency)	Resolution RDC 185 and RDC 40, leading to Cadastro or Registro submissions and approval depending on the classification
Argentina	Administración Nacional de Medicamentos, Alimentos y Tecnología Médica (ANMAT, National Administration of Drugs, Foods and Medical Devices)	MERCOSUR[a] Technical Regulation for Registration of Medical Devices; ANMAT disposition 2318
India	The Drug Controller General of India (DCGI) within the Central Drugs Standard Control Organization (CDSCO)	Medical Device Rules, under the India's Drugs and Cosmetic Act and Rules (DCA)
China	National Medical Products Administration (NMPA) (previously CFDA, China Food and Drug Administration)	Regulations for the Supervision and Administration of Medical Devices
South Africa	South African Health Products Regulatory Authority (SAHPRA)	General Regulations relating to Medical Devices and In Vitro Diagnostic Medical Devices, published in the Government Gazette No. 40480; December 2016

(Continued)

TABLE 7.3 (*Continued*)

Country	Regulatory body/competent authority	Regulations followed
Russia	Roszdravnadzor (RZN)	Resolution 1416, expected to transit to the Eurasian[b] Medical Device Registration Rules (ERR) by the end of 2021
Saudi Arabia	Saudi Food and Drug Authority (SFDA)	Medical Devices Interim Regulation 4/16/1439; National Provisions and Requirements for Medical Devices SA-001

[a] MERCOSUR: Also referred to as the Southern Common Market is a South American trade group consisting of Argentina, Brazil, Paraguay and Uruguay, with associate countries Bolivia, Chile, Colombia, Ecuador, Guyana, Peru and Suriname, and suspended member Venezuela.

[b] Eurasian Medical Device Regulation: harmonisation for members of the Eurasian Economic Union, Russia, Armenia, Belarus, Kazakhstan and Kyrgyzstan.

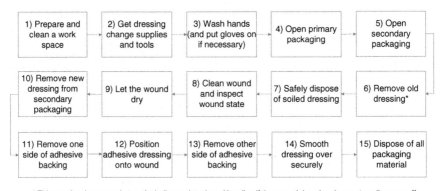

* This may involve several steps including moistening with saline if the wound dressing does not easily come off

FIGURE 7.2
An adhesive dressing change journey

while bearing in mind the practitioner and his/her challenges during the task. The term HF is sometimes used interchangeably with ergonomics or usability engineering (UE), although it is arguable that there are slight nuances within each of those terms. The three are defined in Table 7.4. HF and UE, which are more commonly interchangeably used, are more focused on the safety aspects and risk mitigation, whereas ergonomics tend to focus more on optimisation of performance. Broadly speaking, while UE seems to be more user-focused, HF tends to encompass a wider all-encompassing perspective of the optimal use of a product, considering the behaviour of individuals, their interaction with each other and with their environment.

HF in its recent, integrated form, has evolved in the last couple of decades or so, advancing from basic usability studies. Early references to usability

TABLE 7.4

Human factors, ergonomics and usability engineering

Human factors (HF)	Ergonomics	Usability engineering (UE)
"Enhancing clinical performance through an understanding of the effect of teamwork, tasks, equipment, workspace, culture and organisation on human behaviour and abilities and application of that knowledge in clinical settings."	"… the scientific discipline concerned with the understanding of interactions among humans and other elements of a system, and the profession that applies theory, principles, data and methods to design in order to optimise human well-being and overall system performance."	"Process… (that) permits the manufacturer to assess and mitigate risks associated with correct use and use errors i.e., normal use."
Cited by Catchpole (NHS England National Quality Board, 2013)	International Ergonomics Association (Chartered Institute of Ergonomics and Human Factors, n.d.)	International Standard IEC 62366-1 (IEC, 2015)

and HF in medical devices seemed to be mostly concerned with electronic, mechanical or durable devices referring to displays, set up, input, output, alarms, and so on. The scope is today well accepted to encompass all aspects of wound care, not just devices, and that includes flexible dressings too. The objectives go beyond making sure that a product is easy to use (by the user). They are to ensure patient and practitioner safety, minimise errors, improve quality of care, and clinical experience, particularly given that the hospital, surgery and home care environments can be very different, dynamic, often with high stress levels and significant time pressures. HF also aims to do so not by requiring users to change their behaviour, but by modifying the design of the systems instead; it is not about eliminating human error, but creating systems that are resilient to such errors (Russ et al., 2013).

There is some evidence that utilising principles of HF in healthcare generally can lead to many positive patient-related and practitioner-related outcomes, such as better perceived teamwork, positive perceptual changes, better-observed team skills, better satisfaction with care, improved compliance with briefings, better processes, reduced error rates and better organisational perceptions (Catchpole, 2013). On the product development side, applying HF principles during the design and development phases can assist in enabling the establishment of the principles during use. This has been reflected in the changes in regulatory requirements. In Europe for example, where previously the Medical Device Directive (MDD) required consideration of usability in only a handful of areas, the new MDR has significantly more reference to HF, including sections on designing for lay people, ergonomic displays, controls and indicators and disposal. In the wound dressing development context, as with any other product development process, HF

TABLE 7.5

Examples of human factors (HF) analyses and evaluation methods and validation testing

Analysis and evaluation		
Analytical	**Empirical**	**Validation testing**
FMEA	Contextual inquiry	Simulated-use
FTA	Interviews	Testing of modified designs
Identification of known use-related problems	Formative evaluations	Actual use testing (clinical)
Task analysis		
Heuristic analysis		
Expert review		

Source: FDA (2016a).
FMEA, failure mode effects analysis; FTA, failure tree analysis.

should be considered as early as possible, and fully developed and implemented in the development stage before the design is validated.

Some tools that can be used in implementing HF throughout the product development stages are summed up in Table 7.5 (FDA, 2016a). Analysis and evaluation methods essentially offer ways of identifying potential risks and putting in place a risk mitigation plan. The most effective and the preferred way of eliminating or reducing the risks is to modify the design or include protective or preventative measures within the product or the packaging. However, it is acknowledged that not all risks can be mitigated in such ways, and there may be some residual risks that can only be highlighted in printed matter (labelling, instructions for use) or during training. HF validation testing can be done under conditions of simulated use, or in actual clinical use.

Catchpole (2013) pointed out that in general, there are several challenges to consider for the implementation of HF principles in healthcare: device design, task design, communication, training and incident reporting systems. All of these can be addressed in the development of a wound care product. In the design of the product, attention could be paid to the minimisation of user error and misuse (e.g., for dressings with different layers, it needs to be clear to users as to which layer should be in contact with the wound bed). Importantly, advanced wound dressings and wound care solutions need to be developed not just with minimal risk of error or misuse, but in the context of the whole wound care journey, from the time the product is introduced to the practitioner to the time it is fully disposed of. This is partly exemplified in Figure 7.2, and with the additional steps of pre-use training and information gathering and further tasks associated with disposal. Communication about the product and training should be clear and consistent, with no ambiguity or potential misinterpretation of information by the practitioner. Each step of the task of changing the dressing should be carefully observed and considered, and where risks of misuse, error, unsafe practices, etc. are identified, the product design, communication or training should be amended. In healthcare, these all pose extra challenges as standardisation to a detailed level may not be possible, given the vast range of wounds and practices. Adverse events are also rarely investigated or acted upon, except when the consequences have been serious or indeed tragic. So, in many cases, a range of improvements could be done to a product but is not.

7.3.2 Voice of the Customer and Other Market Research Techniques

In the wound care sector, some consider the 'customer' to be the patient. Certainly, they are the recipient of the treatment, and it is absolutely right that they are situated at the centre of wound care. The key requirements of patients have been discussed in Section 3.2. However, one can also argue that the customers are not only the patients, but also the care practitioners and care givers, i.e., the people who are conducting the dressing changes and who are looking after the patient. They are at the front line to deal with the application of fresh dressings, the removal and disposal of soiled dressings, the consequences of dressings that fall off or leak onto clothing and bedding, helping with pain management, and so on. They are also the main point of contact for any queries from the patient on all aspects of dressing use. Importantly, they may be the decision maker or influencer in the choice of dressing to be used for the wound and patient type. Therefore, the opinion of care practitioners on the product is critical in order to gain support for use. Some essential considerations are briefly outlined in Section 3.5. However, going beyond the basics to ensure that the voice of the clinician is also heard is likely to lead to better product development or new product launches in the future, and better life cycle management of existing products.

Voice of the customer (VoC) is mentioned here as an example approach. However, any other market research and innovation activities, where the clinician's experience, opinions and feedback are taken into consideration are to be considered. A number of VoC methods that can be used to capture the preferences, aversions, expectations, wants and needs of healthcare practitioners are summed up in Table 7.6 (Cooper & Dreher, 2010). These methods can be used at all the stages of product development, with different objectives. Utilising VoC methods early in the concept phase may lead to new idea generation. In the feasibility phase, it could help narrow down technical options. In the development phase, it could be used to verify and validate some of the design features and benefits. In the pre-launch/launch stage it can assist in early feedback of the finished product. In the post-market surveillance stage, it is essential to understand the product's benefits and problems, after repeated use. Market research with clinicians can be a two-way relationship, beneficial for both parties. On the one hand, a product developer can gain

TABLE 7.6

VoC methods in wound care

Methods	Brief description
Ethnographic research	Observing clinicians and patients for extended periods of time as they use and wear the products
Customer visit teams	In-depth and structured interviews with a user (clinician or patient), ideally in their environment
Focus groups	Structured discussions with small groups of users
Lead user analysis	Workshop with a small group of users identified as being innovative
Customer helps design product	Clinicians and/or patients are invited to help the product developer design the next new product
Customer brainstorming	Brainstorming of new ideas or of problems and their solutions with small groups of users
Customer advisory board	Regular discussions with a panel of users
Community of enthusiasts	Generally refers to an online community of users who discuss the product category, identifying problems and potential solutions

Source: Cooper and Dreher (2010).

essential insights into the use of their product, and develop new ones which take on board those insights for the optimal performance of the user. On the other hand, the user gains from a better-suited product, and through the development of a relationship, gains trust with the developer.

7.4 Innovation in Wound Dressings

Innovation is a highly complex topic that cannot be discussed in its whole depth in this book. It is a topic in this chapter because it determines the future of wound care and the introduction of new wound dressings in the market. On a very simplistic level, innovation is about developing and launching something new. In the wound care sector, the term is frequently used quite narrowly to describe new products. However, on a broader scale, innovation also encompasses new clinical practice around wound care, new related services and after-services, new business models, different training and communication strategies, and even alternative technology, manufacturing, and supply solutions.

Innovation can be incremental, semi-radical or radical. Incremental innovation is limited to a small step change in an existing solution or product. Semi-radical innovation involves significant changes to existing solutions

TABLE 7.7

Examples of wound dressing projects with different levels of innovation – from incremental to radical

Innovation type	Example projects
Incremental: Modifications and improvements to existing product lines (life cycle management)	Change of size of existing dressing Minor change of shape of existing dressing Change of packaging of existing dressing Change of adhesive type or release liner Improvement of tensile properties of a wet dressing
Incremental: Additions to existing product line	New sizes of dressings (e.g., extra-large, paediatrics) New shapes of dressings (e.g., sacral, heels, face, hands) Addition of new product range for a specific indication, using the same product line and minor changes (e.g., surgical range, burns range, trauma range) Addition of an extra feature, e.g., incorporation of antimicrobial or other actives to an existing product, or the addition of an extra barrier or contact layer Addition of new accessories to the product pack
Semi-radical: New product lines	New materials developed into a new product, or new previously unused combination of materials (e.g., the first alginate, first hydrogel, first haemostatic, first carboxymethylcellulose fibre dressings, first foam dressing, first barrier film dressing) A product range new to the business (but not new to market)
Radical: Breakthrough innovation	New approach to a problem that is already being solved in a different way, e.g., NPWT, skin substitutes, biologics, bioelectric dressings

to a customer need. Radical or breakthrough innovation offers a completely alternative way of addressing a need, generally requiring a technological change and a business model change simultaneously. All are important in a business portfolio to be able to maintain current market share and profitability, and secure long term launches and future markets. Some examples of innovation and product development projects in the area of wound dressings are given in Table 7.7.

It has been observed that breakthrough innovation – where the proposed idea is completely new to the world – is declining (Cooper & Dreher, 2010; Cooper, 2011). A breakdown of the type of projects in the portfolio of a range of businesses between the 1990s and the 2010s indicate that the number of new product lines was also on a decreasing trend. Instead, there has been greater focus on incremental innovations such as additions to existing product lines and improvements and modifications to existing products (also termed life cycle management). This trend is partially driven by management practices in large corporations and partly by external factors such as

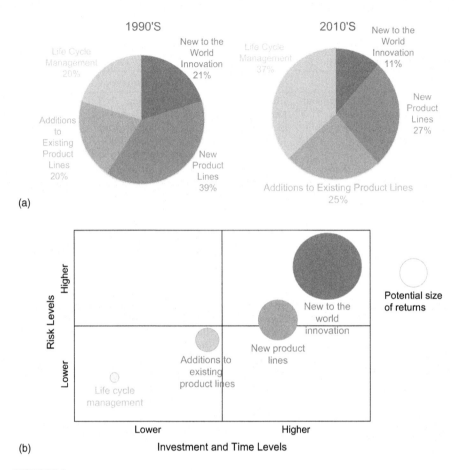

FIGURE 7.3
A simplification of project types, breakdown, risks, investment and returns (a) Breakdown of projects in the 1990s and the 2010s, adapted from Cooper and Dreher (2010), (b) Comparison between project types in terms of risks, investment and rewards

stricter regulatory requirements on new product launches, and the fact that markets are now mature and already well served with a range of products. A very similar scenario is likely to be applicable for the wound dressing sector. Unsurprisingly, the two types of innovation where investment is proportionately low per company (new idea and new product line) are the most time-, effort- and cash-demanding with the highest risks, but potentially the highest rewards (Figure 7.3). Some of these rewards can even be intangible: for example, being at the forefront of innovation could strengthen the reputation of a business as a market leader, not only creating more direct revenues, but also adding value to the business name and its brands. However, more effort and investment are being put on smaller projects with faster turnaround, easy sales, and building on existing market presence. It is estimated that most companies spend over 80% of their total innovation budget on incremental innovation (Davila et al., 2009). Depending on the innovation mindset in the organisation, incremental or semi-radical innovation could simply be called new product development and life cycle management of existing products. They may even be managed by completely different teams from different reporting lines within the organisational structure.

7.4.1 Technology-Based or Customer-Driven, or Other?

In wound care, innovation has sprouted from both technology-led solutions and the requirements of the patients/clinicians, i.e., the customer. Customer-driven[2] innovations often stem from a pain-point observed for the patient or the practitioner. Market research techniques such as those outlined in Section 7.3.2 help to identify unmet needs, and in some cases, can help identify the potential solutions too. Often, customer-driven new product development takes the format of problem-solution, where a problem is identified and a solution is developed. As the market gets more mature and most 'problems' get solved, this type of approach becomes limited and other 'delighters' need to be identified to offer solutions to unknown or unnoticed issues.

One simple example of basic customer-driven innovation is the development of atraumatic silicone adhesives. This was driven by the need to reduce pain upon removal of the dressing, a common concern which can have an interplay on human factors. Indeed, a survey on pain and trauma at dressing changes revealed that 47% of respondents felt that they needed to prevent trauma during dressing changes, and 34% felt that they needed to avoid causing pain (Hollinworth & Collier, 2000). While other solutions are possible to address this issue, e.g., irrigating the wound dressing with saline or sterile water to make it easier and less painful to remove, or the use of analgesics, the development of atraumatic adhesives also addressed the clinician's need to have a shorter and simpler task of changing the dressing. Another example is the development of superabsorbent dressings. On the one hand, they meet the patient's need of better management of excess fluids so their quality of life can improve. On the other hand, they also address the issue of clinicians having to change dressings too frequently and the carer's need to often have to change soiled clothing and bedding. In some cases, innovation is driven by clinical and clinical management needs. The prevention of infection after surgery is an example. In order to increase the likelihood of post-surgery healing without any complications and delays, and hence minimising time and costs, the need for a reduction in the risk of surgical site infections has led to the development of a number of post-operative antibacterial dressings.

Technology-driven innovation occurs when a new technology or material is developed first and then it is matched to unmet needs, sometimes in different industries. Technology-driven companies tend to be businesses that have (or will end up having) a broad portfolio of products spanning different industries, but utilising and adapting a core technology (or several core technologies) and their associated knowledge. An example of a large technology-driven, science-based company is 3M, with offerings in a range of industries from wound care, architecture and home improvement, traffic, and even the aerospace and aircraft sector. One technology-driven innovation in wound care is the development of hydrogel wound dressings. First developed as contact lenses in the 1960s, hydrogels first found their way as potential wound dressings in the early 1990s when the concept of moist wound healing had already gained momentum (Caló & Khutoryanskiy, 2015). For the majority of technology-driven wound dressing innovation, the technologies were not new to the world, but are transferred and modified from other industries to meet the needs of the wound care sector.

Technology can also be used as a way to drive the ideation process, even in non-technology driven businesses. One technique is to analyse the trends in upcoming new technologies, identify the properties and performance of the outputs, correlate them with customer needs and ideate around ways of utilising them in a new product line or breakthrough innovation. The rapid development of electrospinning to create nano structure and nano morphologies can be used as an example where an emerging technology has found potential use in wound care. While this is still in its infancy in the context of wound dressings, a multitude of electrospun polymers have been explored as biodegradable and drug-releasing conduits in the last two decades.

A variation of technology-driven wound dressing innovation is one that is driven from an understanding of the properties of base materials, and their potential performance in wound care. Materials-led companies, such as Dow Corporate or Dupont, are technology-driven science-based companies that acquire an in-depth understanding of their materials and develop evidence of its efficacy in the field of their choice. Eventually, they branch out into a range of industries for expansion and developing other adjacent materials. The combination of materials and blends of materials with different technologies opens up a large arena for play in the wound dressing innovation sector. New product developments rely on the success of the right combination of materials and technology, successfully meeting the right consumer needs, and at the right time.

7.4.2 The Innovation Pipeline or Roadmap

The starting point for any business to fill an innovation pipeline or roadmap meaningfully, coherently and with intent is to have a clear overall business strategy. Ideally an innovation strategy, which takes into account the business's current product ranges, competitive status and market share, is also required. Without a clear forward strategy, businesses tend to become more reactive to market events and subsequently become driven to quickly follow

and catch-up the competitors. While this does not exclude commercial success (and indeed while this may actually be a business strategy), the outputs of the business are more likely to be variations of other products on
the markets and 'me-too's. Conversely, a strategy cannot be too rigid and a
degree of flex is essential to adapt, where deemed necessary, to significant
market changes and competitor pressures. The innovation strategy should
clarify where and how the business wants to position itself with regard to the
competitors, whether it will pursue radical innovation ideas or not and how
frequently new launches need to occur.

Large businesses in the wound care sector are under pressure to provide
new news annually at major conferences and trade events. A new product
launch or an improved version of an existing products are reportable hap-
penings at such events. New product launches provide an opportunity for
penetrating new markets. Improvements of existing products give an opportunity for increasing market share. Both of these occurrences contribute to
growth and the strengthening of the business reputation. Small technology
start-ups do not have the same public-relation pressures, but they are driven
by the requirement for financial growth and expansion. Their pipelines will
look considerably different to those of large established businesses.

The development of a pipeline therefore needs to take all the above into
consideration, and provide a clear road map for the business for a period
of 3–5 years. An example of a new product pipeline is given in Figure 7.4.
Maintaining a healthy pipeline needs it to be reviewed and modified regularly (e.g., annually), identifying predictable impactful events such as
changes in regulation, and expected launches from competitors. Existing
projects and their estimated launches provide the initial framework; from
this, gaps can be identified and longer-term plans can be put in place.
A healthy pipeline contains a balance of different types and size of projects,

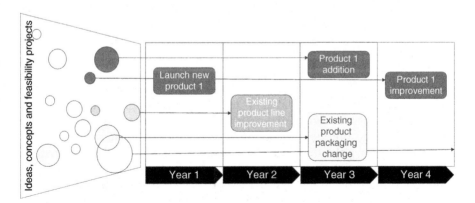

FIGURE 7.4
An example of a new product development pipeline

including lifecycle management and new products. It should help a business understand the resource requirements for various parts of the business – research, development, supply, marketing, and so on. Feeding into the pipeline should be a range of concepts, ideas, and projects in the feasibility and assessment stages.

7.4.3 Sources and Management of Ideas

There are various sources of ideas for new products or product improvements – internal, external and collaborative. Each source has its own benefits and disadvantages. Many wound dressing businesses therefore rely on a combination of the three sources to come up with a range of new projects. The selection of the right idea and its transition to a viable project are important aspects that determine the success of a new launch. It is quite fair to say that ideas are easy to generate in volumes and that many ideas are not unique. If two independent and separate groups of people are tasked with brainstorming on the same specific topic or problem, it is highly likely that the majority of ideas generated will be similar or overlap. Generating novel ideas with potential commercial success is a much harder process, which requires more work than a single brainstorming session, but is more likely to provide a better quality of output. There are many ways of generating ideas aside from brainstorming, e.g., story boarding, mind mapping, sketching, Thinking Hats, reverse thinking, SCAMPER technique, role playing, synectics, peripheral visioning, forced relationships, observations and ethnographic studies, focus groups, lead user analysis, patent mining, etc. A study of various methods showed that those that involve the user, whether through observation or interactions (particularly ethnography, lead user analysis, focus groups and customer visits) were the most effective for creating game-changing ideas (Cooper & Edgett, 2008).

The management of ideas does not focus only on generating them, but on the identification and progression of the winning ones. Three basic elements always need to be considered: user needs, technical feasibility and potential profit margin. Ideas need to meet an unmet or unsatisfactorily met need at the right value; they need to be able to be turned into a product or service that is deliverable reliably and consistently, and they need to provide a profit margin that is acceptable for the company. Supplementary to these, each business has its own evaluation criteria to add on to, such as fit to the business strategy, uniqueness and intellectual property profile, profit margin minimum limits, potential market size and growth opportunity, competitive advantage, etc. At its early stage, an idea does not come with all the information required for it be properly evaluated. Hence, it is important to give ideas time and resources to incubate, to be visualised, to be developed to a certain extent to understand its value to customers. Incubated ideas turn into clearer concepts with a good starting point for a business case. Those that pass the business benchmarks then need to have the right support in place to be developed further as a feasibility project, and subsequently go through the business's product development stage gates.

7.4.3.1 Internal Sources of Ideas – Building An Innovative Mindset

Most new product developments originate from internal ideas. Some of these ideas are generated spontaneously, e.g., when an employee has an idea unprompted, based on observation or experience. Some are created in organised workshops or innovation sessions on a particular topic using any manner of idea generation techniques. A structured internal innovation workshop could involve individuals from different teams, e.g., marketing, manufacturing and R&D. It focuses the participants' interactions and discussions on a topic and leads to many potential solutions and ideas. Innovation workshops are normally organised because there is a business objective further down the line that needs to be met. As such, the outputs of these workshops are likely to receive more attention and traction to move forward into concept ideas, feasibility projects and patent filings. The development of ideas within a group also naturally gives it more 'buy-in', as several people could have contributed into the final output.

By contrast, the generation and development of spontaneous ideas by employees can sometimes not get sufficient attention. Selling an idea internally can be a time-consuming effort, and if there is no encouragement or reward to do so, employees with potentially good ideas may simply just put them aside. Internal unsolicited ideas can only be developed where there is sufficient support and incentive for employees, and that includes having time to think, tinker, innovate and having a positive and encouraging innovative mindset and system within the organisation across all levels. Organisational enablers for developing, capturing and evaluating such ideas include for instance regular personal innovation time, innovation training (including how to develop and sell an idea internally), internal databases of ideas, regular review of employee ideas, a reward system for ideas progressed into projects, a positive approach to innovation from senior management, effective metrics and objectives imbedded with innovation targets, and so on. Even without an official organisational system, the important thing is to enable employees to develop their ideas, to let them mature to where they seem viable, and communicate them to where it can generate support by management.

Internal sources of ideas are largely successful for incremental and semi-radical innovation, because the people involved in developing a concept – employees of the business – often have an excellent understanding of the product category and the competitor landscape. They may even have received feedback, complaints or suggestions from users on the market. They are therefore able to identify obvious product or market problems and find potential solutions that can be turned into product modifications, line extensions or even a new product launch. Internal ideas are also comparatively cheap to generate, without the organisational costs of involving external parties or sharing IP with them. The downside of relying solely on internal ideas is that employees can sometimes be too knowledgeable and too focused on certain aspects of a problem, which can narrow down their perspective on a solution. Over time, internal ideas also start to become repetitive and predictable unless a fresh perspective can be included in the developmental equation.

7.4.3.2 External Sources of Ideas

Like internal ideas, external sources of ideas can also be solicited or unsolicited. For wound care businesses that are well established and well known, customers or general members of the public can submit unsolicited ideas or suggestions for consideration at any time. Some businesses have a system for capturing these ideas, e.g., an online form that customers can fill. Others rely on direct communication with clinicians and patients, online or during discussions with sales representatives. These ideas mostly tend to be improvements or modifications to existing product ranges and tend to be dealt with reactively rather than proactively. For instance, in the case of wound dressings, suggestions about different sizes, shapes and packaging, or even about the development of an antimicrobial version of an existing product are expected unsolicited suggestions. These are useful feedback information to take into consideration in the life cycle management of a product.

Customer ideas can also be solicited in a proactive structured approach, through an advisory board or from requested feedback. Starting ideas can be obtained through open innovation, focus groups, advisory board meetings, innovation workshops and ethnographic studies with patients, clinicians and caregivers. They can then be used as a basis for further concept development internally. Where only early-stage ideas are required, further input from the initial participants is not expected. However, where a collaborative approach is followed instead, some customers may be asked to continue to participate in the development of an idea, for example by providing feedback and improvement suggestions on prototypes and by participating in studies and trials.

Collaborative idea development is also done with external bodies such as technology providers, market research organisations, design and innovation businesses and universities. Where the business collaboratively generates ideas with such external suppliers, the concepts can benefit from thinking from outside the traditional comfort zones of the business. Internal participants in the process on the other hand are able to ensure that the ideas are strategically aligned and that they fit in with their understanding of the business propositions. They are also here to ensure that their customer needs will be met and that ideas generated are positioned advantageously in the competitive landscape. In some cases, ideation is completely outsourced, with an external party (or parties) given a brief and background information to work from. The danger of such an approach is that many of the ideas may not fit with the business's overall expectations; however, the opportunity of something completely different to what could have been generated internally is attractive. One challenge in this and other collaborative approaches is the allocation of intellectual property, which needs to be clearly defined at the onset of any ideation project.

7.4.4 Breakthrough Innovation

The concept of breakthrough innovation has a different time perspective in wound dressings as it would, for example in the consumer goods industry. Breakthrough innovation – where the idea is seemingly new to the world – is an offering where the product solves a big problem in a different way that is already practised. In wound care, this can sometimes take years to take off, one example being NPWT, the application of negative pressure to assist in wound closure. The use of modern negative pressure has been known since the mid-1980s, but this approach only gained momentum with KCI's efforts since the mid-1990s (Miller, 2012; Acelity, 2020). Today, most major wound care companies have launched new product lines to try to get a share of the growing market, previously forecasted to be a USD 2.7 billion industry by the mid-2020s (Fortune Business Insights, 2020).

Breakthrough innovation is essential for wound care for the basic reason that it can advance the quality and outcome of care for patients and clinicians. In order to achieve any breakthrough innovation, there are two important aspects to consider. Firstly, in identifying a real 'big problem', an in-depth understanding of the customers and his/her requirements and wishes is critical. This favours innovation techniques that include the voice of the customer. Secondly, in finding a 'big solution', a business must be open to the fact that the technological solution may sometimes have to be found elsewhere – with a need to partner. The most financially successful breakthrough innovations come when a business has managed to identify a big problem, and already has the expertise in-house to supply an elegant and appealing solution.

From a business perspective, investing in potential breakthrough projects helps a business to stay at the forefront of innovation, giving it the best chance of capturing and maintaining a new market share for longer. Any successful proposition will always be followed by a series of 'me-too's from competitors, gradually eroding the market share. But, if well prepared the leading innovator can delay the success of competitors, e.g., through a robust IP strategy and foreward-thinking innovation pipeline. For those who do not invest in exploring their own breakthrough, a significant amount of time, effort and money is subsequently spent anyway on playing catch up and finding ways around IP barriers. This chase is made more pressurised with a need to catch up and grab a share of the market before it is too late. It is true that not all breakthrough innovation will be highly successful ones. The key to success is identifying which one might be and investing into the project, while building a strong business case, doing solid foundation work and due diligence and mitigating the risks.

One challenge for many businesses is overprotecting weak ideas and the resulting inability for specific departments (e.g., R&D or marketing, where the ideas generally come from) to treat their ideas objectively as real business cases and business opportunities. Instead, they may (perhaps inadvertently) invest a lot of time and effort in building a theoretical business case to make the idea fit the selection criteria. In other words, stage gates are considered simply an administrative task for record keeping. Teams are busy doing projects rather than doing the right project. Successful culling of ideas is critical and equally as important as the generation of ideas, particularly in the context of trying to identify a big breakthrough one. The rigour of the stage-gate decision process is therefore absolutely critical, and stage-gating should be considered a strict business activity without vested interest rather than a progress report.

Linked to the above, another challenge is to have an effective portfolio management. A poor evaluation and prioritisation system for projects, too much risk aversion and a lack of business acuity by the decision makers could all – independently or in combination – result in a wasteful portfolio. The consequences can stretch in two opposing directions – an inability to cull projects that are not significant enough, or an inability to invest more money into the right idea. The overall outcome is an imbalance of the distribution of resources, for example, leaning too far into the low-risk zones of life cycle management and additions to existing product lines. The problem is compounded by the fact that bolder innovations cannot use the same evaluation criteria as other smaller projects. The number of unknowns is higher in the former case, and their financial projections can be inaccurate.

To sum up this section on breakthrough innovation, Cooper's five vectors to drive innovation are worth sharing briefly (Cooper, 2011). Firstly, an innovation strategy focussing on opportunity-rich areas is essential. Secondly, the right organisational climate must be in place, led by example by senior executives. Thirdly, a system for generating, capturing and handling of ideas is required. Fourth, a robust stage-gate system that can deal with breakthrough innovation needs to be in place. Fifth and finally, strong business cases must be built in order to be able to pick the winning projects.

Notes

1 pDADMAC: poly(diallyl dimethyl ammonium chloride).
2 Customer-driven is a term also interchangeably used with consumer-driven.

References

Acelity. (2020). *Negative Pressure Wound Therapy Technology*. Retrieved September 9, 2020, from Acelity: https://www.acelity.com/healthcare-professionals/history-of-innovation/negative-pressure-wound-therapy-technology

Caló, E., & Khutoryanskiy, V. V. (2015, April). Biomedical Applications of Hydrogels: A Review of Patents and Commercial Products. *European Polymer Journal, 65*, 252. doi:10.1016/j.eurpolymj.2014.11.024

Catchpole, K. R. (2013, October). Spreading Human Factors Expertise in Healthcare: Untangling the Knots in People and Systems. *BMJ Quality & Safety, 22*, 793. doi:10.1136/bmjqs-2013-002036

Chartered Institute of Ergonomics and Human Factors. (n.d.). *What Is Ergonomics?* Retrieved August 6, 2020, from: https://www.ergonomics.org.uk/Public/Resources/What_is_Ergonomics_.aspx

Cooper, R. G. (2011). The Innovation Dilemma – How to Innovate When the Market Is Mature. *Journal of Product Innovation Management, 28*(S1), 2.

Cooper, R. G., & Dreher, A. (2010, Winter). Voice-Of-Customer Methods: What Is the Best Source of New Product Ideas? *Marketing Management Magazine*, p. 39.

Cooper, R. G., & Edgett, S. J. (2008). Ideation for Product Innovation: What Are the Best Sources? *Visions, 32*(1), 12.

Davila, T., Epstein, M. J., & Shelton, R. (2009). *Making Innovation Work: How to Manage It, Measure It, and Profit from It*. New Jersey: Wharton School Publishing.

FDA. (2016a, February 3). *Applying Human Factors and Usability Engineering to Medical Devices: Guidance for Industry and Food and Drug Administration Staff*. Retrieved August 10, 2020, from https://www.fda.gov/regulatory-information/search-fda-guidance-documents/applying-human-factors-and-usability-engineering-medical-devices

FDA. (2016b). *Executive Summary: Classification of Wound Dressings Combined with Drugs*. Retrieved September 14, 2020, from http://www.fda.gov/media/100005/download

FDA. (2018, September 14). *Medical Device Overview*. Retrieved September 11, 2020, from US Food and Drug Administration: https://www.fda.gov/industry/regulated-products/medical-device-overview

FDA. (2019, April 1). *CFR-Code of Federal Regulations Title 21*. Retrieved September 14, 2020, from U.S. Food and Drug Administration: https://www.accessdata.fda.gov/scripts/cdrh/cfdocs/cfcfr/CFRSearch.cfm?fr=860.3

Fortune Business Insights. (2020, January 21). *Negative Pressure Wound Therapy Market to Reach $2.74 Billion by 2026; Rising Prevalence of Chronic Wounds to Accelerate Growth*. Retrieved September 9, 2020, from https://www.fortunebusinessinsights.com/press-release/negative-pressure-wound-therapy-npwt-market-9517

Hollinworth, H., & Collier, M. (2000). Nurses' Views about Pain and Trauma at Dressing Changes: Results of a National Survey. *Journal of Wound Care, 9*(8), 369. doi:10.12968/jowc.2000.9.8.26282

IEC. (2015). *IEC 62366-1: 2015 Medical Devices – Part 1: Application of Usability Engineering to Medical Devices*.

Lamph, S. (2012, April). Regulation of Medical Devices Outside the European Union. *Journal of the Royal Society of Medicine, 105*(Suppl. 1), S12. doi:10.1258/jrsm.2012.120037

Medical Device Regulation. (2017a, May 5). *Annex VIII – Classification Rules*. Retrieved from Medical Device Regulation: https://www.medical-device-regulation. eu/2019/08/08/annex-viii/

Medical Device Regulation. (2017b, May 5). *MDR: Article 2 – Definitions*. Retrieved from Medical Device Regulation: https://www.medical-device-regulation.eu/ download-mdr/

Miller, C. (2012, September). The History of Negative Pressure Wound Therapy (NPWT): From "Lip Service" to the Modern Vacuum System. *Journal of the American College of Clinical Wound Specialists*, 4(3), 61. doi:10.1016/j. jccw.2013.11.002

NHS England National Quality Board. (2013). *Human Factors in Healthcare: A Concordat from the National Quality Board*. NHS England National Quality Board. Retrieved August 6, 2020, from http://www.england.nhs.uk/wp-content/ uploads/2013/11/nqb-hum-fact-concord.pdf

Report Linker. (2019). *Wound Care Market – Global Outlook and Forecast 2019–2024*. Report Linker. Retrieved August 4, 2020, from https://www.reportlinker.com/ p05822880/?utm_source=GNW

Russ, A. L., Fairbanks, R. J., Karsh, B.-T., Militello, L. G., Saleem, J. J., & Wears, R. L. (2013). The Science of Human Factors: Separating Fact from Fiction. *BMJ Quality & Safety*, 22(10), 802. doi:10.1136/bmjqs-2012-001450

8

Looking Towards the Future

8.1 The Key Influencers for the Future of Wound Care

Wound care, being at the interface between people and carers, is influenced by both sides (Figure 8.1). One the one side, there are people-related factors, such as population health trends, demographics and purchasing power, discussed in Chapter 1. These are the engines of growth, generating opportunities and business for the wound care sector. On the other 'care' side, the healthcare practitioners, their suppliers, the technology, medical advances and regulatory issues surrounding their profession are the major influencers in the direction in which the care takes in order to satisfy the patient needs. The regulatory aspects and the importance of addressing the needs of the care practitioner have been discussed in Chapter 7. These are influencing factors in the development of new wound dressings. Chapters 4, 5 and 6 discussed various science- and technology-based routes and some of the latest technological progress reported in relation to wound dressings, including the use of biologics and nanotechnology in wound care. In this final part of the book, we take a look at what may lie ahead in technological advances and business requirements, and discuss in particular the role of artificial intelligence in wound dressings and the business challenges which could inform the short- and long-term future of wound dressing development.

8.2 The Impact of Artificial Intelligence (AI)

Artificial intelligence has been a growing technology for many years. It comes as no surprise to see it gradually permeating the medical sector, and even the wound dressing side of this sector. In healthcare in general, it is predicted that in the next decade or so, AI will be able to access a range of data from different networked settings and devices, reveal patterns in health conditions, predict risks of certain diseases developing, suggest prevention strategies,

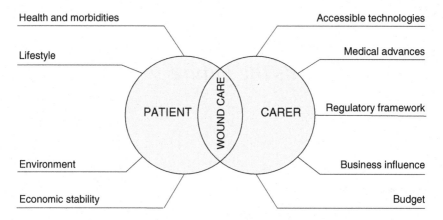

FIGURE 8.1
Wound care influencers

treatment and care, and help improve efficiency and waiting times in care settings (Kriwet, 2020). The integration of AI in healthcare, as in wound care, happens slowly, in small incremental steps and for a full working system to be in place, all stakeholders (government, private and public healthcare providers, businesses and care settings) must align their efforts.

In wound care, the integration of AI has also started in very small steps, beginning with the objective characterisation of wounds with digital imaging to minimise human error and the development of biosensors integrated in a dressing. The goal of AI in wound care would ultimately be to assist in faster patient recovery, whether this is through early reliable characterisation, assisting in diagnosis, monitoring progress, or even suggesting a suitable treatment regime. Figure 8.2 illustrates some of the potential steps in that journey in the context of wound care. Some of these steps have initially started without any data transfer and analysis, but are essential building blocks towards AI in wound care. In addition, as shown in Figure 8.2, the 'sensing' activities can be separate to the 'actuating' activities, but in some cases, the two do merge, and we have the possibility of a continuous loop of wound monitoring and treatment delivery.

Not strictly part of wound dressings *per se*, but a related area, which has witnessed many developments and is worth mentioning, is the objective measurements of wounds. Using imagery, videos, and AI, wound length, width, surface area and depth can be calculated, and wound tissue can even be characterised. This data can already be obtained automatically from a handheld device, transferred, stored and tracked over time, and work is ongoing on its use for analysis and treatment suggestions, all part of steps S1–S4 in Figure 8.2. A large number of these digital wound measurement devices are already on the market, enabling clinicians to view the progress of the wound more objectively and supporting the digitalisation of wound care

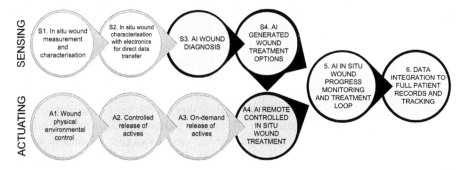

FIGURE 8.2
The gradual integration of AI in various aspects of wound care

---

BOX 8.1   EXAMPLES OF DIGITAL WOUND MEASUREMENT DEVICES

- MolecuLight i:X (MolecuLight)
- Woundworks inSight® (Woundworks)
- WoundZoom (Perceptive)
- Swift Skin and Wound (Swift Medical)
- Silhouette® (Aranz Medical)
- Digital Wound Management (Healthy.io)

---

with electronic medical records (EMR). Many of the devices have claims of reducing nurse visit times, enabling faster documentation and/or leading to less errors in taking dimensions. Some examples are given in Box 8.1.

More pertinent to wound dressings, we are already witnessing significant research activities in the integration of sensors for generating *in situ* data to monitor the wound environment and in the controlled released and on-demand delivery of certain actives. Some examples of these, mostly non-AI controlled but essential steps in the AI journey, are discussed in Sections 5.7.4 and 5.7.5. Integrated pH sensors with visual cues have been ideal starting points for the detection of infection; this type of research progress is situated in S1 of Figure 8.2. From the actuating side, examples of steps A1–A3 of Figure 8.2 are the use of rapid biodegradable polymers to gradually release actives in the wound bed and voltage-actuated release of actives. In these early stages, if any visual or otherwise measurable cues are to be inputted into an AI network or closed loop, a manual operation using a separate device (e.g., a mobile phone or other handheld device) is generally necessary, but it is not long before this step can be automated.

Recently, the remote monitoring of the *use* of a therapy (as opposed to the monitoring of a wound) and its benefits, has been demonstrated. A study of patients receiving NPWT in a home setting with a remote therapy monitoring system showed how use of the device could be monitored and how patient compliance could be improved with a call from trained professionals, should usage levels drop to below a certain limit (Griffin & Casillas, 2018a, 2018b). Several commercialised NPWT systems are now available with connectivity technologies for remotely capturing data on the use of the devices. Remote continuous patient monitoring in general is likely to become a big part of the future of healthcare. Accounting for all types of patient monitoring (including remote glucose monitoring, sleep disorders, cardiovascular disorders, etc.), the global remote monitoring market was expected to grow at just over 14% CAGR from USD 786 million in 2019 to USD 2.1 billion in 2027, prior to the occurrence of the global pandemic (RD Reports and Data, 2020). The wound care aspect was barely represented in this prediction and therefore, when fully developed, and after the global recovery, may also follow similar trends.

The miniaturisation of electronics, fluidics and wireless data transfer has now initiated some important experimental work in step A4 of Figure 8.2, towards the first stages of AI in wound dressings. There have already been several early-stage developments of smart dressings and bandages that can measure parameters from a wound, send and receive data directly, without any manual inputting required. This has been done for the purpose of wound monitoring, or to deliver a specific treatment at a specific time, or for both sensing and triggering a treatment within the same dressing. An example of developmental work on biosensing with data transmission is given by Kassal et al. (2015), who use a screen-printed amperometric biosensor paired with a printed catalytic Prussian blue transducer to detect uric acid. Elevated amounts of uric acid have been linked to chronic wound severity. The uric acid sensor interfaces with a wearable potentiostat that wirelessly transfers data on the uric acid status to a nearby device, from which a clinician can take the necessary action. Another example is that of Mostafalu et al. (2015), who developed an elastomeric dressing with cavities to incorporate a flexible oxygen sensor and its associated electronics system that enables oxygen data readout and wireless transmission. Parducho et al. (2018) for their part described their moisture monitoring dressing with potential for data access through Bluetooth connection. On the actuating side, Derakhshandeh et al. (2020) demonstrated the wirelessly-controlled delivery of actives through minuaturised needle arrays integrated in a flexible bandage.

Several research teams have presented proof-of-concept works on developing a dressing with both a sensing and an actuating function and potential for integrating AI into a closed loop or network. For example, Ochoa et al. (2018) described a dressing incorporating a printed optical oxygen sensor, and patterned catalytic oxygen generating regions that are connected to a flexible microfluidic system. When oxygen levels are deemed low, fresh oxygen can be generated by the decomposition of hydrogen peroxide pumped through the channels, when it contacts the catalytic printed areas. More recently, Pang et al. (2020) developed a smart flexible electronics-integrated wound dressing aiming to detect infection via temperature changes and release an antibiotic from a hydrogel layer when required. The dressing consists of two layers, the upper layer integrating the temperature sensor and UV light-emitting diodes; the lower wound contact layer being a UV-responsive hydrogel that releases the actives when the diodes are on.

These early experimental efforts on the topic suggest that there could be many opportunities for the future of wound care, but there are many challenges that lie ahead before AI can be fully integrated and accepted into standard wound care. To start with, the range of wound types and the variability of wounds, and the range of wound dressings make it practically unrealistic to try to develop a generic wound dressing with both integrated sensors and actuators for the right treatment. The integration of all the steps in Figure 8.2 into one seamless multi-functional dressing is still far from being at our doorstep, and may never be. Instead, developments, particularly initially, have to focus on a very narrow field (e.g., a specific marker from the wound bed, a specific wound type, a specific treatment only) and on a chosen substrate/dressing. This narrowness makes it difficult to get early buy-in by clinicians, as the complexities of wound diagnosis are difficult to boil down to one or two markers. The chosen substrate or dressing onto which the sensor or actuator are attached may also not be the material of choice that the clinician believes is the most suitable for the wound. Integrating sensors and data transfer systems onto a substrate that can be used in parallel with other dressings, without interfering with the wound healing functions of said dressing, may provide a more flexible approach for the monitoring of the status of a wound. Additionally, developing a system that complements and supplements face-to-face nursing and care may also be more favourably seen than one that replaces the human aspect of care.

One big challenge with AI is that by its very nature, its goal is to remove human error and reduce human input and intervention. Some believe that objectives such as remotely triggering the delivery of an active ingredient, or minimising clinical checks with the use of on online monitoring – both of which reduce human interaction – are likely to be part of the future of wound care. The argument is that by eliminating unnecessary human intervention, time and money can be saved and human error could be reduced. With the continuous monitoring option, many may feel reassured that there is a constant, albeit online connection between patient and care giver, including the possibility of accessing past data. However, wound and healthcare specialists, and patients, would argue that the human interaction part is an essential part of wound care. While there are clear benefits in reducing misdiagnoses caused by human error or in selecting the best possible treatment, or in continuous monitoring or indeed in identifying early signs of wound issues before a clinician is able to see the wound, fully sub-contracting the care giving and treatment aspect to an AI system may be met with some resistance, except under certain circumstances (for example, when a patient is located in a remote and difficult to reach location, or during an infectious pandemic, as witnessed in 2020, where social contact is minimised).

Concerns can also be raised on private data protection, on the reliability of any AI system (including power sources, sensor and network stability) and on what the consequences of malfunctions or technical errors could be. For example, the malfunction of any part of the remote system could lead to clinicians not being made aware of an important issue in a timely manner, leading to the degeneration of a wound. The appropriate backing systems or infrastructure would need to be in place to mitigate these risks. The right policies and procedures also need to be developed, taking into account the cyber risks. So, while it is inevitable that AI will gradually permeate wound care, our complete dependence on it for wound diagnosis and treatment is a long while away. What is more likely to be accepted, and therefore present more opportunities for businesses in the near future are (1) continuous wound care monitoring solutions (for both healthcare professionals and patients, who may wish to see their wound progress on their personal devices), (2) the generation of data and development of algorithms for assisting professionals in better understanding, diagnosing wounds and treating wounds and (3) the ability to develop personalised care platforms and improved engagement with patients (Figure 8.3).

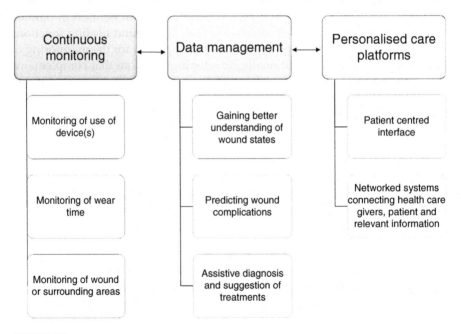

FIGURE 8.3
Areas of opportunity in AI for wound care

Data generation, transmission and management are going to be both the challenge and the big opportunity arising from the integration of sensors and progression of AI. There is a danger that too much data is collected and that this data then becomes unmanageable or difficult to store, filter, interpret and make use of. Data management becomes therefore an essential aspect of the future of wound care, particularly when wound monitoring systems and EMR start to gain more momentum. The important questions are: which data need to be collected, for how long, under what frequency, what is the data going to be used for, how long should the data be kept, where is the data going to be stored, who can access the data, how can the data be accessed and used, who owns the data, and so on. Out of this, businesses may have an opportunity to harness critical information, convert data into intelligence, from which future products and services may be developed in a business-to-business (B2B) or business-to-customer (B2C) context. Safe and effective remote data transfer is particularly key for building these essential B2B and B2C relationships, enabling businesses to be closer to the market.

8.3 Business Practices and Their Effects On the Wound Care Landscape

A big part of what shapes the wound care industry is what businesses do and offer to their customers – caregivers and patients. Naturally, businesses are also equally influenced by their customers, so the relationship normally flows both ways. However, as they are the suppliers of products and services, and as the industry is heavily regulated, businesses have an important role in shaping how wound care evolves, or whether it stagnates. Businesses are mainly driven by the balance sheet, so it does happen that if a medical need does not have sufficient demand to cover development costs and generate profits, there is unlikely to be a high business drive to deliver a solution to the problem. The profit carrot also indicates that other than minimum volumes, the potential maximum volumes and pricing have key roles in business decisions.

8.3.1 The Changing Face of Business Propositions

Pricing is a major driver for any business and across the world, governments are trying to control the growing cost of healthcare, particularly as far as spending is concerned in public hospitals. In today's global marketplace, the differences in labour and overhead costs in different countries have been central in driving costs down in many industries, including the wound care sector. In order to escape the price battles, advanced wound care businesses need to demonstrate the value of their products and innovate in different ways, offering not only better products, but also additional value and benefits linked to the use of the products. We have seen how some products are being developed not just to heal wounds, but to heal wounds with better outcomes for the patient (e.g., less pain, less scarring, less time to be spent in hospital, more mobility, etc.). It is likely that a greater focus will be placed on such added benefits in the future, even if the wound healing performance still remains core. Furthermore, added value around a dressing could also be in the form of intelligence (or in its crude form, data) or offering of associated services, including personalised care options, related to the overall care and well-being of the patient. The future of wound dressing development could be influenced by these drivers and innovation may need to integrate broader aspects of patient care, and not just focus on healing wounds. The traditional model, delivering value through the manufacture and selling of products, is being challenged, and greater emphasis will be expected to be placed on further-reaching healthcare offerings, on better B2B services, and on engaging B2C relationships (van den Heuvel et al., 2018). The role of AI starts to become essential in the integration of such new added value.

Another aspect of wound care that could change the industry is the importance that businesses place on prevention. In healthcare in general, it is widely accepted that prevention is better than cure. To a large extent, the wound care industry has responded to this in multiple ways. For example, the prevention of unnecessary infection is done with the use of dressings with either barrier or antimicrobial properties for surgical wounds or burns. There have been attempts at preventing scar formation, for example, with the early use of pressure garments. Compression bandages are a common tool in the management of venous leg disease to prevent the formation of leg ulcers, or even treat the early stages of the wound to prevent it from degenerating further.

On the other hand, in general, the advanced wound care market has been benefiting hugely from providing large volumes of products for potentially preventable wounds. Amongst the growth drivers for the industry, discussed in Chapter 1, diabetes and obesity are the two large preventable morbidities that contribute to the size of the wound care market, as they are high-risk factors for the development of chronic wounds. Successful prevention programmes on these two health issues may thus have a huge impact on the shape of the chronic wound care industry. Closer to the advanced wound dressing business itself, there are opportunities in the prevention of wound formation, in early diagnostics and in the prevention of the progression of wounds into more advanced degenerative stages. In anticipation or in participation towards these goals, some advanced wound care businesses may look at shifting their priorities and develop new products or services aligning with a prevention strategy, and offering a total care solution from prevention to treatment. This will become a shift from always reactively responding to a demand to proactively engaging in prevention, early diagnosis and treatment.

8.3.2 The Influence of Competition

Competition is normally a natural occurrence in any economy and market, leading to innovation in all aspects, pricing moderation, economic growth, employment, and wealth. Competition does not only drive down pricing and increase value propositions, but it also creates opportunities and new market segments. It is therefore quite common for governments across the world to have policies and programmes in place to encourage the development of new ideas and new start-ups in order to create healthy competition in the market. However, the potential high costs involved in the development and approval of advanced wound care products create a scenario where, due to challenging investment requirements, a large number of these competing small and medium-sized businesses become service providers (R&D or manufacturing) to the bigger corporations rather than their true competitors, or they become developmental partners, or eventually, potential acquisitions.

In a trend that is likely to continue, many businesses have started to increase their collaboration with other businesses, universities and research institutes. The bigger players in the advanced wound dressing industry in particular have been reaping the benefits of collaborations with smaller more nimble businesses to get new products to market more quickly, and to access a range of external innovation fast. It is a mutually beneficial collaboration: the larger companies bring in their experience, existing on-market presence, and finance. The smaller partner brings in a new technology, and/or streamlined R&D, which can boost the speed to market, and which may otherwise never have sufficient investment to be commercialised. Partnerships, co-development and acquisitions are also part of new growth strategies, and the old model of inventing everything in-house is no longer sustainable. While the current dynamics still encourage innovation and the development of new technologies at the base R&D level, the difficulties and competition in getting new ideas to market due to lack of further investment still limit the availability of new technologies at commercial level. In addition, because larger corporations tend to have bigger budgets, only technologies and innovations that match the strategic objectives of these big players, tend to make it to market. In this sense, competition only thrives at the pre-commercialisation stage and is limited at the point of use.

8.3.3 Investments

According to a Deloitte report (Snyder et al., 2017), investment and start-up activities in the medical technologies sector have been declining, putting future innovation at risk. The issues that have been identified in the report are a lack of capital investment due to the time required to get a meaningful return, and increased reimbursement and commercialisation risks for new products. In Chapter 7, it was also highlighted that there has been a general fall in breakthrough projects at the benefit of incremental innovation (not specific to the healthcare industry, but likely reflective of). This also contributes to the observed reduction in investment in this sector. Businesses have become more risk averse, only moderately investing in areas they are comfortable in, leading to more incremental and semi-radical innovations. One of the ways of managing this risk aversion has been, as mentioned above, collaborations, co-developments, partnerships and mergers and acquisitions. This enables two or more entities to share the financial burden, expertise, and risks, while also in some cases enabling access to a new market or market segment.

Another strategy is to focus the investment into an area of maximum return, for example, by investing into platform technologies, i.e., technologies and associated expertise that can be used to support a range of parallel business models in different sections of a business. Silver technologies are good examples of platform technologies that businesses have invested in in the last three decades. Typically, once a business has developed or acquired a silver technology, it tends to have several of its product lines incorporating the same technology, sustaining a healthy pipeline for a number of years. Other examples of potential platform technologies are AI-related technologies. In particular, sensors, data collecting, sharing and management, and customer interfaces are all technologies that can be used to digitalise a range of products or services a business may have on offer. Platform technologies also provide more opportunities for consistent branding of features within a product.

How businesses invest and the level of investment therefore have an important effect on the type of new solutions to be launched in the advanced wound care market. With small investments, it is likely that only small step changes will be offered in the future. Bigger investments, whether in partnership or from a single organisation, are likely to indicate a bigger step change in the wound care picture. However, any breakthrough change in wound care needs to be driven both by healthcare practitioners and businesses together. Without clinical buy-in or business investment, ideas cannot take off.

8.4 Conclusions

The advanced wound care market has evolved hugely since the second half of the 20th century, both from a technological and care perspective. Technologically, we have witnessed a boom in the development and/or processing of many natural and man-made polymers suitable for wound care. There have also been big leaps in the technical ways of forming, structuring and layering these polymers into a flexible form suitable for the wound bed, and in methods of encompassing additives, actives, sensors and actuators into these structures. The merging of previously distinct areas of technology, particularly in recent years, continues to create new developments in this field. Incorporating engineered mechanical and features into a dressing system (for example, in NPWT or bioelectrical dressings) is an example of the convergence of technologies for a common goal. Other adjacent areas such as advanced cosmetic and skincare are also likely to be a source of technological inspiration influencing the development of wound dressings with enhanced skin healing outcomes. An area that also needs to be watched for the future is how AI will be integrated into wound dressing structures, and how data management will be utilised.

From a care perspective, advanced wound care solutions have followed the care best practices as they evolved. For example, the realisation that a moist wound environment is essential for better wound healing was quickly followed by a range of dressings that prevent desiccation of the wound. Care has evolved from simply protecting a wound and letting nature take its course to creating the right environment to assist the healing process, and then to optimising this environment to speed up healing. The need for solutions that prevent complications such as infections, scarring and recurrence of a wound has been part of this gradual journey to assist and speed up healing. More recently, the importance of other holistic aspects of patient health and well-being has increased, for example, quality of life, pain, mobility, dignity, mental health and so on. In addition, wherever possible, more patients are being cared for at home rather than in a hospital setting. Advanced wound dressings have evolved in accordance to these trends, offering additional benefits to the core dressing functions. Many wound dressings, even those used with NPWT, can now be used reliably in a home setting, staying securely in place for several days, enabling patients to wash, move and feel comfortable, whilst performing their core wound healing functions in the background.

The future trends in wound care point towards more care at home scenarios, with increasingly less funding. Self-care and prevention are also likely to be high on the agenda, as are the digitalisation of care and use of transferable EMR, all of which leading to greater monitoring of health and wound variables. If these trends firm up, traditional wound dressing businesses may naturally start to divide into two categories – those that offer a product only, and need to compete on benefits, volume and price, and those that offer products and associated services or support, which compete more on benefits and added value. The advanced wound care market as we know it seems quite mature already and evolves in incremental steps. There may still be opportunities for radical game-changing innovation; however, this needs to be driven both from the care-giving side and the technological side simultaneously.

References

Derakhshandeh, H., Aghabaglou, F., McCarthy, A., Mostafavi, A., Wiseman, C., Bonick, Z., Ghanavati, I., Harris, S., Krekemeier-Bower, C., Basri, S. M. M., Rosenbohm, J., Yang, R., Mostafulu, P., Orgill, D., & Tamayol, A. (2020, March 24). A Wirelessly Controlled Smart Bandage with 3D-Printed Miniaturized Needle Arrays. *Advanced Functional Materials, 30*(13), 1905544. doi:10.1002/adfm.201905544

Griffin, L., & Casillas, L. L. (2018a, March). Evaluating the Impact of a Patient-Centered Remote Monitoring Program on Adherence to Negative Pressure Wound Therapy. *Wounds, 30*(3), E29. Retrieved from https://www.woundsresearch.com/article/evaluating-impact-patient-centered-remote-monitoring-program-adherence-negative-pressure

Griffin, L., & Casillas, L. M. (2018b, August). A Patient-Centered Remote Therapy Monitoring Program Focusing on Increased Adherence to Wound Therapy: A Large Cohort Study. *Wounds, 30*(8), E81. Retrieved from https://www.woundsresearch.com/article/patient-centered-remote-therapy-monitoring-program-focusing-increased-adherence-wound

Kassal, P., Kim, J., Kumar, R., de Araujo, W. R., Murković Steinberg, I., Steinberg, M. D., & Wang, J. (2015, July). Smart Bandage with Wireless Connectivity for Uric Acid Biosensing as an Indicator of Wound Status. *Electrochemistry Communications, 56*, 6. doi:10.1016/j.elecom.2015.03.018

Kriwet, C. (2020, January 7). *World Economic Forum*. Retrieved November 24, 2020, from Here Are 3 Ways AI Will Change Healthcare by 2030: https://www.weforum.org/agenda/2020/01/future-of-artificial-intelligence-healthcare-delivery/

Mostafalu, P., Lenk, W., Dokmeci, M. R., Ziaie, B., Khademhosseini, A., & Sonkusale, S. R. (2015, October). Wireless Flexible Smart Bandage for Continuous Monitoring of Wound Oxygenation. *IEEE Transactions on Biomedical Circuits and Systems, 9*(5), 670. doi:10.1109/TBCAS.2015.2488582

Ochoa, M., Rahimi, R., Zhou, J., Jiang, H., Yoon, C. K., Oscai, M., Jain, V., Morken, T., Oliveira, R. H., Maddipatla, D., Narakathu, B. B., Campana, G. L., Zieger, M. A., Sood, R., Atashbar, M. Z., & Ziaie, B. (2018). A Manufacturable Smart Dressing with Oxygen Delivery and Sensing Capability for Chronic Wound Management. *SPIE Defense + Security, 10639*, 106391C. doi:10.1117/12.2306083

Pang, Q., Lou, D., Li, S., Wang, G., Qiao, B., Dong, M., Ma, L., Gao, C., & Wu, Z. (2020, March 18). Smart Flexible Electronics-Integrated Wound Dressing for Real-Time Monitoring and On-Demand Treatment of Infected Wounds. *Advanced Science, 7*(6), 1902673. doi:10.1002/advs.201902673

Parducho, D., Pujol, A., Ylanan, M., Peralta, N., Ramos, C., Baldovino, R., Bedruz, R., Agueda, J. S., Bandala, A., & Vicerra, R. R. (2018). *Smart Wound Dressing with Arduino Microcontroller. 2018 IEEE 10th International Conference on Humanoid, Nanotechnology, Information Technology, Communication and Control, Environment and Management (HNICEM).* Baguio City. doi:10.1109/HNICEM.2018.8666281

RD Reports and Data. (2020). *Remote Patient Monitoring Market by Product (Vital Sign Monitors and Special Monitors), by Application, and by End-Use (Hospital-Based Patients, Home Healthcare, Ambulatory Patients), Forecasts to 2027.* New York: RD

Reports and Data. Retrieved November 18, 2020, from https://www.report-sanddata.com/report-detail/remote-patient-monitoring-market

Snyder, G., Arboleda, P., & Sha, S. (2017). *Out of the Valley of Death: How Can Entrepreneurs, Corporations, and Investors Reinvigorate Early-Stage Medtech Innovation?* Deloitte Development LLC. Retrieved November 24, 2020, from https://www2.deloitte.com/content/dam/Deloitte/us/Documents/life-sciences-health-care/us-lshc-medtech-innovation.pdf

van den Heuvel, R., Stirling, C., Kapadia, A., & Zhou, J. (2018). *Medical Devices 2030*. KPMG. Retrieved November 23, 2020, from https://advisory.kpmg.us/content/dam/institutes/en/healthcare-life-sciences/pdfs/2018/medical-devices-2030.pdf

Index

Page numbers in *Italics* refer to figures; **bold** refers to table and page number

Printed in the United States
by Baker & Taylor Publisher Services